Covid-19 and its Impact on Cardiovascular Health

Covid-19 and its Impact on Cardiovascular Health

Edited by Robin Davidson

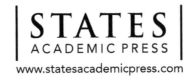

www.statesacademicpress.com

States Academic Press,
109 South 5th Street,
Brooklyn, NY 11249, USA

Visit us on the World Wide Web at:
www.statesacademicpress.com

ISBN: 978-1-63989-766-7

Cataloging-in-Publication Data

Covid-19 and its impact on cardiovascular health / edited by Robin Davidson.
     p. cm.
Includes bibliographical references and index.
ISBN 978-1-63989-766-7
1. Cardiovascular system--Diseases. 2. COVID-19 (Disease). 3. Cardiovascular system--Diseases--Treatment.
4. Cardiovascular system--Diseases--Prevention. 5. Heart--Diseases. I. Davidson, Robin.
RC667 .C683 2023
616.1--dc23

Table of Contents

Preface

Coronavirus disease (Covid-19) refers to an infectious disease caused by the SARS-CoV-2 virus. It spreads when an infected person exhales droplets and very small particles containing the virus. The signs and symptoms of Covid-19 might vary but commonly include headache, breathing difficulties, loss of taste, fever, loss of smell, coughing and exhaustion. The primary presenting symptom of Covid-19 has been reported to be heart palpitations in patients who do not have a cough or fever. The Covid-19 virus has been recently shown as a major risk factor for cardiovascular disorders including myocarditis, myocardial injury, coagulation abnormalities, pericarditis, cardiac arrest, arrhythmias and heart failure in patients. This book provides significant information to help develop a good understanding of Covid-19 and its impact on cardiovascular health. It aims to shed light on some of the unexplored aspects of this disease. A number of latest researches have been included to keep the readers up-to-date with the global concepts in this medical condition.

The information shared in this book is based on empirical researches made by veterans in this field of study. The elaborative information provided in this book will help the readers further their scope of knowledge leading to advancements in this field.

Finally, I would like to thank my fellow researchers who gave constructive feedback and my family members who supported me at every step of my research.

Editor

Two Case Reports of Acute Myopericarditis after mRNA COVID-19 Vaccine

Carlotta Sciaccaluga[1]*, Flavio D'Ascenzi[1], Matteo Cameli[1], Maddalena Gallotta[1], Daniele Menci[1], Giovanni Antonelli[1], Benedetta Banchi[2], Veronica Mochi[1], Serafina Valente[1] and Marta Focardi[1]

[1] Division of Cardiology, Department of Medical Biotechnologies, University of Siena, Siena, Italy, [2] Unit of Diagnostic Imaging, University Hospital Santa Maria alle Scotte, Siena, Italy

*Correspondence:
Carlotta Sciaccaluga
carlotta.sciaccaluga@gmail.com

Background: Cases of myocarditis and myopericarditis after mRNA COVID-19 vaccines have been reported, especially after the second dose and in young males. Their course is generally benign, with symptoms onset after 24–72 h from the dose.

Case Summary: We report two cases of myopericarditis after the second dose of the mRNA-1273 COVID-19 vaccine in two young males. Both the patients were administered the mRNA-1273 COVID-19 vaccine from the same batch on the same day and experienced fever on the same day of the vaccine, and symptoms consisted of myopericarditis 3 days after the dose.

Discussion: Myopericarditis is usually considered an uncommon adverse reaction after various vaccinations, reported also after the mRNA COVID-19 vaccine. Several explanations have been proposed, including an abnormal activation of the immune system leading to a pro-inflammatory cascade responsible for myocarditis development. Both patients experienced the same temporal onset as well as the same symptoms, it is also useful to underscore that both vaccines belonged to the same batch of vaccines. However, despite these cases, vaccination against COVID-19 far outweighs the risk linked to COVID-19 infection and remains the best option to overcome this disease.

Keywords: case report, myocarditis, myopericarditis, mRNA vaccine, COVID-19

INTRODUCTION

The safety profile of mRNA vaccines for the prevention of COVID-19 disease has been demonstrated in several trials (1–3). Systemic reactions, generally mild and transient, are described mainly after the second dose of vaccine and especially in young people. Few cases of myocarditis post-mRNA vaccine (both BNT162b2 and mRNA-1273 vaccines) have also been reported (4, 5), typically with a benign course. In most case series, symptoms arose 24–72 h after the second dose, whereas only rare cases occurred after 1-week post-vaccine (4).

CASE DESCRIPTION

We report two cases of myopericarditis after the second dose of the mRNA-1273 COVID-19 vaccine, from the same batch of vaccines, administered on the same day. Two young males, 20-years old and 21-years old, with no past medical history, experienced fever (38 and 40°C, respectively) on the same day of the second dose of mRNA-1273 COVID-19 vaccine and chest pain, exacerbated with breathing, 3 days later, for which they were admitted to the emergency department. On admission, both patients had normal vital signs with no fever. Nasopharyngeal SARS-CoV2 polymerase chain reaction was negative in both patients. The 12-lead resting electrocardiograms on arrival showed sinus rhythm, normal atrioventricular conduction, incomplete right bundle

branch block and no ventricular repolarization abnormalities (**Figure 1**). Both chest x-rays revealed no significant findings. Blood tests revealed a C-reactive protein = 1.9 mg/dL in both cases, with white blood count within normal limits and increased levels of high-sensitivity troponin (211 and 366 ng/L, respectively). Due to the clinical presentation and the elevation of high-sensitivity troponin, a complete transthoracic echocardiographic exam was performed. In the first case, transthoracic echocardiography showed no pericardial effusion, a mild inferolateral wall thickness (12 mm) with normal biventricular function, absence of wall motion abnormalities and no significant heart valve disease. The echocardiographic examination of the 21-year-old patient showed a minimal pericardial effusion (2 mm) with hyperreflective pericardial

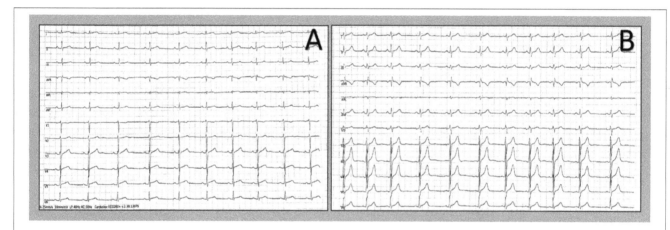

FIGURE 1 | Twelve-lead resting electrocardiograms collected at the hospital admission. Patients' electrocardiograms on admission: 20-year-old patient **(A)** and 21-year-old patient **(B)**. The resting ECGs showed sinus rhythm, normal atrioventricular conduction, incomplete right bundle branch block and no ventricular repolarization abnormalities.

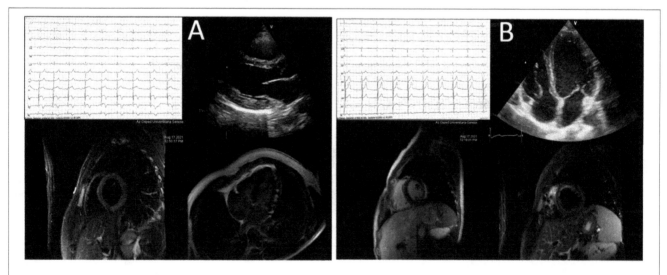

FIGURE 2 | **(A,B)** Central illustration. The picture summarizes the main non-invasive findings in the two patients experiencing acute myopericarditis after mRNA-1273 COVID-19 vaccine. See text for details.

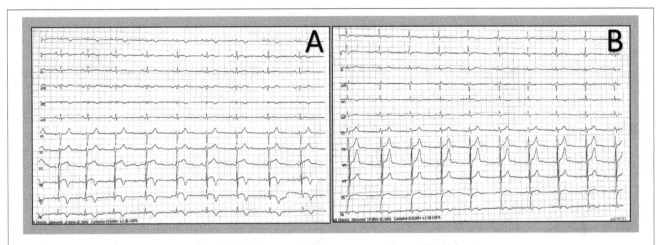

FIGURE 3 | T-wave inversion showed by twelve-lead resting electrocardiograms. Patients' electrocardiograms on day 2 from admission show T-wave inversion in the anterolateral leads in the 20-years old patient **(A)**, whereas in the other patient, the T-wave inversion occurred in the lateral leads **(B)**.

layers, normal biventricular function and no significant heart valve disease. Due to the temporal correlation between the symptom onset and the second dose vaccine, the hypothesized diagnosis was acute myopericarditis as an adverse reaction to the mRNA-1273 COVID-19 vaccine. Therefore, on the day after hospital admission, both patients underwent cardiac magnetic resonance (CMR), which confirmed the diagnosis of acute myopericarditis, with evidence of myocardial oedema and late gadolinium enhancement (LGE) with subepicardial pattern (**Figure 2A**). In particular, in the 20-year old patient, myocardial oedema was found in the middle inferolateral wall, whereas LGE involved the subepicardial region of the lateral wall, inferior basal wall, and anterior apical septum, with left ventricular ejection fraction (LVEF) = 55%. The CMR of the 21-year-old patient revealed myocardial oedema in the mid-basal lateral wall and LGE in the subepicardial region of the basal inferolateral wall and mid-basal lateral wall with LVEF 52% (**Figure 2B**). The disease course was benign in both patients, and only one patient presented rare ventricular arrhythmias on the admission day (isolated ventricular ectopic beats, 3 couplets and 1 triplet). Due to the patients' low-risk profile and the clear etiology of the myocarditis, we decided not to perform an endomyocardial biopsy. Both patients were treated with low doses of beta-blockers, angiotensin-converting enzyme, and antagonists of mineralocorticoid receptors. Non-steroidal anti-inflammatory drugs were introduced to control chest pain, whereas colchicine was not introduced due to the prevalent myocardial involvement. Serial electrocardiograms showed T-wave inversion in the anterolateral leads in the 20-years old patient, whereas in the other patient, the T-wave inversion occurred in the lateral leads, both occurred 2 days later from admission (**Figures 3A,B**). Blood tests revealed an initial increase in markers of myocardial injury (peak high-sensitivity troponin 2,474 and 1,414 ng/L and isozyme creatin-kinase MB 80.4 and 50 ng/ml respectively) and C-reactive protein levels (peak 1.9 and 2.16 mg/dl respectively), with a decreasing trend until complete normalization before the

hospital discharge. They were both discharged on the 9th day of the in-hospital stay. **Figure 4** shows the timeline of these two patients from the day of the vaccine and symptoms onset to discharge. One month after hospital discharge, both patients were asymptomatic and were evaluated by clinical examination, resting ECG and echocardiograms which were all within normal limits. In particular, resting ECG showed almost complete resolutions of repolarization abnormalities (**Figure 5**).

Their 48-h Holter ECG did not show any brady- or tachyarritmias as well as ST-T dynamic changes. CMR was scheduled at 3 months from the acute event.

DISCUSSION

Myopericarditis is usually considered an uncommon adverse reaction after various vaccinations (5–7), and few cases have also been described after the mRNA COVID-19 vaccine, both after BNT162b2 and mRNA-1273 COVID-19 vaccines (4, 8). Both vaccines encode the stabilized prefusion spike glycoprotein of SARS-CoV2, and they were recommended as a 2-dose schedule. In certain individuals with genetic predisposition, nucleoside modifications of mRNA might trigger the immune system and the abnormal activation of both innate and acquired immune response (9), leading to a pro-inflammatory cascade responsible for myocarditis development. Besides mRNA immune reactivity, antibodies cross-reaction between SARS-CoV2 spike glycoproteins and myocardial proteins might play a role in post-vaccine myocarditis (10). Furthermore, both age and sex could be factors involved in the development of this adverse reaction (10). In fact, according to several case reports (11) and the large retrospective analysis conducted in Israel (12), the incidence of myocarditis after BNT162b2 mRNA vaccine is significantly higher in young male subjects, hinting that hormonal differences might play a central role in modulating

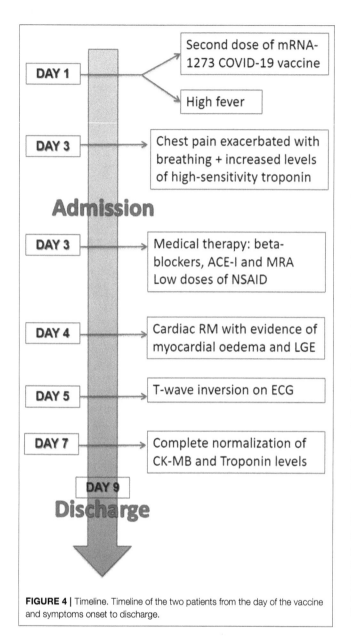

the immune response. Within the Vaccine Adverse Event Reporting System (VAERS), 1,226 reports of myocarditis after mRNA vaccination during the first 6 months of 2021 (13). Furthermore, it has been widely demonstrated that the rate of adverse reactions to the vaccine is significantly lower compared to the rate of complications related to SARS-CoV2 infection (14), also in young individuals (15). In particular, Barda et al. showed that the risk of developing myocarditis after mRNA vaccine is much lower than after SARS-CoV2 infection (2.7 events vs. 11.0 events per 100,000 persons respectively) (16). In line with these results, the Italian Society of Cardiology still recommends vaccination against COVID-19 even in patients that developed myopericarditis after mRNA vaccine (17). However, it recognizes that these patients represent a vulnerable population and therefore some precautions might be taken such as prolonging the interval between the two doses and perhaps choosing a different vaccine for the second dose (17). The two cases we presented showed clinical characteristics in line with the other documented cases and the latest report by Rosner et al. (18): prevalence of male sex, symptoms onset 48–72 h after the second dose of vaccine, and uncomplicated course with mild symptoms. Indeed, both patients, of approximately the same age, were administered mRNA-1273 COVID-19 vaccine on the same day and in the same hospital, and both experienced fever on the same day and symptoms consisted of myopericarditis 3 days after the dose. Furthermore, it is useful to underscore that both vaccines belonged to the same batch of vaccines, questioning whether problems in vaccines storage may be at least in part responsible for these adverse reactions. To the best of our knowledge there are no clear reports linking a storage problem with the onset of systemic adverse reactions, either for COVID-19 vaccine or for other anti-viral vaccines. However, it is well-known that mRNA vaccines require specific handling which might be particularly challenging such as the need to guarantee a correct temperature (19). We actually cannot know whether there had been any problems with the transportation, storage or administration of this batch of vaccine and whether this might have had affected the onset of myocarditis, but it is important to stress this aspect for raising awareness of a possible correlation

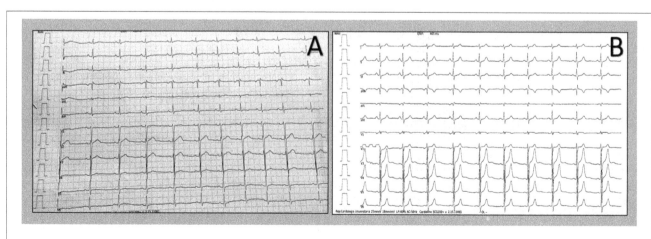

FIGURE 5 | Resting electrocardiograms after hospital discharge. Patients' electrocardiograms after one month from hospital discharge show almost complete resolution of repolarization abnormalities in both patients [in the 20-years old patient **(A)** and in the 21-year old patient **(B)**].

between these problems and the onset of side effects, which might therefore be explained with a possible toxic effect rather than an immunological pathophysiology.

CONCLUSIONS

We reported two cases of acute myopericarditis in two young males who developed chest pain three days after the second dose of the mRNA-1273 COVID-19 vaccine. Due to several cases of myocarditis after mRNA COVID-19 vaccination, clinical suspicion should be high, especially in young males. However, despite these cases, vaccination against COVID-19 far outweighs the risk linked to COVID-19 infection and remains the best option to overcome this disease.

AUTHOR CONTRIBUTIONS

CS, DM, VM, and BB collected the data upon which the manuscript was based. CS, FD'A, GA, and MG wrote the manuscript, while MC, SV, and MF critically revised it. All authors contributed to the article and approved the submitted version.

REFERENCES

1. Polack FP, Thomas SJ, Kitchin N, Absalon J, Gurtman A, Lockhart S, et al. Safety and efficacy of the BNT162b2 mRNA Covid-19 vaccine. *N Engl J Med.* (2020) 383:2603–15. doi: 10.1056/NEJMoa2034577

2. Walsh EE, Frenck Jr RW, Falsey AR, Kitchin N, Absalon J, Gurtman A, et al. Safety and immunogenicity of two RNA-based Covid-19 vaccine candidates. *N Engl J Med.* (2020) 383:2439–50. doi: 10.1056/NEJMoa2027906

3. Oliver SE, Gargano JW, Marin M, Wallace M, Curran KG, Chamberland M, et al. The advisory committee on immunization practices' interim recommendation for use of Pfizer-BioNTech COVID-19 vaccine—United States, December 2020. *MMWR Morb Mortal Wkly Rep.* (2020) 69:1922–4. doi: 10.15585/mmwr.mm6950e2

4. Mouch SA, Roguin A, Hellou E, Ishai A, Shoshan U, Mahamid L. et al. Myocarditis following COVID-19 mRNA vaccination. *Vaccine.* (2021) 39:3790–3. doi: 10.1016/j.vaccine.2021.05.087

5. Abbasi J. Researchers investigate what COVID-19 does to the heart. *JAMA.* (2021) 325:808–11. doi: 10.1001/jama.2021.0107

6. Cassimatis DC, Atwood JE, Engler RM, Linz PE, Grabenstein JD, Vernalis MN. Smallpox vaccination and myopericarditis: a clinical review. *J Am Coll Cardiol.* (2004) 43:1503–10. doi: 10.1016/j.jacc.2003.11.053

7. Eckart RE, Love SS, Atwood JE, Arness MK, Cassimatis DC, Campbell CL, et al. Incidence and follow-up of inflammatory cardiac complications after smallpox vaccination. *J Am Coll Cardiol.* (2004) 44:201–5. doi: 10.1016/j.jacc.2004.05.004

8. García B, Ortega P, JA BF, León C, Burgos R, Dorta C. Acute myocarditis after administration of the BNT162b2 vaccine against COVID-19. *Rev Esp Cardiol.* (2021) 74:812–4. doi: 10.1016/j.recesp.2021.03.009

9. Bozkurt B, Kamat I, Hotez PJ. Myocarditis with COVID-19 mRNA vaccines. *Circulation.* (2021) 144:471–84. doi: 10.1161/CIRCULATIONAHA.121.056135

10. Heymans S, Cooper LT. Myocarditis after COVID-19 mRNA vaccination: clinical observations and potential mechanisms. *Nat Rev Cardiol.* (2021) 2021:1–3. doi: 10.1038/s41569-021-00662-w

11. Diaz GA, Parsons GT, Gering SK, Meier AR, Hutchinson IV, Robicsek A. Myocarditis and pericarditis after vaccination for COVID-19. *JAMA.* (2021) 326:1210–2. doi: 10.1001/jama.2021.13443

12. Mevorach D, Anis E, Cedar N, Bromberg M, Haas EJ, Nadir E, et al. Myocarditis after BNT162b2 mRNA vaccine against Covid-19 in Israel. *N Engl J Med.* (2021) 385:2140–9. doi: 10.1056/NEJMoa2109730

13. Shimabukuro TT, Nguyen M, Martin D, DeStefano F. Safety monitoring in the vaccine adverse event reporting system (VAERS). *Vaccine.* (2015) 33:4398–405. doi: 10.1016/j.vaccine.2015.07.035

14. Inciardi RM, Lupi L, Zaccone G. Cardiac involvement in a patient with coronavirus disease 2019 (COVID-19). *JAMA Cardiol.* (2020) 5:819–24. doi: 10.1001/jamacardio.2020.1096

15. Cavigli L, Frascaro F, Turchini F, Mochi N, Sarto P, Bianchi S, et al. A prospective study on the consequences of SARS-CoV-2 infection on the heart of young adult competitive athletes: Implications for a safe return-to-play. *Int J Cardiol.* (2021) 336:130–6. doi: 10.1016/j.ijcard.2021.05.042

16. Barda N, Dagan N, Ben-Shlomo Y, Kepten E, Waxman J, Ohana R, et al. Safety of the BNT162b2 mRNA Covid-19 vaccine in a nationwide setting. *N Engl J Med.* (2021) 385:1078–90. doi: 10.1056/NEJMoa2110475

17. Sinagra G, Porcari A, Merlo M, Barillà F, Basso C, Ciccone MM, et al. Myocarditis and pericarditis following mRNA COVID-19 vaccination. Expert opinion of the Italian Society of Cardiology. *G Ital Cardiol.* (2021) 22:894–9. doi: 10.1714/3689.36747

18. Rosner CM, Genovese L, Tehrani BN, Atkins M, Bakhshi H, Chaudhri S, et al. Myocarditis temporally associated with COVID-19 vaccination. *Circulation.* (2021) 144:502–5. doi: 10.1161/CIRCULATIONAHA.121.055891

19. Uddin MN, Roni MA. Challenges of storage and stability of mRNA COVID-19 vaccines. *Vaccines.* (2021) 9:1033. doi: 10.3390/vaccines9091033

2

Acute Fulminant Myocarditis after ChAdOx1 nCoV-19 Vaccine

Chia-Tung Wu[1], Shy-Chyi Chin[2] and Pao-Hsien Chu[1]*

[1] Department of Cardiology, Linkou Medical Center, Chang Gung Memorial Hospital, Taoyuan City, Taiwan, [2] Department of Medical Imaging and Intervention, Chang Gung Memorial Hospital, Linkou Medical Center and Chang Gung University College of Medicine, Taoyuan City, Taiwan

Correspondence:
Pao-Hsien Chu
taipei.chu@gmail.com

According to recent literatures, myocarditis is an uncommon side effect of mRNA vaccines against COVID-19. On the other hand, myocarditis after adenovirus based vaccine is rarely reported. Here we report a middle-aged healthy female who had acute fulminant perimyocarditis onset 2 days after the first dose of ChAdOx1 vaccine (AstraZeneca) without any other identified etiology. Detailed clinical presentation, serial ECGs, cardiac MRI, and laboratory data were included in the report. Possible mechanisms of acute myocarditis after adenoviral vaccine was reviewed and discussed. To our knowledge, a few cases of myocarditis after Ad26.COV2.S vaccine were reported, and this is the first case report after ChAdOx1 vaccine.

Keywords: COVID-19, vaccine, adenovirus, ChAdOx1, myocarditis

INTRODUCTION

Growing evidence has shown that acute myocarditis is a rare complication after mRNA COVID-19 vaccinations, with an estimated incidence of ~2 per 100,000 persons after BNT162b2 mRNA vaccine (1, 2), and the risk is higher in adolescent males. Typically, acute myocarditis occurs within 5 days after mRNA vaccination, and the mechanism is still unclear. Myocarditis after adenovirus or protein-based vaccines has seldom been reported. Here, we report the case of a 44-year-old female who had acute fulminant perimyocarditis following the first dose of ChAdOx1 nCoV-19 vaccine with no other identified etiology.

CASE DESCRIPTION

A previously healthy 44-year-old Taiwanese female hairdresser (153 cm, 63 kg), without any documented systemic disease, received first dose of ChAdOx1 nCoV-19 vaccine (AstraZeneca) on August 6, 2021. She denied taking any long-term or short -term medication, and had no fever, sore throat, or other symptoms suggesting viral infection within 2 weeks before vaccination. She started to feel persistent stabbing chest pain and breathless approximately 48 h after vaccination. Because the symptoms progressed, she visited the emergency department at another hospital on August 11. Initial troponin I was 17 ng/mL and D-dimer was 1020 ng/mL FEU. ECG showed diffuse low QRS voltage and 1 mm convex ST elevation over V1 and V2 (**Figure 1A**). Coronary angiography revealed patent coronary arteries, and no pulmonary embolism was found on enhanced CT. She had nausea, vomiting, and abdominal distension after admission. Hypotension developed on August 12, and echocardiography showed poor left ventricular function. Norepinephrine was infused, and she was transferred to our intensive care unit for further management on August 13.

On arrival, her vital signs included temperature 37.2°C, heart rate 108/min, blood pressure 96/77 mmHg (under norepinephrine 0.3 μg/kg/min), respiration 20/min, and O2 saturation 93% under O2 nasal cannula. Fine crackles were heard over bilateral basal lung fields and there was no audible pleural or pericardial friction rub. ECG showed sinus tachycardia, diffuse low QRS voltage, and convex ST elevation over V1 to V3 (**Figure 1B**). Chest X-way revealed acute pulmonary edema, and echocardiography showed left ventricular diameter 47/39 mm, left ventricular ejection fraction (LVEF) about 35%, and small amount of pericardial effusion. Initial laboratory data on August 13 showed elevated troponin I (8.1 ng/mL), BNP (399 pg/mL), D-dimer (3,815 ng/mL FEU), and ALT (100 U/L). Her creatinine (0.6 mg/dL) and lactate (19 mg/dL) were normal. Complete blood cell count showed leukocytosis (WBC 11,700/μL with segment 88%) with normal hemoglobin (12.4 g/dL) and platelets (251 K/μL). Other relevant in-hospital laboratory results were presented in **Supplementary Table 1**.

We checked COVID-19, influenza A/B, adenovirus, coxsackievirus, mycoplasma, CMV, EBV, HIV, and markers for autoimmune disease. The results were all negative except for reactive CMV IgG with negative CMV IgM and low C3 66 mg/dL (reference 90~180). Myocardial biopsy was suggested but she refused. Because D-dimer level increased from 3,815 to 6,433 ng/mL FEU and history of ChAdOx1 vaccination, anti-PF4 antibody level was checked on August 16, and it was 0.15 optical density (normal < 0.4 OD). There was no detectable venous thrombosis by chest CT and peripheral Doppler. Post-vaccine acute fulminant myocarditis is impressed. Since there is no established treatment protocol for post-vaccine myocarditis, we offered the patient standard therapy for heart failure and perimyocarditis.

Initial medication included furosemide, ivabradine, colchicine, and norepinephrine to keep mean arterial pressure above 65 mmHg. After above treatment for 2 days, her appetite and orthopnea gradually improved, and norepinephrine was discontinued on August 16. Her pulmonary edema resolved and troponin I level decreased (daily troponin I 8.1, 6.8, 5.6, 2.1 mg/mL from August 13 to 16). Spironolactone was added and she was transferred to ward on August 18.

Cardiac MRI on August 19 showed global LV hypokinesia with LVEF 41.6% and markedly increased LV T1 and T2 signal values (**Figure 2**). Late Gadolinium enhancement (LGE) images depict the patchy enhancements sparsely distributed in the mid-layer and subepicardium, and subendocardial enhancement in the antero-septal subendocardium of LV mid-cavity. On August 23, her LVEF was 45% by echocardiography and ECG showed evolutionary changes including higher QRS voltage and diffuse T wave inversion (**Figure 1C**). She was discharged on August 24 with colchicine, losartan, ivabradine, and spironolactone. She had mild dyspnea on exertion and tingling chest pain at discharge, and the symptoms gradually disappeared after discharge. Her latest echocardiography on January 17 2022 showed normal LV diameter (45/31 mm), LVEF 60%, and no pericardial effusion. ECG showed normal sinus rhythm without ST-T changes (**Supplementary Figure 3**). There was a complete recovery of her fulminant perimyocarditis.

DISCUSSION

Acute perimyocarditis is an uncommon side effect after vaccination in the pre-COVID-19 era. In the US Vaccine Adverse Event Reporting System (VAERS), total 708 reports met the definition as perimyocarditis from 1990 to 2018 (3). It occurs more commonly in males (79%) than in females, and the most frequently reported vaccines are smallpox (59%), anthrax (23%), and typhoid (13%) vaccines. There is growing evidence that myocarditis is a rare side effect of mRNA vaccines against COVID-19 (1, 2, 4–6). Considering the background incidence of viral myocarditis [about 10–22 per 100,000 individuals per year (7)], a nationwide study in Israel reported a calculated risk ratio of 2.35-fold of acute myocarditis between BNT162b2 (Pfizer) vaccinated and unvaccinated persons (2), and the risk ratio was higher in adolescent males. Most cases of myocarditis occurred within 5 days (median 2 days) following the second dose (1, 2, 8).

While clinical and basic researchers are working on the relationship between myocarditis and mRNA vaccines, myocarditis after adenovirus or protein-based COVID-19 vaccines has seldom been reported. In a recent review of post-COVID-19 vaccination myocarditis (9), only one of the 61 cases received Ad26.COV2.S adenoviral vaccine (Johnson and Johnson) while the other cases all received mRNA vaccine. In another case report of fulminant myocarditis after Ad26.COV2.S vaccine, the patient expired within 24 h despite of ECMO support (10). Autopsy revealed lymphohistocytic myocarditis. In our report, because the patient refused myocardial biopsy, the diagnosis of myocarditis is based on diagnostic criteria from European Society of Cardiology Working Group on Myocardial and Pericardial Diseases (**Table 1**) (11). All diagnostic criteria include abnormal ECG and echocardiography, elevated Troponin I, and myocardial damage by cardiac MRI were met and coronary angiography showed patent coronary arteries. Because her symptoms onset 2 days after the first dose of ChAdOx1 nCoV-19 vaccine without any other identified etiology, vaccine-related myocarditis was highly suspected. Currently there is no established test to confirm the causal relationship. According to the report from VAERS, rates of post-vaccine myocarditis for females aged 40–49 years was 0.1/1.1 per 1 million doses after first/second dose of BNT162b2 and 0.2/1.4 after first/second dose of mRNA-1273 vaccine (Moderna) (12). The reported incidence of myocarditis after mRNA vaccines is quite low at her age as well. A phase 3 study of ChAdOx1 nCoV-19 vaccine enrolled 32,451 participants, and the number was still underpowered to detect uncommon side effects such as vaccine-induced immune thrombotic thrombocytopenia (VITT). Although no myocarditis was reported in either group, two cases with cardiac disorders were reported as medically attended adverse events in the ChAdOx1 group compared to 0 events in the placebo group (13).

Our patient had negative anti-PF4 antibody, so the pathophysiology was different from VITT. There are several possible mechanisms that may lead to myocarditis after ChAdOx1 vaccination. First, adenovirus is an established cause of acute myocarditis (14). Adenovirus can enter cardiomyocytes by binding to a common transmembrane receptor [coxsackievirus

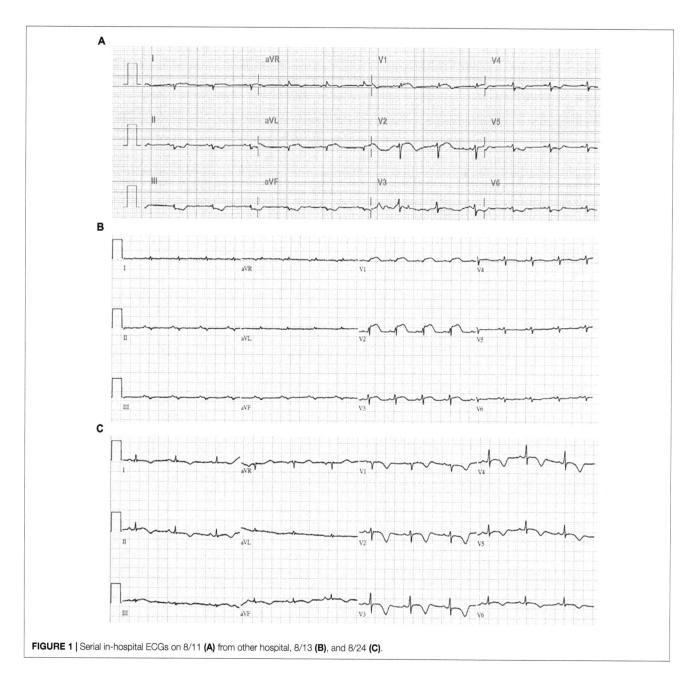

FIGURE 1 | Serial in-hospital ECGs on 8/11 **(A)** from other hospital, 8/13 **(B)**, and 8/24 **(C)**.

and adenovirus receptor (CAR)], induce direct myocardial injury, and trigger an uncontrolled immune response even after viral clearance (15). The genes of dsDNA adenovirus are classified into early genes (E 1–4) which encode proteins for DNA replication and late genes (L 1–5) which encode structural proteins. The viral vector of ChAdOx1 vaccine is a chimpanzee adenovirus (ChAd), which can evade pre-existing human immunity. The ChAd was vectorized by deleting E1/E3 and modifying E4 to reduce virulence and replication in human body (16). In an animal study on rhesus macaques, virus replication in the respiratory tract was limited after vaccination with ChAdOx1 (17). This may explain why a throat swab for adenoviral antigen was negative in our patient.

Another potential mechanism is the molecular similarity between SARS-CoV-2 spike protein and human antigens. Commercially available mouse monoclonal antibodies against SARS-CoV-2 spike protein have been shown to cross-react with some human protein sequences, including α-myosin and actin (18). Repeated antigen exposure may also trigger a dysregulated host response in certain individuals, resulting in polyclonal B-cell expansion, immune complex formation, and inflammation. Induction of anti-idiotype antibodies (antibody 2 against antibody 1) is another possible mechanism for myocarditis after SARS-CoV-2 infection or vaccination (19). Post-vaccination myocarditis bears some similarities to anti-idiotype antibody related myocarditis

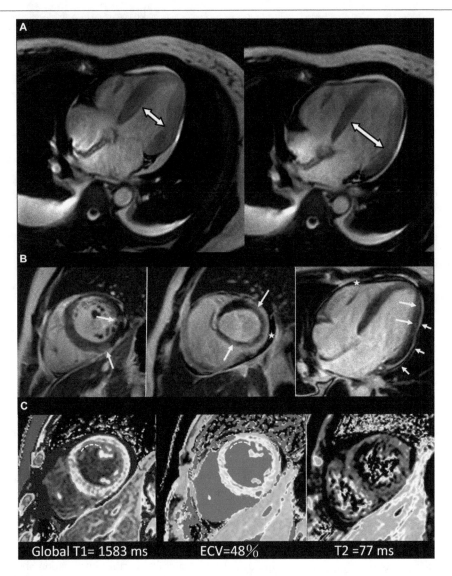

FIGURE 2 | Cardiac MRI of the patient. **(A)** Cardiac MR 4-chamber cine end-systolic (left) and end-diastolic (right) images show the limited LV dimensional change, indicative of the impaired LV systolic function. **(B)** Cardiac MR late Gadolinium enhancement images of short-axis (left, middle) and 4-chamber (right) view. Yellow arrows depict the patchy enhancements sparsely distributed in the mid-layer and subepicardium in a non-ischemic pattern, arrowheads depict pericardial enhancement and stars depict pericardial effusion. The curved dashed line depicts the subendocardial enhancement in the antero-septal subendocardium of LV mid-cavity which is within the LAD territory. **(C)** T1 map (left), ECV map (middle) and T2 map (right) in short-axis views show elevated T1, ECV, and T2 values, indicating acute myocardial injury (global T1 = 1,583 ms, ECV = 48%, T2 = 77 ms; institution-specific cut-off values for abnormal myocardium: T1 global ≥ 1,250 ms, T2 global ≥ 60 ms). CMR findings meet updated 2018 Lake Louise criteria for acute myocarditis (25). The curved dashed lines depict the focally elevated T1 and ECV values in the antero-septal subendocardium, equivalent to the enhanced area depicted in **(B)**.

after viral infections (20). These autoimmune hypotheses can explain the higher incidence of myocarditis after second dose comparing to first dose.

The cardiac MRI in our patient showed increased LV T1 and T2 signal values, indicating acute myocardial injury. Patchy enhancements in the mid-layer and subepicardium by LGE can be observed in the infarction-caused fibrosis and also myocardial damage/necrosis such as myocarditis. These changes are similar to the finding from other myocarditis cases after mRNA vaccination (9). An unusual finding is the enhancement in the antero-septal subendocardium of LV by LGE image,

and the pattern is compatible with myocardial infarction with non-obstructive coronary arteries (MINOCA) (21). Common causes of MINOCA are coronary dissection, coronary artery or microvascular spasm, Takotsubo cardiomyopathy, and myocarditis (22). The MRI abnormalities may be related to the degree of myocardial damage, but cannot explain the etiology. Clinically, most cases of myocarditis following mRNA vaccination have been reported to be mild. In a report from Israel, 41 of the 54 cases were mild, one case received ECMO support, and one case died of unknown cause after discharge (1).

TABLE 1 | Diagnostic criteria for clinically suspected myocarditis from European society of cardiology working group on myocardial and pericardial diseases (11).

Clinical presentations

1. Acute chest pain, pericarditic, or pseudo-ischemic.
2. New-onset (days up to 3 months) or worsening of: dyspnea at rest or exercise, and/or fatigue, with or without left and/or right heart failure signs
3. Sub-acute/chronic (> 3 months) or worsening of: dyspnea at rest or exercise, and/or fatigue, with or without left and/or right heart failure signs
4. Palpitation, and/or unexplained arrhythmia symptoms and/or syncope, and/or aborted sudden cardiac death
5. Unexplained cardiogenic shock

Diagnostic criteria

1. ECG/Holter/stress test: Newly abnormal 12 lead ECG and/or Holter and/or stress testing, any of the following: I to III degree atrioventricular block, or bundle branch block, ST/T wave change (ST elevation or non ST elevation, T wave inversion), sinus arrest, ventricular tachycardia or fibrillation and asystole, atrial fibrillation, reduced R wave height, intraventricular conduction delay (widened QRS complex), abnormal Q waves, low voltage, frequent premature beats, supraventricular tachycardia.
2. Myocardiocytolysis markers: Elevated TnT/TnI
3. Functional and structural abnormalities on cardiac imaging (Echo/Angio/CMR): New, otherwise unexplained LV and/or RV structure and function abnormality (including incidental finding in apparently asymptomatic subjects): regional wall motion or global systolic or diastolic function abnormality, with or without ventricular dilatation, with or without increased wall thickness, with or without pericardial effusion, with or without endocavitary thrombi
4. Tissue characterization by CMR: Edema and/or LGE of classical myocarditic pattern

Clinically suspected myocarditis if ≥ 1 clinical presentation and ≥ 1 diagnostic criteria from different categories, in the absence of: (1) angiographically detectable coronary artery disease (coronarystenosis ≥ 50%); (2) known pre-existing cardiovascular disease or extra-cardiac causes that could explain the syndrome (e.g., valve disease, congenital heart disease, hyperthyroidism, etc.). Suspicion is higher with higher number of fulfilled criteria.
If the patient is asymptomatic ≥ 2 diagnostic criteria should be met.

According to Australian Guidance on Myocarditis and Pericarditis after mRNA COVID-19 Vaccines (23), initial evaluation of post-vaccine myocarditis/pericarditis was similar to that of typical myocarditis, including history taking, 12-lead ECG, chest X-ray, and Troponin level. Suspected cases require referral to a cardiologist for further investigations including echocardiogram, coronary angiography, and cardiac MRI. Endomyocardial biopsy is rarely indicated, as determined by cardiologist. Often supportive treatment is all that is required. Another important issue is about the subsequent COVID-19 vaccines after post-vaccine myocarditis. According to a recent report about the risk of a second COVID-19 vaccine in 40 patients with VITT after first dose of ChAdOx1 nCoV-19 vaccine (5 patients received ChAdOx1 nCoV-19 again, 2 received mRNA-1273, and 33 received BNT162b2), none of the 40 patients had relapse of symptoms or severe adverse reactions (24). To date, there is no published report about the risk of subsequent vaccine on patients with post-vaccine myocarditis. The Canadian National Advisory Committee on Immunization recommends that individuals who had myocarditis/pericarditis after a first dose of mRNA vaccine should wait to receive a second dose until more information is available. In our case, the patient decided to postpone the schedule of second vaccine.

CONCLUSION

Acute pericarditis/myocarditis is a rare but existing side effect after mRNA COVID-19 vaccination, and the incidence is higher among young and adolescence males. Our report demonstrated the possibility of acute myocarditis after ChAdOx1 nCoV-19 vaccine, and the pathophysiology is different from VITT. The risk of post-vaccine myocarditis has affected the public policy in some countries. For example, Finland and Sweden have limited the use of mRNA-1273 vaccine in young people since October 2021. Although myocarditis is potentially lethal, benefits of COVID-19 vaccination (9) still far outweigh this uncommon side effect. Without appropriate evidences, policies about vaccine should be made carefully. Further information about the mechanism and long-term clinical outcome of post-vaccine myocarditis is needed for physicians to manage and give advice about subsequent vaccination on these affected individuals.

AUTHOR CONTRIBUTIONS

C-TW took care of the patient and wrote the report. S-CC performed cardiac MRI and provided the image. P-HC revised the report. All authors contributed to the article and approved the submitted version.

REFERENCES

1. Witberg G, Barda N, Hoss S, Richter I, Wiessman M, Aviv Y, et al. Myocarditis after covid-19 vaccination in a large health care organization. *N Engl J Med.* (2021) 385:2132–9. doi: 10.1056/NEJMoa2110737
2. Mevorach D, Anis E, Cedar N, Bromberg M, Haas EJ, Nadir E, et al. Myocarditis after BNT162b2 mRNA vaccine against Covid-19 in Israel. *N Engl J Med.* (2021) 385:2140–9. doi: 10.1056/NEJMoa2109730
3. Su JR, McNeil MM, Welsh KJ, Marquez PL, Ng C, Yan M, et al. Myopericarditis after vaccination, vaccine adverse event reporting system (VAERS), 1990-2018. *Vaccine.* (2021) 39:839–45. doi: 10.1016/j.vaccine.2020.12.046
4. Verma AK, Lavine KJ, Lin CY. Myocarditis after covid-19 mRNA vaccination. *N Engl J Med.* (2021) 385:1332–4. doi: 10.1056/nejmc2109975
5. Li M, Yuan J, Lv G, Brown J, Jiang X, Lu ZK. Myocarditis and pericarditis following COVID-19 vaccination: inequalities in age and vaccine types. *J Pers Med.* (2021) 11:1106. doi: 10.3390/jpm11111106

6. Miqdad MA, Nasser H, Alshehri A, Mourad AR. Acute myocarditis following the administration of the second BNT162b2 COVID-19 vaccine dose. *Cureus.* (2021) 13:e18880. doi: 10.7759/cureus.18880

7. Olejniczak M, Schwartz M, Webber E, Shaffer A, Perry TE. Viral myocarditis-incidence. Diagnosis and management. *J Cardiothorac Vasc Anesth.* (2020) 34:1591–601. doi: 10.1053/j.jvca.2019.12.052

8. Gargano JW, Wallace M, Hadler SC, Langley G, Su JR, Oster ME, et al. Use of mRNA COVID-19 vaccine after reports of myocarditis among vaccine recipients: update from the advisory committee on immunization practices – United States, June 2021. *MMWR Morb Mortal Wkly Rep.* (2021) 70:977–82. doi: 10.15585/mmwr.mm7027e2

9. Bozkurt B, Kamat I, Hotez PJ. Myocarditis with COVID-19 mRNA vaccines. *Circulation.* (2021) 144:471–84. doi: 10.1161/circulationaha.121.056135

10. Ujueta F, Azimi R, Lozier MR, Poppiti R, Ciment A. Lymphohistocytic myocarditis after Ad26.COV2.S viral vector COVID-19 vaccination. *Int J Cardiol Heart Vasc.* (2021) 36:100869. doi: 10.1016/j.ijcha.2021.10 0869

11. Caforio AL, Pankuweit S, Arbustini E, Basso C, Gimeno-Blanes J, Felix SB, et al. Current state of knowledge on aetiology, diagnosis, management, and therapy of myocarditis: a position statement of the European society of cardiology Working group on myocardial and pericardial diseases. *Eur Heart J.* (2013) 34:2648a–2648a. doi: 10.1093/eurheartj/eht210

12. Su JR. *Myopericarditis Following COVID-19 Vaccine: Updates from the VACCINE ADVERSE Events Reporting System (VAERS).* Atlanta GA: Centers for Disease Control and Prevention (2021).

13. Falsey AR, Sobieszczyk ME, Hirsch I, Sproule S, Robb ML, Corey L, et al. Phase 3 safety and efficacy of AZD1222 (ChAdOx1 nCoV-19) Covid-19 vaccine. *N Engl J Med.* (2021) 385:2348–60. doi: 10.1056/NEJMoa2105290

14. Woodruff JF. Viral myocarditis. A review. *Am J Pathol.* (1980) 101:425–84.

15. Badorff C, Lee GH, Lamphear BJ, Martone ME, Campbell KP, Rhoads RE, et al. Enteroviral protease 2A cleaves dystrophin: evidence of cytoskeletal disruption in an acquired cardiomyopathy. *Nat Med.* (1999) 5:320–6. doi: 10.1038/6543

16. Mendonca SA, Lorincz R, Boucher P, Curiel DT. Adenoviral vector vaccine platforms in the SARS-CoV-2 pandemic. *NPJ Vaccines.* (2021) 6:97. doi: 10. 1038/s41541-021-00356-x

17. van Doremalen N, Haddock E, Feldmann F, Meade-White K, Bushmaker T, Fischer RJ, et al. A single dose of ChAdOx1 MERS provides protective immunity in rhesus macaques. *Sci Adv.* (2020) 6:eaba8399. doi: 10.1126/sciadv. aba8399

18. Vojdani A, Kharrazian D. Potential antigenic cross-reactivity between SARS-CoV-2 and human tissue with a possible link to an increase in autoimmune diseases. *Clin Immunol.* (2020) 217:108480. doi: 10.1016/j.clim.2020.108480

19. Murphy WJ, Longo DL. A possible role for anti-idiotype antibodies in SARS-CoV-2 infection and vaccination. *N Engl J Med.* (2021) 386:394–6. doi: 10. 1056/NEJMcibr2113694

20. Paque RE, Miller R. Autoanti-idiotypes exhibit mimicry of myocyte antigens in virus-induced myocarditis. *J Virol.* (1991) 65:16–22. doi: 10.1128/JVI.65.1. 16-22.1991

21. Abdu FA, Mohammed AQ, Liu L, Xu Y, Che W. Myocardial infarction with nonobstructive coronary arteries (MINOCA): a review of the current position. *Cardiology.* (2020) 145:543–52. doi: 10.1159/000509100

22. Scalone G, Niccoli G, Crea F. Editor's choice- pathophysiology, diagnosis and management of MINOCA: an update. *Eur Heart J Acute Cardiovasc Care.* (2019) 8:54–62. doi: 10.1177/2048872618782414

23. Australian Government. *Guidance on Myocarditis and Pericarditis after mRNA COVID-19 Vaccines.* (2021). Available online at: https: //www.health.gov.au/resources/publications/covid-19-vaccination-guidance-on-myocarditis-and-pericarditis-after-mrna-covid-19-vaccines (accessed December 2, 2021).

24. Lacy J, Pavord S, Brown KE. VITT and second doses of covid-19 vaccine. *N Engl J Med.* (2022) 386:95. doi: 10.1056/NEJMc2118507

25. Ferreira VM, Schulz-Menger J, Holmvang G, Kramer CM, Carbone I, Sechtem U, et al. Cardiovascular magnetic resonance in nonischemic myocardial inflammation: expert recommendations. *J Am Coll Cardiol.* (2018) 72:3158–76. doi: 10.1016/j.jacc.2018.09.072

3

Serial Cardiovascular Magnetic Resonance Studies Prior to and after mRNA-Based COVID-19 Booster Vaccination to Assess Booster-Associated Cardiac Effects

Claudia Meier, Dennis Korthals, Michael Bietenbeck, Bishwas Chamling,
Stefanos Drakos, Volker Vehof, Philipp Stalling and Ali Yilmaz*

Division of Cardiovascular Imaging, Department of Cardiology I, University Hospital Münster, Münster, Germany

Correspondence:
Ali Yilmaz
Ali.Yilmaz@ukmuenster.de

Background: mRNA-based COVID-19 vaccination is associated with rare but sometimes serious cases of acute peri-/myocarditis. It is still not well known whether a 3rd booster-vaccination is also associated with functional and/or structural changes regarding cardiac status. The aim of this study was to assess the possible occurrence of peri-/myocarditis in healthy volunteers and to analyze subclinical changes in functional and/or structural cardiac parameters following a mRNA-based booster-vaccination.

Methods and Results: Healthy volunteers aged 18–50 years ($n = 41$; $m = 23$, $f = 18$) were enrolled for a CMR-based serial screening before and after 3rd booster-vaccination at a single center in Germany. Each study visit comprised a multi-parametric CMR scan, blood analyses with cardiac markers, markers of inflammation and SARS-CoV-2-IgG antibody titers, resting ECGs and a questionnaire regarding clinical symptoms. CMR examinations were performed before (median 3 days) and after (median 6 days) 3rd booster-vaccination. There was no significant change in cardiac parameters, CRP or D-dimer after vaccination, but a significant rise in the SARS-CoV-2-IgG titer ($p < 0.001$), with a significantly higher increase in females compared to males ($p = 0.044$). No changes regarding CMR parameters including global native T1- and T2-mapping values of the myocardium were observed. A single case of a vaccination-associated mild pericardial inflammation was detected by T2-weighted CMR images.

Conclusion: There were no functional or structural changes in the myocardium after booster-vaccination in our cohort of 41 healthy subjects. However, subclinical pericarditis was observed in one case and could only be depicted by multiparametric CMR.

Keywords: COVID-19, vaccination, CMR, MRI, myocarditis, t1-mapping, t2-mapping

INTRODUCTION

Without any doubt, COVID-19 vaccines are a blessing and prevented many millions of people world-wide from becoming either very ill or even dying due to a COVID-19 infection. Nevertheless, various reports showed that particularly mRNA-based COVID-19 vaccines are associated with rare but sometimes serious cases of acute peri-/myocarditis (1, 2). We still need to better understand why some people show cardiac adverse events following vaccination.

Magnetic resonance imaging (MRI) is the non-invasive gold standard in the diagnosis of myocardial inflammation (3). In this context, some impressive case reports presented severe myocardial damage on cardiovascular magnetic resonance imaging (CMR) even without functional impairment (4, 5), and the true number of COVID-19 vaccine-associated peri-/myocarditis may even be underreported since CMR is still not widely available.

So far, there are only limited data available regarding the frequency of vaccine-associated peri-/myocarditis following a 3rd booster vaccination for COVID-19 and regarding the value of CMR (6, 7). Hence, the aim of this prospective study was (a) to assess the possible occurrence of peri-/myocarditis following a mRNA-based booster vaccination in healthy volunteers and (b) to also analyze whether there are subclinical changes in functional and/or structural cardiac parameters possibly triggered by the preceding booster vaccination.

METHODS

Healthy volunteers aged 18–50 years were enrolled for a CMR-based serial screening before and after 3rd booster vaccination in the CMR-Center of University Hospital Muenster, Germany. Each study visit comprised a CMR scan, blood analyses with cardiac markers, markers of inflammation and SARS-CoV-2-IgG antibody titers, resting ECGs and a questionnaire regarding clinical symptoms. After their baseline examination, the study subjects received their 3rd booster dose of a mRNA-based COVID-19 vaccine with either mRNA-1273 (Moderna) or BNT162b2 (Pfizer-BioNTech) within 1–10 days. The follow-up examination was performed 4–10 days after booster vaccination.

Cardiovascular magnetic resonance imaging was performed on a 1.5 T-scanner (Philips Healthcare, Best, Netherlands) with a modified standard protocol used in clinical practice for suspected myocarditis (8). The protocol included high resolution cine, native T1- as well as T2-mapping, T2-STIR imaging and flow measurements. Contrast agent administration with additional late-gadolinium-enhancement (LGE) imaging was only intended if the native scan showed clear signs of active myocardial inflammation. Native T1- and T2- times were measured on three short axis views using pixelwise maps. All subjects gave their written informed consent to the study.

Skewed variables are expressed as median and interquartile range (IQR). Categorical variables are expressed as frequency with percentage. A p-value ≤ 0.05 was considered statistically significant.

RESULTS

Between November 2021 and January 2022, we prospectively examined 41 healthy, individuals with a median age of 35 years before (median 3 days) and after (median 6 days) their 3rd booster vaccination. The subjects (56% male) had no history of any cardiac disease or prior COVID-19 infection. There was one loss of follow up, because one participant experienced a COVID-19 infection in the interval between the third vaccination and the follow-up appointment. 30% of the subjects received mRNA-1273 (Moderna) and 70% received BNT162b2 (BioNTech) for booster (**Table 1**). No association between the subjective burden of symptoms and the respective increase in SARS CoV-2-IgG titer was observed.

There was no pathological elevation and no significant change in serum markers such as CK, CK-MB, high-sensitive troponin T, NT-proBNP, CRP or D-dimer before and after the 3rd booster vaccination (**Table 2**). As expected, there was a highly significant rise in the SARS-CoV-2-IgG titer ($p < 0.001$) in our study population. In addition, females showed a significantly higher increase in SARS-CoV-2-IgG titer ($p = 0.044$) compared to males.

In general, the assessment of both functional as well as structural CMR parameters showed highly consistent and reproducible values when the respective CMR parameters measured before and after the booster vaccination were compared. In particular, there was no change in biventricular function and volumes, in global longitudinal strain and in myocardial mass (**Table 2**). Moreover, the global native T1- and T2-mapping values remained unchanged (988 vs. 983 ms in T1

TABLE 1 | Subject characteristics.

Parameter			
Age, years		35 (31–38)	
Male/female, n (%)		23/18 (56%/44%)	
BMI, kg/m^2		23.2 (22.2–24.4)	
Time between BL-CMR and booster vaccination, days		3.0 (1.3–6.0)	
Time between FUP-CMR and booster vaccination, days		(5.3–7.8)	
Vaccine for 3rd vaccination			
- BioNTech (BNT162b2)		28 (70%)	
- Moderna (mRNA-1273)		12 (30%)	
Allergies, n (%)		14 (34%)	
Symptoms after 3rd vs. 2nd vaccination	n	n	p^*
- Local	34	22	**0.008**
- Fever	9	10	0.08
- Palpitations	4	1	0.27
- Chest pain	1	1	0.31
- Dyspnea	2	1	0.65
- Fatigue	22	24	0.67
- No symptoms	6	12	**0.011**

*If not stated otherwise all data are expressed as median (interquartile range). *Calculated for duration of symptoms not frequency among subjects. BMI, body mass index; BL-CMR, cardiac magnetic resonance at baseline; FUP-CMR, cardiac magnetic resonance at follow-up. The variables in bold show the significant correlations at a significance level of p.*

TABLE 2 | Cardiac magnetic resonance (CMR)-findings, laboratory, and ECG parameters.

Parameter	Pre booster	Post booster	p-Value
➤ **CMR findings**			
LV-EF,%	60 (55–63)	61 (57–64)	0.05
LV-EDVi, ml/m^2	87 (80–95)	86 (90–94)	0.24
LV- GLS,%	−16.2 (−17.2 to −15.0)	−15.9 (−17.1 to −14.6)	0.75
RV-EF,%	55 (50–59)	54 (51–57)	0.85
RV-EDVi, ml/m^2	92 (83–102)	91 (80–100)	0.48
LV-mass, g/m^2	47 (42–54)	47 (42–54)	0.61
Global native T1, ms	988 (964–1,011)	983 (970–1,024)	0.90
No. of segments with elevated T1 Mapping value > 1,060 ms, n (%)	0 (0%)	0 (0%)	
Global T2, ms	50 (49–51)	50 (49–51)	0.40
No. of segments with elevated T2 Mapping value > 59 ms, n (%)	0 (0%)	0 (0%)	
Presence of edema in T2 weighted images,			
- myocardial, n (%)	0 (0%)	0 (0%)	
- pericardial, n (%)	2 (1.6%)	3 (2.6%)	
➤ **Biochemistry marker**			
CK, U/l	113 (83–187)	99 (78–133)	0.07
CK-MB, U/l	14 (12–16)	14 (12–17)	0.50
Troponin T, ng/l	3.0 (3.0–4.7)	3.0 (3.0–4.3)	0.59
NT-pro-BNP, pg/ml	30 (13–58)	21 (11–52)	0.26
D-dimer, mg/l	0.27 (0.27–0.27)	0.27 (0.27–0.28)	0.39
CRP, mg/dl	0.5 (0.5–0.5)	0.5 (0.5–0.5)	0.32
SARS CoV-2-IgG, AU/ml	1,319 (681–1,788)	16,077 (10,312–32,540)	**<0.001**
SARS CoV-2-IgG in male, AU/ml	1,807 (601–2,485)	15,643 (9,129–19,650)	**<0.001**
SARS CoV-2-IgG in female, AU/ml	2,076 (691–1,717)	24,271 (11,092–40,000)	**<0.001**
Δ SARS CoV-2-IgG, AU/ml	*Male*	*Female*	
	13,388 (8,873–15,927)	20,640 (9,332–38,637)	**0.044**
➤ **ECG parameters**			
Heart rate, bpm	67 (60–75)	71 (64–78)	0.06
ST-elevation			
- minor < 0,1 mV, n	14 (34%)	12 (30%)	
- significant ≥ 0,1 mV, n	0 (0%)	0 (0%)	
ST-depression ≥ -0,1 mV, n	0 (0%)	0 (0%)	

If not stated otherwise all data are expressed as median (interquartile range); All biochemistry marker (with exception of SARS CoV-2-IgG) are in normal range of values. LV-EF, left ventricular ejection fraction; LV-EDVi, indexed left ventricular end-diastolic volume; LV-GLS, left ventricular global longitudinal stain; RV-EF, right ventricular ejection fraction; RV-EDVi, indexed right ventricular end-diastolic volume; CK, creatinine kinase; CK-MB, creatinine kinase isoenzyme MB; NT-pro BNP, N-terminal -pro brain natriuretic peptide; CRP, C-reactive protein; SARS CoV-2-IgG, anti-severe acute respiratory syndrome coronavirus 2 -immunoglobulin G. Δp – significance between the changes among IgG rise in male and female. p < 0.05 is considered as significant. The variables in bold show the significant correlations at a significance level of p.

and each 50 ms in T2). There was one female who demonstrated a new "pericardial" T2-STIR-weighted hyperintensity in the basal to midventricular inferolateral pericardium and also a new pleural effusion (**Figure 1**). In the absence of any symptoms or signs of other diseases, we interpreted these findings as a vaccination-associated form of very mild pericardial inflammation. There was no known clinical characteristic or laboratory parameter that could provide a predisposition to pericarditis in this case.

DISCUSSION

Although the pivotal approval studies, sponsored by the respective pharmaceutical companies, did not show an increased risk of myocarditis following COVID-19 vaccination (9, 10), today there is no doubt that mRNA-based COVID-19 vaccination can cause peri-/myocarditis particularly in young males (1, 11, 12). It has also been shown that the risk of myocarditis is predominantly increased after the second vaccination dose. Assuming an autoimmune-mediated process, it is still unknown whether a 3rd booster vaccination is also associated with a non-neglectable risk of peri-/myocarditis.

To the best of our knowledge, our present study is the first one that used multi-parametric serial CMR studies prior to and after mRNA-based COVID-19 booster vaccination to carefully assess potential booster-associated cardiac effects. Our major findings can be summarized as follows:

First, the present data show that no relevant myocardial changes could be observed by CMR following the 3rd booster vaccination. Our data support current recommendations regarding booster vaccinations that should not be withheld for fear of adverse cardiac events in healthy subjects aged <50 years (considering that there is no vaccination with mRNA-1273

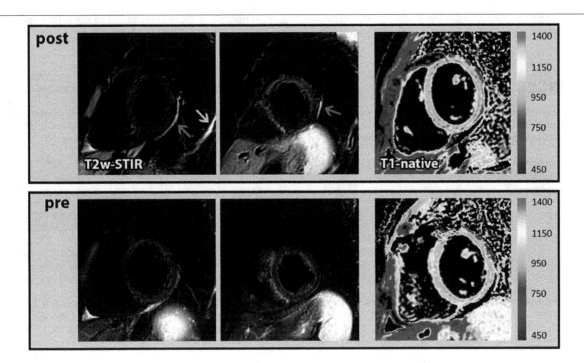

FIGURE 1 | Cardiac magnetic resonance (CMR) images of pericarditis. *First row*: T2-STIR-weighted short-axis images with the occurrence of pericardial hyperintensity as indication for edema/mild pericardial inflammation (red arrow) and a new pleural effusion (green arrow) following the 3rd COVID-19 vaccination. In addition, corresponding T1 mapping without signs of myocardial impairment. *Second row*: Corresponding images at baseline (prior to 3rd COVID-19 vaccination) from the same subject without any pathological findings.

(Moderna) in subjects <30 years since cases of peri-/myocarditis were more frequently observed after Moderna vaccination in this age group).

Second, subclinical pericarditis was observed in 1 out of 40 subjects following a 3rd booster vaccination whereas no cases of myocarditis were observed in the present study. Importantly, multi-parametric CMR imaging was the only diagnostic modality that allowed to depict such a mild pattern of pericardial inflammation. In line with this findings, a large descriptive study, based on reports to the VEARS (Vaccine Adverse Event Reporting System) reported only 17% of abnormal findings based on echocardiograms (in the cohort of myocarditis patients younger than 30 years), but abnormalities were reported in >70% by CMR (1).

Today, CMR is well-known and robust modality for the non-invasive diagnosis of myocarditis that does not only detect regional dysfunction, but allows also to depict edema and other subtle structural changes based on elevated T1- and T2-mapping values and/or characteristic patterns of LGE (13, 14). Therefore, the Lake Louise criteria for CMR-based diagnosis of myocardial inflammation were already established in 2009 and updated in 2018 (15, 16). Since the diagnosis of vaccine-associated myocarditis is important for symptom management, for exercise recommendations, for further cardiomyopathy monitoring and future (e.g., booster) vaccination decisions (3), physicians should be aware of the potential of multi-parametric CMR.

Last but not least, our present data clearly show that a 3rd booster vaccination leads to a substantial increase in the SARS CoV-2-IgG antibody titer – and interestingly to a higher increase in females compared to males. Hence, gender-based differences should be evaluated more carefully in future studies.

CONCLUSION

The present serial CMR data support current recommendations regarding the safety of 3rd booster vaccinations since no functional or subtle structural changes were observed in the myocardium – as long as current vaccination recommendations are followed. However, subclinical pericarditis was observed in one case and could only be depicted by multiparametric CMR.

AUTHOR CONTRIBUTIONS

CM devised the project, performed CMR examinations, performed major analyses of the CMR data, and drafted the manuscript. DK performed the CMR analyses and participated in the interpretation of results. MB participated in the design of the study, performed CMR examinations, and statistical analyses. BC participated in the design of the study, CMR exams, and critically reviewed the manuscript. SD participated in the CMR exams and in the analysis of the CMR data. VV and PS performed CMR examinations and participated in the analysis of clinical data. AY provided the main conceptual idea, supervised the work, provided critical feedback and helped shape the research, analysis, and

manuscript. All authors contributed to the article and approved the submitted version.

REFERENCES

1. Oster ME, Shay DK, Su JR, Gee J, Creech CB, Broder KR, et al. Myocarditis cases reported after mRNA-Based COVID-19 vaccination in the US From December 2020 to August 2021. *JAMA*. (2022) 327:331–40. doi: 10.1001/jama.2021.24110

2. Albert E, Aurigemma G, Saucedo J, Gerson DS. Myocarditis following COVID-19 vaccination. *Radiol Case Rep*. (2021) 16:2142–5.

3. Tschöpe C, Ammirati E, Bozkurt B, Caforio ALP, Cooper LT, Felix SB, et al. Myocarditis and inflammatory cardiomyopathy: current evidence and future directions. *Nat Rev Cardiol*. (2021) 18:169–93. doi: 10.1038/s41569-020-00435-x

4. Chamling B, Vehof V, Drakos S, Weil M, Stalling P, Vahlhaus C, et al. Occurrence of acute infarct-like myocarditis following COVID-19 vaccination: just an accidental co-incidence or rather vaccination-associated autoimmune myocarditis? *Clin Res Cardiol*. (2021) 110:1850–4. doi: 10.1007/s00392-021-01916-w

5. Kim HW, Jenista ER, Wendell DC, Azevedo CF, Campbell MJ, Darty SN, et al. Patients with acute myocarditis following mRNA COVID-19 vaccination. *JAMA Cardiol*. (2021) 6:1196–201. doi: 10.1001/jamacardio.2021.2828

6. Atmar RL, Lyke KE, Deming ME, Jackson LA, Branche AR, El Sahly HM, et al. Homologous and heterologous Covid-19 booster vaccinations. *N Engl J Med*. (2022) 386:1046–57. doi: 10.1056/NEJMoa2116414

7. Shiyovich A, Witberg G, Aviv Y, Kornowski R, Hamdan A. A case series of myocarditis following third (Booster) Dose of COVID-19 vaccination: magnetic resonance imaging study. *Front Cardiovasc Med*. (2022) 9:839090. doi: 10.3389/fcvm.2022.839090

8. Kramer CM, Barkhausen J, Bucciarelli-Ducci C, Flamm SD, Kim RJ, Nagel E. Standardized cardiovascular magnetic resonance imaging (CMR) protocols: 2020 update. *J Cardiovasc Magn Reson*. (2020) 22:17. doi: 10.1186/s12968-020-00607-1

9. Food and Drug Administration [FDA], Center for Biologics Evaluation and Researc [CBER]. *Vaccines and Related Biological Products Advisory Committee December 17, 2020 Meeting Briefing Document - FDA, CBER, Biologics,COVID-19 FDA Briefing Document Moderna COVID-19 Vaccine: Published online December 17, 2020*. Silver Spring, MD: Food and Drug Administration (2020).

10. Covid PB. *Pfizer-Biontech COVID-19 Vaccine (BNT162, PF-07302048) Vaccines and Related Biological Products Advisory Committee Briefing Document*. Silver Spring, MD: Food and Drug Administration (2020). p. 92

11. Montgomery J, Ryan M, Engler R, Hoffman D, McClenathan B, Collins L, et al. Myocarditis following immunization with mRNA COVID-19 vaccines in members of the US Military. *JAMA Cardiol*. (2021) 6:1202–6. doi: 10.1001/jamacardio.2021.2833

12. Castiello T, Georgiopoulos G, Finocchiaro G, Claudia M, Gianatti A, Delialis D, et al. COVID-19 and myocarditis: a systematic review and overview of current challenges. *Heart Fail Rev*. (2022) 27:251–61. doi: 10.1007/s10741-021-10087-9

13. Yilmaz A, Ferreira V, Klingel K, Kandolf R, Neubauer S, Sechtem U. Role of cardiovascular magnetic resonance imaging (CMR) in the diagnosis of acute and chronic myocarditis. *Heart Fail Rev*. (2013) 18:747–60. doi: 10.1007/s10741-012-9356-5

14. McDonagh TA, Metra M, Adamo M, Gardner RS, Baumbach A, Böhm M, et al. 2021 ESC Guidelines for the diagnosis and treatment of acute and chronic heart failure. *Eur Heart J*. (2021) 42:3599–726.

15. Friedrich MG, Sechtem U, Schulz-Menger J, Holmvang G, Alakija P, Cooper LT, et al. Cardiovascular magnetic resonance in myocarditis: a JACC White Paper. *J Am Coll Cardiol*. (2009) 53:1475–87. doi: 10.1016/j.jacc.2009.02.007

16. Ferreira VM, Schulz-Menger J, Holmvang G, Kramer CM, Carbone I, Sechtem U, et al. Cardiovascular magnetic resonance in nonischemic myocardial inflammation: expert recommendations. *J Am Coll Cardiol*. (2018) 72:3158–76. doi: 10.1016/j.jacc.2018.09.072

4

Women and COVID-19: A One-Man Show?

Jef Van den Eynde[1*], Karen De Vos[2*], Kim R. Van Daalen[3] and Wouter Oosterlinck[1]

[1] Department of Cardiovascular Diseases, University Hospitals Leuven, Leuven, Belgium, [2] Faculty of Law, KU Leuven, Leuven, Belgium, [3] Cardiovascular Epidemiology Unit, Department of Public Health and Primary Care, University of Cambridge, Cambridge, United Kingdom

*Correspondence:
Jef Van den Eynde
jef.vandeneynde@student.kuleuven.be
Karen De Vos
karen.devos@student.kuleuven.be

Keywords: COVID-19, gender equality, human rights, public health, women

Coronavirus disease 2019 (COVID-19) severity and mortality have consistently been higher in men compared to women. The possible biological and behavioral factors underlying this difference have recently been analyzed by Capuano et al. (1). The ideas raised by the authors define a clear need for a more adequate approach to sex differences in case fatality rate. The higher mortality rate in men has indeed been described extensively in literature (2–4). However, the impact of the current pandemic reaches far beyond mortality rates. To tackle this pandemic effectively, an integrated response is essential (5). That is why in this article, we would like to draw attention to some of the main structural, psychological, social and economic impacts this pandemic has on women, as observed by academics, practitioners and international organizations.

Although we acknowledge gender to be complex, social, and non-binary, we will mainly focus on the impact of the current pandemic on women and refer to other publications about the impact on transgender and non-binary populations (6–8).

THE CURRENT LACK OF SEX-DISAGGREGATED DATA

Sex- and gender-disaggregated data on COVID-19 confirmed cases are important in order to address gender disparities in COVID-19 health outcomes and ensure a gender-responsive approach. However, sex disaggregated data is lacking for most countries and gender disaggregated data is nearly absent. As of August 3, 2020, 18.07 million cases were reported worldwide. Data presented in **Figure 1** ($n = 8{,}587{,}718$ sex-disaggregated cases), therefore, represent only 47.5% of all reported cases, highlighting the current lack of these valuable data. Furthermore, a striking difference in the percentage of women among confirmed cases is seen, with 60% in countries such as Belgium, the United Kingdom, and Canada, to 20% in countries such as the Central African Republic, Uganda, and India. Indeed, recent data show that among all persons tested for COVID-19 in the Central African Republic, only 26% were women.

INFECTION RISK AMONG THE HEALTHCARE WORKFORCE

Women face a higher risk of becoming infected during a pandemic because of their position in society as reported by the United Nations (UN) and the World Health Organization (WHO) (9–11). As doctors, nurses, midwives, and community health workers, women are overrepresented at the frontlines, making up 70% of the global health and social workforce (11). Particular issues are the global lack of personal appropriate protective equipment (PPE) and the fact that most PPE are

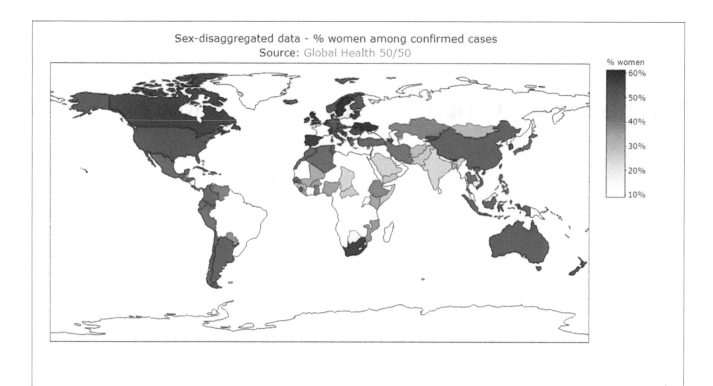

FIGURE 1 | Sex-disaggregated data (Source: Global Health 50/50, https://globalhealth5050.org/covid19/sex-disaggregated-data-tracker/, 15/08/2020) Data are reported from the date that sex-disaggregated data was last available. The map was created using R Statistical Software (version 4.0.2. 2020-06-22, Foundation for Statistical Computing, Vienna, Austria), "plotly" package.

based on a *"default man"* size providing a suboptimal barrier to most women and leaving them more exposed (12). Data from several outbreaks Ebola outbreaks and the SARS outbreak of 2003 demonstrate that nurses and other caretakers have been heavily infected in comparison to other groups in society (13).

SOCIAL IMPACT

As a result of traditional social roles and stereotypes, women still act as the primary caregiver in households, globally spending three to four times more time on unpaid domestic work than men [The International Labor Organization (ILO)] (14). The additional care burden associated with childcare and homeschooling during lockdowns and the care for sick family members can lead to considerable health impacts including e.g., psychological stress. Usual coping mechanisms are limited, given the reduced contact with peers and the disruption of supportive networks. This especially hits single-parent households, of which the majority are headed by women (21% of households with children in the United States compared to 4% by men) (15). Furthermore, as a result, having less time for education, paid work, and career advancement, women can experience increased social inequality during this pandemic (15, 16). Stay-at-home measures together with financial and security concerns can put considerable strain on families, which in some situations can lead to domestic abuse and sexual violence. UN-reports show that

violence against women and girls has increased by 25% in several countries and even doubled in some countries since the outbreak of COVID-19 (17).

ECONOMIC IMPACT

Across the globe, women and girls earn less, have less access to educational opportunities, more often hold insecure jobs, and have limited access to financial resources and digital technology (18). Apart from deepening these existing inequalities, multiple studies show that the COVID-19 pandemic has a disproportionately large economic effect on women because the sectors in which they are most active are hard-hit (19). First of all, the manufacturing-and-retail industry has experienced large fallbacks in export and sales because of lockdown and distancing measures. The World Trade Organization (WTO) reports that female employees represent 80% of the workforce in ready-made garment production in Bangladesh, in which industry orders declined by 81% in April alone (20). Moreover, a larger share of women than men work in tourism and business travel which are highly disrupted by travel restrictions and will require a long recovery period (16, 18). Relying on face-to-face interactions, these occupations do not lend themselves to teleworking. Finally, this economic downturn will also be felt by female start-up entrepreneurs who are increasingly finding their way to micro, small and medium enterprises

TABLE 1 | Recommendations for a more gender-sensitive approach to pandemics.

Issue	Recommendation
Lack of sex-disaggregated data	States, their partners and research institutions should collect, report, and analyze data on confirmed COVID-19 cases and deaths that are disaggregated by sex and age (10). The WHO provides global and national surveillance guidelines (10).
Higher risk of infection	Employers should be aware of the higher risk women face in the health and social domain and provide safe and decent working conditions. This can be monitored by workplace representatives, trade unions, and mutual control between employers (12).
Social impact	There should be more social awareness about the social impacts of pandemics. (In)formal protection and support services should be in place together with innovative solutions such as online fora and hotlines (16). Core health and education services and systems should be maintained (26).
Economic impact	Apart from tackling existing economic inequalities, (financial) support measures for businesses should be provided to prevent an economic downfall (16). Moreover, the value of women's unpaid care work should be recognized by including it in the formal labor market and redistributing unpaid family care equally.
Human rights	Decision-makers should be aware that outbreaks affect groups differently and ensure a gender-responsive intersectional response to the COVID-19 pandemic (that recognizes the realities of different genders and addresses these) in policies, program development, implementation etc. Increased participation of women in decision-making will help establish adaptive responses to these realities (27). Inclusivity and diversity in decision-making should be ensured reflecting the population they represent. Existing women's and youth rights networks should be engaged to support connectivity and vital information flow (26).

(MSMEs) (21). MSMEs tend to be the first businesses impacted in times of recession. Given the long-term economic impact that COVID-19 will have, protecting female entrepreneurship should be on the priority list of governments in order to build a faster and more inclusive growth during the economic recovery period.

HUMAN RIGHTS

The Secretary General of the Council of Europe put it best: "While the virus is resulting in the tragic loss of life, we must nonetheless prevent it from destroying our way of life" (22). Human rights reflect the minimum standards necessary for people to live with dignity. While the COVID-19 crisis is fast becoming a socio-economic crisis it adds pressure on human rights. For women and girls, the problems identified form an undeniable increased threat to their right to life and right to health (23). Various international law instruments [e.g., The Universal Declaration of Human Rights, Art. 25 (24)] recognize the right to health as an inclusive right, encompassing a wide range of factors that help humans lead a healthy life (25). These factors include safe drinking water, safe food, sanitation, but also health-related education and information, the right to access to health care, and gender equality. As the UN state in their latest Policy Brief, the economic impact and prevalence of poverty among women, their experience of violence, their position in society, the limited power many women have over their sexual and reproductive lives, and their lack of influence in decision-making are social realities that adversely impact women's human rights and that should move to global action (9).

A WAY FORWARD

Prevention and response management is hindered when gendered impacts of outbreaks are ignored obscuring critical trends. In order to minimize these impacts, different steps should be undertaken. In **Table 1** we provide a list of important recommendations made by international organizations.

CONCLUSION

Gendered differences of COVID-19 are present not only at the biological level, but also at the psychological, social and societal level. Although literature shows that men are clearly predisposed to COVID-19 related mortality, women are just as well victimized, albeit in a different way. The current pandemic painfully highlights that gender inequality is still insufficiently addressed in our society. Public health should never be a predominantly men affair mainly focusing on the male body—a one-man show. In contrast, more gender-sensitive approaches that take into account different physical, mental, and social needs across the full gender spectrum are indispensable to guarantee optimal well-being of all.

AUTHOR CONTRIBUTIONS

JV and KD conceived and wrote the manuscript. KV and WO critically revised the manuscript and provided important intellectual contribution. All authors contributed to the article and approved the submitted version.

REFERENCES

1. Capuano A, Rossi F, Paolisso G. Covid-19 kills more men than women: an overview of possible reasons. *Front Cardiovasc Med.* (2020) 7:131. doi: 10.3389/fcvm.2020.00131

2. Gagliardi MC, Tieri P, Ortona E, Ruggieri A. ACE2 expression and sex disparity in COVID-19. *Cell Death Discov.* (2020) 6:37. doi: 10.1038/s41420-020-0276-1

3. Elgendy IY, Pepine CJ. Why are women better protected from COVID-19: clues for men? Sex and COVID-19. *Int J Cardiol.* (2020) 315:105–06. doi: 10.1016/j.ijcard.2020.05.026

4. Agrawal H, Das N, Nathani S, Saha S, Saini S, Kakar SS, et al. An assessment on impact of COVID-19 infection in a gender specific manner. *Stem Cell Rev Rep.* (2020) 1–19. doi: 10.1007/s12015-020-10048-z

5. Wenham C, Smith J, Davies SE, Feng H, Grépin KA, Harman S, et al. Women are most affected by pandemics - lessons from past outbreaks. *Nature.* (2020) 583:194–8. doi: 10.1038/d41586-020-02006-z

6. Salerno JP, Williams ND, Gattamorta KA. LGBTQ populations: psychologically vulnerable communities in the COVID-19 pandemic. *Psychol Trauma.* (2020) 12:S239–42. doi: 10.1037/tra0000837

7. Wang Y, Pan B, Liu Y, Wilson A, Ou J, Chen R. Health care and mental health challenges for transgender individuals during the COVID-19 pandemic. *Lancet Diabetes Endocrinol.* (2020) 8:564–5. doi: 10.1016/S2213-8587(20)30182-0

8. Sevelius JM, Gutierrez-Mock L, Zamudio-Haas S, McCree B, Ngo A, Jackson A, et al. Research with marginalized communities: challenges to continuity during the COVID-19 pandemic. *AIDS Behav.* (2020) 24:2009–12. doi: 10.1007/s10461-020-02920-3

9. United Nations. *The Impact of COVID-19 on Women.* (2020). Available online at: https://www.unwomen.org/-/media/headquarters/attachments/sections/library/publications/2020/policy-brief-the-impact-of-covid-19-on-women-en.pdf?la=en&vs=1406 (accessed November 9, 2020).

10. World Health Organization? *Gender and COVID-19: Advocacy Brief* (2020). Available online at: https://apps.who.int/iris/handle/10665/332080 (accessed November 9, 2020).

11. World Health Organization. *Gender Equity in the Health Workforce: Analysis of 104 Countries.* (2019). Available online at: https://apps.who.int/iris/bitstream/handle/10665/311314/WHO-HIS-HWF-Gender-WP1-2019.1-eng.pdf?ua=1 (accessed August 16, 2020).

12. Trades Union Congress. *Personal Protective Equipment and Women.* (2017). Available online at: https://www.tuc.org.uk/sites/default/files/PPEandwomenguidance.pdf (accessed August 16, 2020).

13. World Health Organization. *Addressing Sex and Gender in Epidemic-Prone Infectious Diseases.* (2007). Available online at: https://www.who.int/csr/resources/publications/SexGenderInfectDis.pdf (accessed August 16, 2020).

14. International Labour Organization. *Care Work and Care Jobs for the Future of Decent Work.* (2018). Available online at: https://www.ilo.org/wcmsp5/groups/public/---dgreports/---dcomm/---publ/documents/publication/wcms_633135.pdf (accessed August 16, 2020).

15. Alon T, Doepke M, Olmstead-Rumsey J, Tertilt M. The impact of COVID-19 on Gender equality. In: *Covid Economics: Vetted and Real-Time Papers.* (2020) 4:62–85.

16. World Bank Group. *Gender Dimensions of the COVID-19 Pandemic.* (2020). Available online at: http://documents1.worldbank.org/curated/en/618731587147227244/pdf/Gender-Dimensions-of-the-COVID-19-Pandemic.pdf (accessed August 16, 2020).

17. UN Women. *COVID-19 and Ending Violence Against Women and Girls.* (2020). Available online at: https://prod.unwomen.org/-/media/headquarters/attachments/sections/library/publications/2020/issue-brief-covid-19-and-ending-violence-against-women-and-girls-en.pdf?la=es&vs=5006 (accessed August 16, 2020).

18. World Trade Organization. *The Economic Impact of COVID-19 on Women in Vulnerable Sectors and Economies.* (2020). Available online at: https://www.wto.org/english/news_e/news20_e/info_note_covid_05aug20_e.pdf?fbclid=IwAR131NFWHhdwPQIOM3GN6_jYpnwae5JTleO9pPqgFVo5sKubCi8NkNxOr6I (accessed August 16, 2020).

19. World Trade Organization. *Trade in Services in the Context of COVID-19.* (2020). Available online at: https://www.wto.org/english/tratop_e/covid19_e/services_report_e.pdf (accessed August 16, 2020).

20. Financial Express. *Bangladesh's RMG Export in April Declines Nearly 85 per cent.* (2020). Available online at: https://www.globaltimes.cn/content/1187514.shtml (accessed August 16, 2020).

21. World Trade Organization. *World Trade Report 2019 – The Future of Services Trade.* (2020). Available online at: https://www.wto.org/english/res_e/booksp_e/00_wtr19_e.pdf (accessed August 16, 2020).

22. Council of Europe. *Speeches 2020 - Saint Petersburg International Legal Forum.* (2020). Available online at: https://www.coe.int/en/web/secretary-general/-/saint-petersburg-international-legal-forum (accessed August 16, 2020).

23. United Nations. *COVID-19 and Human Rights – We are All in This Together.* (2020). Available online at: https://www.un.org/sites/un2.un.org/files/un_policy_brief_on_human_rights_and_covid_23_april_2020.pdf?fbclid=IwAR2ojuGQlNSdbBUOEfG-gsWWtc4FSI8f4KI7-DypyTpGBU_IiPO5R7cOSD0 (accessed August 16, 2020).

24. United Nations. *The Universal Declaration of Human Rights.* (1948). Available online at: https://www.ohchr.org/EN/UDHR/Documents/UDHR_Translations/eng.pdf (accessed August 16, 2020).

25. Office of the United Nations High Commissioner for Human Rights. *The Right to Health, Fact Sheet No. 31.* (2008). Available online at: https://www.ohchr.org/Documents/Publications/Factsheet31.pdf (accessed August 16, 2020).

26. UNICEF. *Five Actions for Gender Equality in the COVID-19 Response.* (2020). Available online at: https://www.unicef.org/media/66306/file/Five%20Actions%20for%20Gender%20Equality%20in%20the%20COVID-19%20Response:%20UNICEF%20Technical%20Note.pdf (accessed on November 9, 2020)

27. Bali S, Dhatt R, Lal A, Jama A, Van Daalen K, Sridhar D. Off the back burner: diverse and gender-inclusive decision-making for COVID-19 response and recovery. *BMJ Glob Health.* (2020) 5:e002595. doi: 10.1136/bmjgh-2020-002595

5

Cardiovascular Complications of COVID-19 Vaccines

Runyu Liu[1†], Junbing Pan[1†], Chunxiang Zhang[2,3,4] and Xiaolei Sun[1,2,3,4,5,6*]

[1] Department of General Surgery (Vascular Surgery), The Affiliated Hospital of Southwest Medical University, Luzhou, China, [2] Key Laboratory of Medical Electrophysiology, Ministry of Education and Medical Electrophysiological Key Laboratory of Sichuan Province, Collaborative Innovation Center for Prevention and Treatment of Cardiovascular Disease of Sichuan Province, Institute of Cardiovascular Research, Southwest Medical University, Luzhou, China, [3] Cardiovascular and Metabolic Diseases Key Laboratory of Luzhou, Luzhou, China, [4] Nucleic Acid Medicine of Luzhou Key Laboratory, Southwest Medical University, Luzhou, China, [5] Department of Interventional Medicine, The Affiliated Hospital of Southwest Medical University, Luzhou, China, [6] King's College London British Heart Foundation Centre of Research Excellence, School of Cardiovascular Medicine and Sciences, Faculty of Life Science and Medicine, King's College London, London, United Kingdom

*Correspondence:
Xiaolei Sun
sunxiaolei@swmu.edu.cn;
xiaolei.sun@kcl.ac.uk

† These authors have contributed
equally to this work

Coronavirus disease 2019 (COVID-19) has become a global public health catastrophe. Vaccination against severe acute respiratory syndrome coronavirus-2 (SARS-CoV-2) is proven to be the most effective measure to suppress the pandemic. With the widespread application of the four vaccines, namely, ChAdOx1, Ad26.COV2.S, BNT162b2, and mRNA-1273.2, several adverse effects have been reported. The most serious type of complication is cardiovascularly related, including myocarditis, immune thrombocytopenia (ITP), cerebral sinus venous thrombosis, among others. All these adverse events undermine the health of the vaccinees and affect the administration of the vaccines. As the distribution of COVID-19 vaccines is surrounded by suspicion and rumors, it is essential to provide the public with accurate reports from trusted experts and journals. Monitoring the safety of COVID-19 vaccines is an important and ongoing process that is also urgent. Thus, we summarized the cardiovascular complications of the major types of COVID-19 vaccines, including mRNA vaccines, which are now generally considered to be innovative vaccines, and the future for vaccination against COVID-19, in addition to the underlying pathogenesis and potential therapeutics.

Keywords: COVID-19, vaccine, cardiovascular, complication, mRNA

INTRODUCTION

Severe acute respiratory syndrome coronavirus-2 (SARS-CoV-2), also known as coronavirus disease 2019 (COVID-19), has spread rapidly throughout the world, leading to acute respiratory distress syndrome (ARDS). COVID-19 has become a global public health catastrophe. Vaccination against SARS-CoV-2 is now proven to be the most effective means of suppressing the pandemic (1). COVID-19 vaccines showed high efficacy against SARS-CoV-2 during the different phases of clinical trials (1). The first four vaccine preparations (i.e., ChAdOx1 and AD26.COV2·S, BNT162b2, and mRNA-1273) have received marketing authorization from the European Medicines Agency (EMA) (2). With the widespread application of these four vaccines, several adverse effects, such as pain at the site of inoculation, fever, and allergic reactions, have been reported (3). The most serious complications are cardiovascularly related, and these complications include myocarditis, immune thrombocytopenia (ITP), cerebral sinus venous thrombosis, and visceral thrombosis. All of these adverse events impair the health of those receiving vaccinations and affect the administration of the vaccines (4, 5). Thus, it is necessary to summarize the cardiovascular complications of the major types of COVID-19 vaccines (**Figure 1**) and review the underlying pathogenesis and potential therapies.

mRNA Vaccines

At present, there are two types of mRNA vaccines used to prevent SARS-CoV-2, namely, Pfizer's BNT162b2 mRNA vaccine and Moderna's mRNA-1273 vaccine. mRNA vaccines use the mRNA that encodes the spike protein of SARS-CoV-2, surrounded by lipid nanoparticles (LNPs). The spike protein induces the body to produce the corresponding antibodies, which causes recipients to develop immunity to SARS-CoV-2. The BNT162b2 mRNA vaccine has been reported to be effective in a variety of COVID-19 clinical trials (6). However, the development of cardiovascular adverse events after the administration of these mRNA vaccines should be seriously considered.

Myocarditis After COVID-19 mRNA Vaccination

A total of 561,197 people in North Carolina were vaccinated from February 1 to April 30, 2021. Later, the Duke University Medical Center in Durham reported 4 cases of myocarditis; in all cases, the patients developed severe chest pain with biomarker evidence of myocardial damage, and all 4 patients were later hospitalized (4). In another case, one Filipino patient was diagnosed with myocarditis 3 days after receiving the second dose of the BNT162b2 mRNA vaccine (7). From January 30 to February 20, 2021, six patients with chest pain were treated in the Hillel Yaffe Medical Center, Israel, soon after vaccination with the BNT162b2 mRNA vaccine. All six of these patients were diagnosed with myocarditis, and one of these patients had received only the first dose of the vaccination (8). As mRNA vaccination becomes more widespread, an increasing number of myocarditis cases have been diagnosed. All patients with mild symptoms can be discharged within 4–8 days after treatment with non-steroidal anti-inflammatory drugs or colchicine (8). As on June 11, 2021, more than 296 million doses of COVID-19 mRNA vaccine had been administered in the United States, of which 52 million were administered to people aged 12–29 years. From December 29, 2020, to June 11, 2021, the Vaccine Adverse Event Reporting System (VAERS) received 1,226 reports of myocarditis after mRNA vaccination. The risk of myocarditis increases within 7 days after the first or second dose of an mRNA vaccine (9). The Centers for Disease Control and Prevention reported two cases of histologically confirmed myocarditis after COVID-19 mRNA vaccination on August 18, 2021. A 42-year-old man developed breathing difficulties and chest pain 2 weeks after receiving the second dose of the mRNA-1273 vaccine. It was also reported that he had no viral prodrome, and his PCR tests were negative for SARS-CoV-2. The patient developed tachycardia and fever. An electrocardiogram (ECG) showed diffuse ST-segment elevation, and Doppler echocardiography showed biventricular dysfunction (ejection fraction, 15%). The patient died of cardiogenic shock 3 days after the visit, and an autopsy revealed biventricular myocarditis (10). The potential

mechanisms of mRNA vaccine-induced myocarditis are still unclear. It has been reported that the mRNA-1273 vaccine can induce a strong CD4 cytokine response involving type 1 helper T (Th1) cells, and CD4 cells are an important factor in myocarditis (11, 12). The detailed mechanisms warrant further clinical and basic research.

Thrombosis With COVID-19 mRNA Vaccination

The Medicines and Healthcare Products Regulatory Agency in the United Kingdom reported that, with the administration of 10.6 million doses of the BNT162b2 mRNA vaccine, there were 24 cases of cerebral venous sinus thrombosis (CVST), 3 cases of cerebral vascular thrombosis, 3 cases of superior sagittal sinus thrombosis, and 1 case of transverse sinus thrombosis (13). Among 4 million doses of mRNA-1273 that have been administered, 5 cases of suspected CVST have been reported (14). The mechanism underlying the association between mRNA vaccination and thrombosis is unelucidated. It is speculated that it is related to the encoding of the SARS-CoV-2 spike protein by mRNA vaccines. The spike protein, which is necessary to allow SARS-CoV-2 to invade human cells, enhances platelet aggregation and promotes the secretion of dense granules from platelets (15). Moreover, as a binding ligand of the ACE2 receptor, the SARS-CoV-2 spike protein induces an inflammatory response in brain endothelial cells and impairs the functional integrity of the blood-brain barrier, which promotes the activation of endothelial cells and the upregulation of leucocyte chemokines, pro-inflammatory cytokines (interleukin (IL)-1β and IL-6), and cell adhesion molecules [intercellular adhesion molecule 1 (ICAM-1) and vascular cell adhesion molecule 1 (VCAM-1)] (16). All of these mRNA vaccine-related pathophysiological activities might initiate the development of thrombosis. Thus, anti-spike protein monoclonal antibodies or recombinant human ACE2 proteins might assist in the treatment of patients with COVID-19 mRNA vaccine-induced thrombosis (15). However, at present, the current clinical treatment of choice is anticoagulation therapy with unfractionated heparin, followed by low-molecular-weight heparin and then warfarin (13).

Vaccine-Induced Thrombocytopenia

One day after receiving the first dose of the mRNA-1273 vaccine, a 60-year-old African-American man developed the symptoms of low-grade fever and chills, followed by the appearance of a severe generalized rash on his skin that quickly spread throughout his body. In addition, he was diagnosed with ITP (17). From mid-February to mid-March, nearly 5 million people in Israel were vaccinated with the BNT162b2 mRNA vaccine, and four patients were diagnosed with acquired thrombotic thrombocytopenic purpura (ATTP) (18). In the United States, more than 20 million people (as on February 2, 2021) have received at least one dose of either of the two available mRNA vaccines, and 20 of these patients developed thrombocytopenia after vaccination. Most of the 20 patients had symptoms, such as bruises or mucosal bleeding. Nine of these patients were vaccinated with the BNT162b2 mRNA vaccine, and 11 of these patients were vaccinated with the mRNA-1273 vaccine (19). Interestingly, in the United States, approximately 50,000 adults are diagnosed with ITP each year. Thus, the incidence rate of mRNA vaccine-related ITP is almost the same as that of the baseline incidence rate for the population (19). However, most of these patients developed ITP symptoms after their first dose of COVID-19 mRNA vaccination; therefore, there seems to be a link between ITP and mRNA vaccine administration. However, the potential mechanism underlying the relationship between mRNA vaccines and ITP is unknown. Vaccines can activate autoimmunity through molecular mimicry, which induces the production of antiplatelet autoantibodies and causes thrombocytopenia (20).

ADENOVIRAL VECTOR VACCINES

At present, the cardiovascular complications that have been observed in association with adenoviral vector vaccines, i.e., the ChAdOx1 nCoV-19 (Oxford-AstraZeneca [AZ]; also known as Vaxzevria) vaccine and AD26.COV2·S (Johnson & Johnson [JJ]) vaccine, are primarily associated with thrombosis with thrombocytopenia syndrome (TTS). The ChAdOx1 nCoV-19 and AD26.COV2·S vaccines are composed of recombinant adenovirus vectors from chimpanzee adenovirus or human adenovirus, which encode the spike protein of SARS-CoV-2 (21). As on April 7, 2021, 34 million people had been vaccinated with ChAdOx1 in the European Economic Area and the United Kingdom, and the EMA reported 169 cases of cerebral venous thrombosis and 53 cases of splanchnic vein thrombosis (SVT) after vaccination (2). Six cases of suspected CVST have been reported among more than 7 million recipients of the AD26.COV2·S adenovirus vector vaccine (14). In the context of a worldwide vaccination campaign, these safety issues should not be ignored. Most patients with thrombosis are positive for anti-PF4 antibodies, which have effects similar to heparin-induced thrombocytopenia (HIT); therefore, this syndrome was named vaccine-induced immune thrombotic thrombocytopenia (VITT) (2, 14). VITT mainly occurs in women under the age of 55 years, often occurs 4–16 days after patients receive an adenovirus-based vaccine, and is associated with a high mortality rate (14, 22). A 35-year-old pregnant woman developed intracerebral hemorrhage in the left temporal lobe associated with VITT 12 days after off-label ChAdOx1 nCoV-19 vaccination. This pregnant woman, who was at 23 weeks of gestation, died on day 17 (after vaccination) of refractory intracranial hypertension despite the use of all available pressure control measures (23).

The activation and depletion of platelets in VITT do not rely on heparin (2, 21, 24). Why, then, do anti-PF4 antibodies appear? It has been reported that the presence of PF4-immunoglobulin G (IgG) antibodies increases with the severity of trauma (25); therefore, the production of PF4 antibodies may be associated with an inflammatory response following adenovirus vector vaccination. As PF4 is released by platelets and forms a complex with heparin in the pathogenesis of HIT, the human body forms an IgG against the PF4-heparin complex. Another hypothesis is that after vaccination, viral proteins and free DNA bind to PF4 and form a new antigen (26). These antibodies can bind to FcγRIIa on platelets, promoting platelet activation and aggregation and thus leading to thrombosis (27). In addition,

the activation of von Willebrand factor (vWF) and P-selectin after the administration of adenoviral vector vaccines plays a key role in complexes of platelets, white blood cells, and endothelial cells and accelerates the activation and clearance of platelets (28, 29). The other underlying mechanism is that the ethylenediaminetetraacetic acid (EDTA) in vaccine preparations may increase vascular permeability at the injection site and may cause the vaccine components to spread through the bloodstream, which may produce a signal that leads to the production of anti-PF4 antibodies in B cells (2).

However, not all adenoviral vector vaccines induce similar symptoms. No VITT-related adverse events have been reported for the AD5 adenovirus vector vaccine produced by CanSino Biologics (2). The principles for the treatment of VITT are the administration of intravenous immunoglobulin, anticoagulation, the avoidance of heparin, and the transfusion of platelets (30). If the platelet levels are $>30 \times 10^9$/L and if fibrinogen is >1.5 g/L, non-heparin anticoagulation, including argatroban, bivalirudin, apixaban, or rivaroxaban, is suggested (20).

INACTIVATED VACCINES

Inactivated vaccines have been extensively studied and have the advantage of being easy to store and transport, making them suitable for many low-income countries (31). The BBIP-CorV inactivated vaccine was produced by Sinopharm in China and developed from the HB02 strain isolated from patients at the Jinyintan Hospital in Wuhan, China. The ZhongkangKewei (WIBP-CorV) inactivated vaccine, developed from the WIVO4 strain, was also isolated from patients at the Jinyintan Hospital (31). The CoronaVac vaccine is produced by Sinovac Life Sciences in China. In the 40,382 recipients of these vaccines, all three inactivated vaccines had a high level of safety and efficacy (>70%), and none of the patients developed serious cardiovascular adverse events related to vaccination (31). However, in Turkey, among more than 7 million vaccinated people, a 41-year-old woman without any cardiovascular risk factors developed symptoms that included facial flushing, chest palpitations, and chest pain 15 min after receiving the first vaccine dose. She was diagnosed with type one Kounis syndrome, which is a combination of acute coronary disease and hypersensitivity. After treatment with oral antihistamine and aspirin, the patient improved and was discharged from the hospital (32). Although this is the first reported case of allergic myocardial infarction secondary to the administration of an inactivated vaccine, more clinical data and research on the underlying mechanism are needed.

The cardiovascular complications associated with COVID-19 vaccines are presented in detail in **Table 1**.

DISCUSSION

The emergence of the delta variant (Pango lineage B.1.617.2) of SARS-CoV-2 has caused a global resurgence of the pandemic. However, fortunately, the latest real-world data have revealed that COVID-19 vaccines, (33) especially the BNT162b2 mRNA

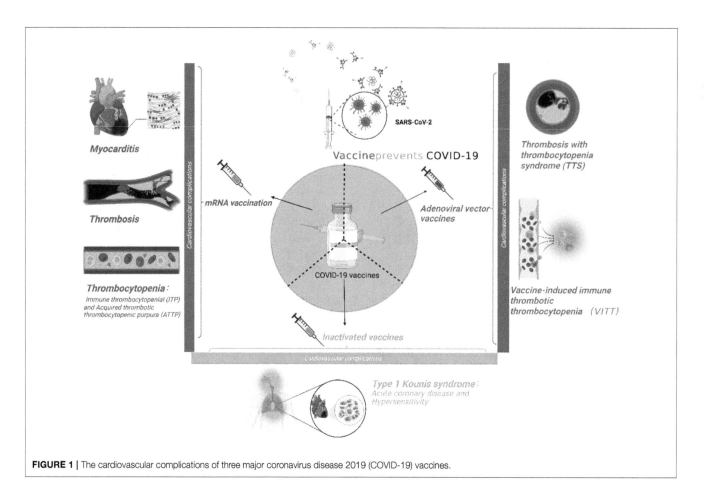

FIGURE 1 | The cardiovascular complications of three major coronavirus disease 2019 (COVID-19) vaccines.

vaccine, still have 88% efficacy for preventing the symptomatic morbidity of the delta variant of SARS-CoV-2 (34). With the increasingly widespread use of COVID-19 vaccines, safety issues associated with the vaccines are gradually becoming the focus of public concern.

Inactivated vaccines have been used for many years to prevent a variety of infectious diseases, and consequently, their safety is generally considered good. However, cardiovascular-related allergic events can occur during vaccination. According to the available literature, the frequency of severe allergic reactions after inactivated vaccine administration appears to be low. However, type one Kounis syndrome is one such rare serious adverse event. Physicians should be aware that Kounis syndrome is a rare but dangerous complication of inactivated coronavirus vaccines. Patients who develop chest pain or severe allergic reactions after vaccination should undergo ECG, echocardiography, and troponin measurement, and these patients should undergo adequate observation or hospitalization if necessary (32).

The VITT, a particularly rare cardiovascular complication, has been observed in adenoviral vector vaccines but not in the other types of vaccines; however, cases of thrombocytopenia after mRNA vaccination have been reported and may be due to an autoimmune mechanism. The key point is whether the VITT/TTS was observed with ChAdOx1 nCoV-19 and AD26.COV2·S vaccinations to represent side effects specific

to adenovirus vector vaccines and the extent to which this may affect the administration of the adenoviral vector vaccines. There have been reports suggesting that the incidence of VITT/TTS may be much higher than previously assumed, and this incidence may further increase as physicians become increasingly aware of the syndrome. The estimated incidence of VITT varies among different reports, from ~1 in 25,000 vaccinated with ChAdOx1 and 1 in more than 500,000 vaccinated with AD26.COV2·S (2). However, these findings should not be used as a reason to discontinue the use of ChAdOx1 nCoV-19 or AD26.COV2·S vaccines. The incidence of VITT complications following adenovirus vector vaccination remains low, while the COVID-19 infection rate and mortality rate are much higher (25).

The mRNA vaccines are innovative vaccines that represent the future of vaccination against COVID-19, and they have the advantages of low production costs and short production cycles. Although the BNT162b2 and mRNA-1273 vaccines were 95% effective after two doses in a phase III clinical trial, (35) the long-term efficacy of these mRNA vaccines is poorly understood. Although mRNA vaccines have been proven to be highly preventive, their cardiovascular side effects should also be seriously considered. Acute myocarditis is a critical adverse event after mRNA vaccination, especially in young males, and these adverse events should be considered in patients who

TABLE 1 | Cardiovascular complications of coronavirus disease 2019 (COVID-19) vaccines.

Vaccine	Data source or region	Time	Complication	Total number administered	Number of events	Complication rate
BNT162B2 (8)	Israel	To 2021.3.24	Myocarditis	More than 4 million	6	1.5/1 million
BNT162B2 (13)	MHRA	2020.12.9–2021.5.26	Thrombosis	10.6 million	33	3.11/1 million
BNT162B2 (13)	Singapore	To 2021.5.31	Thrombosis	1,766,493	3	1.70/1 million
BNT162B2 (14)	EMA	Unknown	Thrombosis	54 million	35	0.65/1 million
mRNA vaccine (19)	VAERS	To 2021.2.2	ITP	20 million	20	1.00/1 million
BNT162B2 (18)	Israel	2021.2–2021.3	ATTP	5 million	4	0.80/1 million
mRNA vaccine (4)	DUMC	2021.2.1–2021.4.30	Myocarditis	561,197	4	7.14/1 million
mRNA vaccine (9)	USA	2020.12.29–2021.6.1	Myocarditis	52 million	1,226	23.58/1 million
mRNA-1273 (14)	EMA	Unknown	Thrombosis	4 million	5	1.25/1 million
mRNA vaccine and ChAdOx1 (13)	VigiBase	2020.12.12–2021.3.16	Thrombosis	Unknown	2,169	Unknown
ChAdOx1 (1)	PRAC	To 2021.4.7	Thrombotic thrombocytopenia	34 million	222	6.53/1 million
ChAdOx1 (21)	UK	To 2021.4.14	Thrombotic thrombocytopenia	21.2 million	168	7.92/1 million
AD26.COV2·S (21)	USA	To 2021.4.13	Thrombosis	6.8 million	15	2.21/1 million
AD26.COV2·S (14)	EMA	Unknown	Thrombosis	More than 7 million	6	0.86/1 million

MHRA, Medicines and Healthcare Products Regulatory Agency of the United Kingdom; EMA, European Medicines Agency; VAERS, Vaccine Adverse Events Reporting System; DUMC, Duke University Medical Center; VigiBase, WHO Global Database for Individual Case Safety Reports; PRAC, the EMA's Pharmacovigilance Risk Assessment Committee.

develop cardiac symptoms after receiving an mRNA vaccine (7). However, the specific mechanism needs to be further explored in larger studies. The cases of mRNA vaccine-secondary ITP following the administration of the BNT162b2 mRNA vaccine or the mRNA-1273 vaccine have been reported and have raised public concern (17, 18). Public panic intensified after the first confirmation of a patient who died of an intracranial hemorrhage (19). The incidence of ITP after mRNA vaccination was actually not far from the estimated baseline annual incidence in the general population; however, post-vaccination ITP remains a possibility, especially in patients with an onset of 1–2 weeks after exposure (19). For patients with cardiovascular complications after mRNA vaccination, such as myocarditis, thrombosis, and ITP, further study is needed to determine whether a second dose of vaccine is needed, whether a different type of vaccine should be used, or whether ITP following the initial dose will exacerbate all of these problems. British researchers launched a phase I clinical trial of a second-generation COVID-19 vaccine on September 20, 2021. The new vaccine, named GRT-R910, (36) is a self-amplified mRNA vaccine. With the global trend of the development of new mRNA vaccines, it is important for researchers to pay increased attention to these possible fatal cardiovascular complications.

The attitudes of people in the community toward vaccination against COVID-19 have been volatile since the end of 2019. People were reluctant to be vaccinated at the initial stage of the application of the new COVID-19 vaccines, as the mid- and long-term data were lacking. As the pandemic worsened in 2020, many people were in favor of being vaccinated. However, as the number of adverse events, especially cardiovascular complications, of these COVID-19 vaccines merged, people became conflicted about whether to be vaccinated, even when the delta variant and the subsequent omicron variant merged. In contrast, due to a lack of scientific and prompt

information and data, people are concerned about the possible complications of these vaccines and refuse to allow themselves or their children to be vaccinated. This contradiction also impacts their normal life, resulting in different degrees of anxiety (37). For countries around the world, spending on nationwide COVID-19 vaccination under the suspicion of these adverse events might have unprecedented budget implications for governments and commercial payers. Governments should focus on expanding health system infrastructure and subsidize payer coverage to deliver these vaccines effectively (38). Since the outbreak of the pandemic in 2019, people have been concerned about the complications of vaccines, which have sparked anti-vaccine movements. It is now most important to raise public awareness of COVID-19 vaccine complications through urgent education to reduce the negative impact of a lack of knowledge of COVID-19 vaccination decisions (39).

Although multiple COVID-19 vaccine-related cardiovascular adverse events have been reported, vaccines are still widely used because they are effective against the virus. Compared with the low incidence of complications, the high efficacy of the vaccines against COVID-19 suggests that COVID-19 vaccines should be widely administered. In fact, the cardiovascular complications caused by vaccines can be effectively treated, and most patients improve quickly. Furthermore, a recent study indicated that SARS-CoV-2 infection is itself a very strong risk factor for myocarditis, and the virus also substantially increases the risk of many other serious adverse events (40). A syndrome called Long-COVID-19 has recently emerged among COVID-19 survivors, which is characterized by persistent, typical acute symptoms accompanied by changes in inflammatory and coagulation parameters caused by endothelial damage. SARS-CoV-2 causes the activation of local and circulating coagulation factors, inducing the production of diffuse coagulation. The similarities and differences between the cardiovascular complications caused by COVID-19 and those caused by mRNA vaccines *via* the spike protein need to be further studied (41). Thus, people should not refuse vaccinations or promote conspiracy theories out of fear of vaccine-related complications.

As the distribution of COVID-19 vaccines is surrounded by suspicion and rumors, it is essential to provide the public with accurate reports from trusted experts, such as medical professionals. Monitoring the safety of COVID-19 vaccines is an important and ongoing process that warrants urgent attention. We propose the establishment of a global database on COVID-19 vaccine adverse events to collect precise and continuous data. In addition, regional regulatory systems should regulate vaccine administration and monitor the occurrence of adverse events and their follow-up in vaccinated people.

AUTHOR CONTRIBUTIONS

All authors listed have made a substantial, direct, and intellectual contribution to the work and approved it for publication.

REFERENCES

1. Greinacher A, Thiele T, Warkentin TE, Weisser K, Kyrle PA, Eichinger S. Thrombotic thrombocytopenia after ChAdOx1 nCov-19 vaccination. *N Engl J Med.* (2021) 384:2092–101. doi: 10.1056/NEJMoa2104840

2. Tsilingiris D, Vallianou NG, Karampela I, Dalamaga M. Vaccine induced thrombotic thrombocytopenia: the shady chapter of a success story. *Metabol Open.* (2021) 11:100101. doi: 10.1016/j.metop.2021.100101

3. Abu-Hammad O, Alduraidi H, Abu-Hammad S, Alnazzawi A, Babkair H, Abu-Hammad A, et al. Side effects reported by jordanian healthcare workers who received COVID-19 vaccines. *Vaccines.* (2021) 9:577. doi: 10.3390/vaccines9060577

4. Kim HW, Jenista ER, Wendell DC, Azevedo CF, Campbell MJ, Darty SN, et al. Patients with acute myocarditis following mRNA COVID-19 vaccination. *JAMA Cardiol.* (2021) 6:1196–201. doi: 10.1001/jamacardio.2021.2828

5. Schultz NH, Sørvoll IH, Michelsen AE, Munthe LA, Lund-Johansen F, Ahlen MT, et al. Thrombosis and thrombocytopenia after ChAdOx1 nCoV-19 vaccination. *N Engl J Med.* (2021) 384:2124–30. doi: 10.1056/NEJMoa2104882

6. Dagan N, Barda N, Kepten E, Miron O, Perchik S, Katz MA, et al. BNT162b2 mRNA Covid-19 vaccine in a nationwide mass vaccination setting. *N Engl J Med.* (2021) 384:1412–23. doi: 10.1056/NEJMoa2101765

7. Habib MB, Hamamyh T, Elyas A, Altermanini M, Elhassan M. Acute myocarditis following administration of BNT162b2 vaccine. *IDCases.* (2021) 25:e01197 doi: 10.1016/j.idcr.2021.e01197

8. Abu Mouch S, Roguin A, Hellou E, Ishai A, Shoshan U, Mahamid L, et al. Myocarditis following COVID-19 mRNA vaccination. *Vaccine.* (2021) 39:3790–3 doi: 10.1016/j.vaccine.2021.05.087

9. Gargano JW, Wallace M, Hadler SC, Langley G, Su JR, Oster ME, et al. Use of mRNA COVID-19 vaccine after reports of myocarditis among vaccine recipients: update from the advisory committee on immunization practices - United States, June 2021. *MMWR Morb Mortal Wkly Rep.* (2021) 70:977–82. doi: 10.15585/mmwr.mm7027e2

10. Koizumi T, Awaya T, Yoshioka K, Kitano S, Hayama H, Amemiya K, et al. Myocarditis after COVID-19 mRNA vaccines. *QJM.* (2021) 114:741–3. doi: 10.1093/qjmed/hcab244

11. Vdovenko D, Eriksson U. Regulatory role of CD4(+) T Cells in Myocarditis. *J Immunol Res.* (2018) 2018:4396351. doi: 10.1155/2018/4396351

12. Anderson EJ, Rouphael NG, Widge AT, Jackson LA, Roberts PC, Makhene M, et al. Safety and immunogenicity of SARS-CoV-2 mRNA-1273 vaccine in older adults. *N Engl J Med.* (2020) 383:2427–38. doi: 10.1056/NEJMoa2028436

13. Fan BE, Shen JY, Lim XR, Tu TM, Chang CCR, Khin HSW, et al. Cerebral venous thrombosis post BNT162b2 mRNA SARS-CoV-2 vaccination: a black swan event. *Am J Hematol.* (2021) 96:E357–61. doi: 10.1002/ajh.26272

14. Cines DB, Bussel JB. SARS-CoV-2 vaccine-induced immune thrombotic thrombocytopenia. *N Engl J Med.* (2021) 384:2254–6. doi: 10.1056/NEJMe2106315

15. Zhang S, Liu Y, Wang X, Yang L, Li H, Wang Y, et al. SARS-CoV-2 binds platelet ACE2 to enhance thrombosis in COVID-19. *J Hematol Oncol.* (2020) 13:120. doi: 10.1186/s13045-020-00954-7

16. Buzhdygan TP, DeOre BJ, Baldwin-Leclair A, Bullock TA, McGary HM, Khan JA, et al. The SARS-CoV-2 spike protein alters barrier function in 2D static and 3D microfluidic in-vitro models of the human blood-brain barrier. *Neurobiol Dis.* (2020) 146:105131. doi: 10.1016/j.nbd.2020.105131

17. Malayala SV, Mohan G, Vasireddy D, Atluri P. Purpuric rash and thrombocytopenia after the mRNA-1273 (Moderna) COVID-19 vaccine. *Cureus.* (2021) 13:e14099. doi: 10.7759/cureus.14099

18. Maayan H, Kirgner I, Gutwein O, Herzog-Tzarfati K, Rahimi-Levene N, Koren-Michowitz M, et al. Acquired thrombotic thrombocytopenic purpura: a rare disease associated with BNT162b2 vaccine. *J Thromb Haemost.* (2021) 19:2314–7. doi: 10.1111/jth.15420

19. Lee EJ, Cines DB, Gernsheimer T, Kessler C, Michel M, Tarantino MD, et al. Thrombocytopenia following Pfizer and moderna SARS-CoV-2 vaccination. *Am J Hematol.* (2021) 96:534–7. doi: 10.1002/ajh.26132

20. Rinaldi M, Perricone C, Ortega-Hernandez OD, Perricone R, Shoenfeld Y. Immune thrombocytopaenic purpura: an autoimmune cross-link between infections and vaccines. *Lupus.* (2014) 23:554–67. doi: 10.1177/0961203313499959

21. Long B, Bridwell R, Gottlieb M. Thrombosis with thrombocytopenia syndrome associated with COVID-19 vaccines. *Am J Emerg Med.* (2021) 49:58–61. doi: 10.1016/j.ajem.2021.05.054

22. Marcucci R, Marietta M. Vaccine-induced thrombotic thrombocytopenia: the elusive link between thrombosis and adenovirus-based SARS-CoV-2 vaccines. *Intern Emerg Med.* (2021) 16:1113–9. doi: 10.1007/s11739-021-02793-x

23. Mendes-de-Almeida DP, Martins-Goncalves R, Morato-Santos R, De Carvalho GAC, Martins SA, Palhinha L, et al. Intracerebral hemorrhage associated with vaccine-induced thrombotic thrombocytopenia following ChAdOx1 nCOVID-19 vaccine in a pregnant woman. *Haematologica.* (2021) 106:3025–8. doi: 10.3324/haematol.2021.279407

24. Dotan A, Shoenfeld Y. Perspectives on vaccine induced thrombotic thrombocytopenia. *J Autoimmun.* (2021) 121:102663. doi: 10.1016/j.jaut.2021.102663

25. Thiele T, Ulm L, Holtfreter S, Schonborn L, Kuhn SO, Scheer C, et al. Frequency of positive anti-PF4/polyanion antibody tests after COVID-19 vaccination with ChAdOx1 nCoV-19 and BNT162b2. *Blood.* (2021) 138:299–303. doi: 10.1182/blood.2021012217

26. Aladdin Y, Algahtani H, Shirah B. Vaccine-induced immune thrombotic thrombocytopenia with disseminated intravascular coagulation and death following the ChAdOx1 nCoV-19 vaccine. *J Stroke Cerebrovasc Dis.* (2021) 30:105938. doi: 10.1016/j.jstrokecerebrovasdis.2021.105938

27. Novak N, Tordesillas L, Cabanillas B. Adverse rare events to vaccines for COVID-19: From hypersensitivity reactions to thrombosis and thrombocytopenia. *Int Rev Immunol.* (2021) 12:1–10. doi: 10.1080/08830185.2021.1939696

28. Othman M, Labelle A, Mazzetti I, Elbatarny HS, Lillicrap D. Adenovirus-induced thrombocytopenia: the role of von Willebrand factor and P-selectin in mediating accelerated platelet clearance. *Blood.* (2007) 109:2832–9. doi: 10.1182/blood-2006-06-032524

29. Handtke S, Wolff M, Zaninetti C, Wesche J, Schonborn L, Aurich K, et al. A flow cytometric assay to detect platelet-activating antibodies in

VITT after ChAdOx1 nCov-19 vaccination. *Blood.* (2021) 137:3656–9. doi: 10.1182/blood.2021012064

30. Bourguignon A, Arnold DM, Warkentin TE, Smith JW, Pannu T, Shrum JM, et al. Adjunct immune globulin for vaccine-induced immune thrombotic thrombocytopenia. *N Engl J Med.* (2021) 385:720–8. doi: 10.1056/NEJMoa2107051

31. Al Kaabi N, Zhang Y, Xia S, Yang Y, Al Qahtani MM, Abdulrazzaq N, et al. Effect of 2 Inactivated SARS-CoV-2 vaccines on symptomatic COVID-19 infection in adults: a randomized clinical trial. *JAMA.* (2021) 326:35–45. doi: 10.1001/jama.2021.8565

32. Ozdemir IH, Ozlek B, Ozen MB, Gunduz R, Bayturan O. Type 1 kounis syndrome induced by inactivated SARS-COV-2 vaccine. *J Emerg Med.* (2021) 61:e71–6. doi: 10.1016/j.jemermed.2021.04.018

33. Lucas C, Vogels CBF, Yildirim I, Rothman JE, Lu P, Monteiro V, et al. Impact of circulating SARS-CoV-2 variants on mRNA vaccine-induced immunity. *Nature.* (2021) 600:523–9. doi: 10.1038/s41586-021-04085-y

34. Tartof SY, Slezak JM, Fischer H, Hong V, Ackerson BK, Ranasinghe ON, et al. Effectiveness of mRNA BNT162b2 COVID-19 vaccine up to 6 months in a large integrated health system in the USA: a retrospective cohort study. *Lancet.* (2021) 397:1819–29. doi: 10.1016/S0140-6736(21)02183-8

35. Sadarangani M, Marchant A, Kollmann TR. Immunological mechanisms of vaccine-induced protection against COVID-19 in humans. *Nat Rev Immunol.* (2021) 21:475–84 doi: 10.1038/s41577-021-00578-z

36. *Early Trial of Multivariant COVID-19 Vaccine Booster Begins in Manchester* (2021). Available online at: https://www.manchester.ac.uk/discover/news/early-trial-of-first-multivariant-covid-19-vaccine-booster-begins-in-manchester (accessed September 20, 2021).

37. Saha K, Torous J, Caine ED, De Choudhury M. Psychosocial effects of the COVID-19 pandemic: large-scale quasi-experimental study on social media. *J Med Internet Res.* (2020) 22:e22600 doi: 10.2196/22600

38. Padula WV, Malaviya S, Reid NM, Cohen BG, Chingcuanco F, Ballreich J, et al. Economic value of vaccines to address the COVID-19 pandemic: a U.S. cost-effectiveness and budget impact analysis. *J Med Econ.* (2021) 24:1060–9. doi: 10.1080/13696998.2021.1965732

39. Abu Hammour K, Abu Farha R, Manaseer Q, Al-Manaseer B. Factors affecting the public's knowledge about COVID-19 vaccines and the influence of knowledge on their decision to get vaccinated. *J Am Pharm Assoc (2003).* (2022) 62:309–16. doi: 10.1016/j.japh.2021.06.021

40. Barda N, Dagan N, Ben-Shlomo Y, Kepten E, Waxman J, Ohana R, et al. Safety of the BNT162b2 mRNA Covid-19 vaccine in a nationwide setting. *N Engl J Med.* (2021) 385:1078–90. doi: 10.1056/NEJMoa2110475

41. Acanfora D, Acanfora C, Ciccone MM, Scicchitano P, Bortone AS, Uguccioni M, et al. The cross-talk between thrombosis and inflammatory storm in acute and long-COVID-19: therapeutic targets and clinical cases. *Viruses.* (2021) 13:1904. doi: 10.3390/v13101904

6

Normalized Cardiac Structure and Function in COVID-19 Survivors Late after Recovery

Yi-Ping Gao, Wei Zhou, Pei-Na Huang, Hong-Yun Liu, Xiao-Jun Bi, Ying Zhu, Jie Sun, Qiao-Ying Tang, Li Li, Jun Zhang, Rui-Ying Sun, Xue-Qing Cheng, Ya-Ni Liu* and You-Bin Deng*

Department of Medical Ultrasound, Tongji Hospital, Tongji Medical College, Huazhong University of Science and Technology, Wuhan, China

*Correspondence:
You-Bin Deng
ybdeng2007@hotmail.com
Ya-Ni Liu
yani.liu@163.com

Background: Coronavirus disease 2019 can result in myocardial injury in the acute phase. However, information on the late cardiac consequences of coronavirus disease 2019 (COVID-19) is limited.

Methods: We conducted a prospective observational cohort study to investigate the late cardiac consequences of COVID-19. Standard echocardiography and myocardial strain assessment were performed, and cardiac blood biomarkers were tested in 86 COVID-19 survivors 327 days (IQR 318–337 days) after recovery. Comparisons were made with 28 age-matched and sex-matched healthy controls and 30 risk factor-matched patients.

Results: There were no significant differences in all echocardiographic structural and functional parameters, including left ventricular (LV) global longitudinal strain, right ventricular (RV) longitudinal strain, LV end-diastolic volume, RV dimension, and the ratio of peak early velocity in mitral inflow to peak early diastolic velocity in the septal mitral annulus (E/e') among COVID-19 survivors, healthy controls and risk factor-matched controls. Even 26 patients with myocardial injury at admission did not have any echocardiographic structural and functional abnormalities. There were no significant differences among the three groups with respect to serum concentrations of N-terminal pro-B-type natriuretic peptide (NT-proBNP) and high-sensitivity cardiac troponin I (cTnI).

Conclusion: This study showed that COVID-19 survivors, including those with myocardial injury at admission and those with severe and critical types of illness, do not have any echocardiographic evidence of cardiac structural and functional abnormalities 327 days after diagnosis.

Keywords: COVID-19, speckle tracking echocardiography, myocardial strain, NT-proBNP, troponin

INTRODUCTION

Coronavirus disease-2019 (COVID-19) is now the deadliest pandemics caused by the novel severe acute respiratory syndrome-coronavirus-2 (SARS-CoV-2) (1). Though it primarily affects the respiratory system, cardiovascular complications are common in COVID-19 (2, 3). Myocardial injury reflected through elevated troponin concentration was reported in the acute stage of COVID-19 (4, 5). Left ventricular (LV) and right ventricular (RV) enlargements and dysfunctions were found with conventional and speckle tracking echocardiography in patients with COVID-19 (6–8). Since most COVID-19 patients recover from the illness, the understanding of the late cardiovascular consequences of infection was important. Until now, there are only a few studies on the cardiac outcome of COVID-19 survivors (9–13). These studies have reported residual cardiac structural and functional abnormalities even after recovery from COVID-19 using cardiac magnetic resonance (CMR) imaging (11–13) and echocardiography (9–11). However, these studies have been limited by their short time interval between COVID-19 diagnosis and follow-up study from 26 to 140 days which may not be long enough for cardiac abnormalities to resolve. Therefore, we performed the present study to examine the myocardial mechanical function with speckle tracking echocardiography as well as cardiac blood biomarkers in COVID-19 survivors 327 days after diagnosis.

METHODS

Study Design and Participants

This is a single-center, prospective observational cohort study undertaken in Tongji Hospital of Huazhong University of Science and Technology, a designated medical unit for treating patients with COVID-19. COVID-19 survivors were identified from the hospital medical record system and recruited through posting recruitment notices. Exclusion criteria were unwillingness to participate, incapability of communication, acute conditions such as infection, organ dysfunction and active autoimmune disease, and other illness requiring hospitalization. Patients with unsatisfactory recordings of echocardiograms were also excluded. Finally, a total of 86 consecutive patients with a history of confirmed SARS-CoV-2 infection using reverse transcription-polymerase chain reaction swab test of the upper respiratory tract were recruited between December 2020 and January 2021. In total, 28 healthy subjects matched for age and sex were recruited as the healthy controls. While the other 30 matched for age, sex, hypertension, diabetes mellitus, smoking, hypercholesterolemia, and coronary artery disease were also recruited as the risk factor-matched controls. All control group subjects were recruited from communities with consent of each participant. Our research was in concordance with the Declaration of Helsinki and the International Conference on Harmonization of Good Clinical Practice. The Tongji Hospital Ethics Committee approved the study (TJ-C20200156) and informed consent was obtained from each participant before their enrollment in the study.

Clinical characteristics, laboratory test results, and treatment for the acute phase of illness were collected from electronic medical records or patient discharge summaries. After recording the present clinical characteristics, all subjects underwent blood sampling, standard echocardiography, and myocardial strain assessment.

Standard Echocardiography and Myocardial Strain Assessment

All participants underwent echocardiographic examinations according to the recommendation of the American Society of Echocardiography using a Vivid E95 digital ultrasound system (GE Medical System, Horten, Norway) equipped with a 1.7–3.4 MHz M5Sc phased array transducer (14). All images were analyzed offline using commercially available software (EchoPac version 203, GE Vingmed, Horten, Norway). LV dimension, wall thickness, and LV mass were obtained from M-mode echocardiography. The biplane Simpson's method was used to calculate LV volume and ejection fraction. Left atrial (LA) volume was measured with the modified Simpson's method. LA volume and LV volume, and mass were indexed to the body surface area. Peak early (E) and late diastolic (A) velocities in mitral inflow, and peak early diastolic velocity (e') in septal mitral annulus were measured, and the E/A and E/e' ratios were calculated. Each parameter was averaged in three cardiac cycles.

Right atrial and RV dimensions and RV area were measured in the apical four-chamber view. RV fractional area change was calculated by dividing the difference between RV end-diastolic and end-systolic areas by the end-diastolic area. The tricuspid annular plane systolic excursion was obtained from the M-mode recording as the systolic displacement of the tricuspid lateral annulus. Tricuspid lateral annular systolic tissue velocity was measured in apical four-chamber view. The presence and severity of tricuspid regurgitation and pulmonary artery systolic pressure were assessed on color Doppler and continuous wave Doppler spectrum according to current guidelines.

Myocardial strain off-line analysis was performed using software (EchoPac version 203, GE Vingmed, Horten, Norway) on the two-dimensional gray-scale image with a frame rate of 70–90 frames/s according to the recommendations of the American Society of Echocardiography and the European Association of Cardiovascular Imaging (15). LV myocardial strain was obtained from the apical four-chamber, apical two-chamber, apical long-axis using a 17-segmental model with speckle tracking echocardiographic method. The LV global longitudinal strain was calculated by averaging peak strain values in 17 LV segments. RV free wall longitudinal strain for basal, mid, and apical segments was obtained in the apical four-chamber view. RV longitudinal strain was calculated by averaging the peak strain values in the three segments of the RV free wall.

Laboratory Examination

Peripheral venous blood samples were drawn at least 30 min before echocardiographic examination. Blood samples were processed using standardized commercially available test kits for analysis of high-sensitivity troponin I [(cTnI), Roche

Diagnostics, Rotkreuz, Switzerland] and N-terminal pro-B-type natriuretic peptide [(NT-proBNP), Abbott, Illinois, USA]. Myocardial injury was defined as a serum cTnI above the upper 99th percentile value. Serum NT-proBNP level was considered elevated according to the age-specific diagnostic threshold for heart failure. The local laboratory cTnI values above the upper 99th percentile counted as a significant increase were 15.6 pg/ml for women and 34.2 pg/ml for men. The age-specific diagnostic thresholds of serum NT-proBNP for heart failure were as follows: <62.9 pg/ml for men and <116 pg/ml for women (18–44 years old); <89.3 pg/ml for men and <169 pg/ml for women (45–54 years old); <161 pg/ml for men and <247 pg/ml for women (55–64 years old); <241 pg/ml for men and <285 pg/ml for women (65–74 years old); <486 pg/ml for men and <738 pg/ml for women (above 75 years old).

Statistical Analysis

Statistical analysis was carried out using SPSS version 21 software (IBM, Armonk, NY, USA). Normality was evaluated using the Shapiro-Wilk test. Categorical variables were expressed as counts and percentage, and continuous variables as mean ± SD or median [interquartile range (IQR)]. Wilcoxon test was utilized for comparisons of the data obtained at the acute phase and recovery of the illness. Unpaired Student's t-test was used to compare clinical data between two groups if normally distributed, and Mann-Whitney U-test if not normally distributed. Comparisons among three groups were performed using one-way ANOVA with Bonferroni corrected $post$-hoc comparisons for normal distribution or Kruskal-Wallis tests for non-normal distribution, as appropriate. Differences in proportions were analyzed with the Chi-square test or the Fisher exact test. A p-value < 0.05 was considered to indicate statistical significance.

RESULTS

Patient Characteristics

A total of 86 patients were enrolled in this study (Table 1). Median (IQR) age was 58 (39–70) years and 32 (37%) were men. Among the 86 patients, 45 (52%) were diagnosed as having moderate-type COVID-19 illness, 27 (31%) as having severe-type, and 14 (17%) as having critical-type from January to February 2020 according to the Diagnosis and Treatment Protocol of Novel Coronavirus issued by the National Health Commission of the People's Republic of China.[1] Furthermore, 78 (91%) patients required hospitalization. Among these 78 hospitalized patients, 1 patient (1%) underwent extracorporeal membrane oxygenation, 6 (8%) underwent mechanical ventilation, and 10 (13%) underwent non-invasive ventilation with positive airway pressure. Nasal cannula oxygen support was needed in 68 (87%) patients. All patients received antiviral and antibiotics therapy. Corticosteroid was used in 41

of 78 hospitalized patients (53%). Histories of cardiovascular conditions included hypertension in 32 (37%) patients, diabetes mellitus in 14 (16%), hypercholesterolemia in 16 (19%), and coronary heart disease in 13 (15%). During hospitalization, serum cTnI and NT-proBNP levels were available in 64 and 45 patients, respectively. Among them, a significant rise in cTnI was detected in 26 patients (26/64, 41%) while an elevated NT-proBNP level was found in 25 patients (25/45, 56%)

Patient characteristics, echocardiographic findings, and cardiac biomarkers on the day of echocardiographic strain are shown in Table 1. The median (IQR) interval between the COVID-19 diagnosis and echocardiographic examination was 327 (318–337) days. Exertional shortness of breath and chest discomfort was reported in 25 (29%) and 33 (38%), respectively, on the day of echocardiographic examination.

Echocardiographic Findings

No difference was found among COVID-19 survivors, healthy controls, and risk factor-matched patients with respect to age, percentage of male subjects, body mass index, body surface area, heart rate, and blood pressure. Hypertension, diabetes mellitus, coronary artery disease, and hypercholesterolemia were more common in COVID-19 survivors than those in healthy controls, but there were no differences between COVID-19 survivors and risk factor-matched patients (Table 1).

There were no significant differences in all echocardiographic structural and functional parameters, including LV global longitudinal strain, RV longitudinal strain among COVID-19 survivors, healthy controls, and risk factor-matched controls (Figures 1A,B, Table 1). There were even no significant differences in echocardiographic structural and functional parameters among groups classified according to disease severity and the presence of myocardial injury at admission, healthy control, and risk-matched control (Figures 1C–G).

Blood Biomarkers

There were no significant differences among the three groups with respect to serum concentrations of NT-proBNP and cTnI (Table 1). In a proportion of survivors with obtainable data in the acute phase, NT-proBNP and cTnI concentrations were both significantly decreased 327 days after diagnosis when compared with those in the acute phase (Figure 2).

DISCUSSION

Our study showed that there were no significant differences in echocardiographic structural and functional parameters among COVID-19 survivors, healthy control, and risk factor-matched control 327 days after diagnosis regardless of the presence of myocardial injury in the acute phase and severity of the illness at admission. In addition, blood biomarkers of myocardial injury and function revealed no significant differences among COVID-19 survivors, healthy and risk-factor matched controls.

Coronavirus disease 2019 is a global pandemic leading to high morbidity and mortality (1). A significant proportion of patients with COVID-19 were reported to suffer from a myocardial injury in the acute phase. Echocardiographic abnormalities, including

---

[1]National Health Commission of the People's Republic of China. Diagnosis and treatment protocol of novel coronavirus (trial version 7th). National Health Commission of the People's Republic of China Website. http://www.nhc.gov.cn/yzygj/s7653p/202003/46c9294a7dfe4cef80dc7f5912eb1989.shtml. Accessed March 4, 2020.

TABLE 1 | Clinical characteristics, echocardiographic findings, and laboratory results of coronavirus disease 2019 (COVID-19) survivors 327 days after diagnosis.

	Healthy control (n = 28)	Risk factor-matched control (n = 30)	COVID-19 (n = 86)	p-value
Patient characteristics				
Age, years	56 (37–65)	62 (39–67)	58 (39–70)	0.392
Male, n%	10 (36%)	11 (37%)	32 (37%)	0.990
Body mass index, kg/m^2	23 ± 3	24 ± 3	24 ±3	0.304
Body surface area, m^2	1.7 ± 0.2	1.7 ± 0.2	1.7 ± 0.2	0.561
Heart rate, beats/min	67 (61–81)	69 (63–73)	73 (65–79)	0.119
Systolic blood pressure, mm Hg	125 ± 12	126 ± 16	131 ± 18	0.132
Diastolic blood pressure, mm Hg	73 (67–82)	72 (67–79)	77 (70–82)	0.228
Oxygen saturation, %	NA	NA	98 (97–99)	NA
Hypertension, n%	0 (0%)	10 (33%)*	32 (37%)*	0.001
Diabetes mellitus, n%	0 (0%)	2 (7%)	14 (16%)*	0.032
Coronary heart disease, n%	0 (0%)	3 (10%)	13 (15%)	0.076
Hypercholesterolemia, n%	0 (0%)	9 (30%)*	16 (19%)*	0.003
Echocardiographic findings				
LA dimension, mm	31 (28–33)	31 (28–33)	32 (29–34)	0.388
LV dimension, mm	45 (43–50)	45 (43–49)	46 (44–49)	0.780
IVS thickness, mm	8 (7–8)	8 (7–9)	8 (7–9)	0.180
LV posterior wall thickness, mm	8 (7–8)	8 (7–8)	8 (7–9)	0.094
LV mass, g/m^2	73 (63–87)	78 (64–86)	80 (67–96)	0.346
LV end-diastolic volume, ml/m^2	47 (43–51)	48 (44–52)	45 (40–54)	0.866
LV end-systolic volume, ml/m^2	18 (15–19)	17 (15–19)	17 (14–21)	0.889
LV ejection fraction, %	63 (61–67)	63 (61–67)	63 (61–68)	0.870
LA volume, ml/m^2	22 (18–26)	22 (18–27)	21 (18–25)	0.750
E/A ratio	1.1 (0.8–1.4)	1.1 (0.8–1.2)	0.9 (0.7–1.3)	0.190
E/e' ratio	8 ± 3	9 ± 4	9 ± 2	0.426
LV GLS, %	21 ± 2	21 ± 2	20 ± 2	0.381
LV GLS < 16%, n%	0 (0%)	0 (0%)	4 (5%)	0.476
RA dimension, mm	34 (30–36)	34 (30–35)	33 (30–38)	0.554
RV dimension, mm	31 (27–33)	30 (27–34)	32 (28–36)	0.217
TAPSE, mm	27 (24–29)	26 (23–28)	26 (24–28)	0.346
RV fractional area change, %	47 ± 9	49 ± 8	51 ± 9	0.158
S', cm/s	14 (13–17)	14 (13–17)	14 (13–16)	0.936
PASP, mm Hg	23 (19–28)	24 (19–28)	25 (21–30)	0.707
RV longitudinal strain, %	30 ± 5	30 ± 6	29 ± 6	0.722
RV longitudinal strain < 20%, n%	1 (4%)	1 (3%)	2 (2%)	1.000
Pericardial effusion, n%	0 (0%)	0 (0%)	1 (1%)	1.000
Laboratory results				
NT-proBNP, pg/mL	36 (15–65)	41 (19–72)	51 (24–104)	0.113
cTnI, pg/mL	1.9 (1.9–2.5)	1.9 (1.9–2.8)	1.9 (1.9–4.9)	0.159

Numbers are given as median (interquartile range) or mean ± standard deviation or as case numbers with percentages in parentheses.

NA, not applicable; LA, left atrium; LV, left ventricle; IVS, interventricular septum; E, peak early diastolic velocity in mitral inflow; A, late diastolic velocity in mitral inflow; e', peak early diastolic velocity in septal mitral annulus; GLS, global longitudinal strain; RA, right atrium; RV, right ventricle; TAPSE, tricuspid annular plane systolic excursion; S', tricuspid lateral annular systolic tissue velocity; PASP, pulmonary artery systolic pressure; NT-proBNP, N-terminal pro-B-type natriuretic peptide; cTnI, high-sensitivity cardiac troponin I.

*p < 0.01, vs. healthy control.

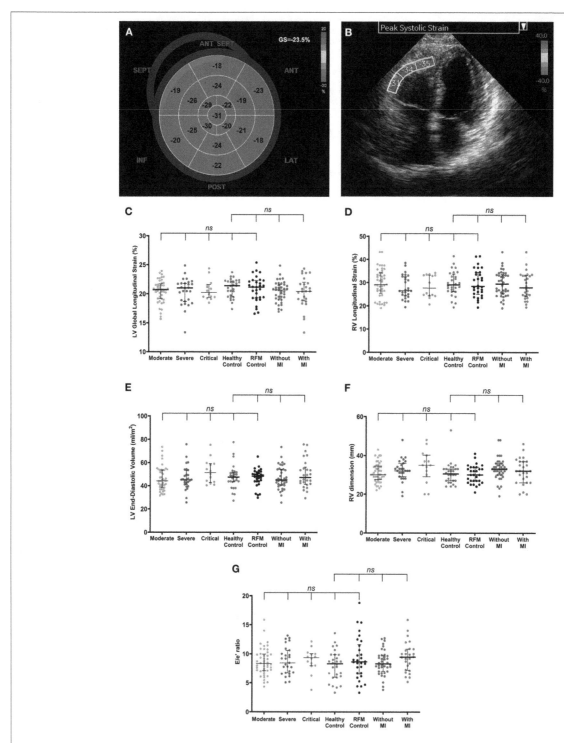

FIGURE 1 | Normalized cardiac structure and function in coronavirus disease 2019 (COVID-19) survivors late after the recovery. **(A,B)** A patient (75–80 years old) with no history of hypertension, diabetes, and/or coronary heart disease was diagnosed with severe-type COVID-19 illness. High-sensitivity troponin I level was 1,137 pg/ml at admission and 4.3 pg/ml on the day of echocardiographic examination (316 days after COVID-19 diagnosis). **(A)** Shows normal left ventricular (LV) global longitudinal strain (GS) and panel B shows normal right ventricular (RV) free wall longitudinal strain for basal, mid, and apical segments. **(C–G)** There were no significant differences in LV global longitudinal strain **(C)**, RV longitudinal strain **(D)**, LV end-diastolic volume **(E)**, RV dimension **(F)**, and the ratio of peak early velocity in mitral inflow to peak early diastolic velocity in the septal mitral annulus [E/e', **(G)**] among groups classified according to disease severity and the presence of myocardial injury at admission, healthy control, and risk-matched control. Longer black lines indicate the medians and shorter black lines indicate the interquartile ranges. Each dot represents a value. ANT, anterior; LAT, lateral; POST, posterior; INF, inferior; SEPT, septum; ANT SEPT, anterior septum; RFM, risk-factor matched; MI, myocardial injury; LV, left ventricular; RV, right ventricular.

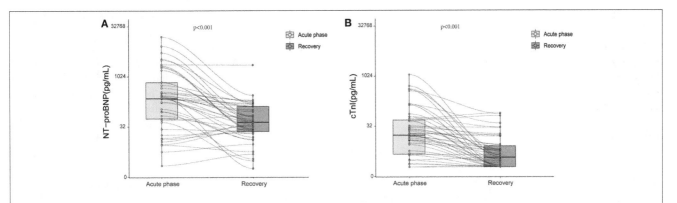

FIGURE 2 | Blood biomarkers obtained at the acute phase and late after the recovery. During hospitalization, serum NT-proBNP **(A)** and cTnI **(B)** levels were available in 45 and 64 patients, respectively. Both were significantly decreased 327 days after diagnosis compared with those in the acute phase (*p* < 0.001). Each small circle represents a value. The top and bottom of the rectangle represent the interquartile range. Bold black lines in the rectangle indicate medians.

global LV dysfunction, regional wall motion abnormalities, diastolic dysfunction, RV dysfunction, and pericardial effusion were detected in patients with COVID-19 in the acute phase and a higher prevalence of echocardiographic abnormalities was found in patients with biomarker evidence of myocardial injury (4). CMR also revealed myocarditis, LV dysfunction, pericarditis, and Takotsubo cardiomyopathy in the acute phase of COVID-19 illness, indicated by abnormalities in T1 and T2 mapping and late gadolinium enhancement images (16–18). Nevertheless, it is still unclear whether the myocardial injury at the acute phase of illness leaves persistent lesions and how significant these abnormalities are in the long run. A few studies on the cardiovascular consequences of COVID-19 with limited follow-up intervals have been published (9–13, 19–24). In a study of cohort patients 71 days after recovery of COVID-19, magnetic resonance revealed cardiac involvement, including myocardial late gadolinium enhancement, raised myocardial native T1 and T2 in 78% of patients independent of preexisting conditions, severity, and overall course of the acute illness (12). Echocardiographic studies showed similar findings. The study of Zhou et al. reported LV dysfunction with decreased LV ejection fraction after a short period of 1–4 weeks following discharge (20). Another study showed that despite normalized blood concentrations of troponin and NT-proBNP, 29% of survivors had an abnormality in echocardiography after 3 months of admission, with reverse RV remodeling in the majority reflected by dilated RV dimension and decreased RV fractional area change (9). To notice, 80% of patients in this study had undergone mechanical ventilation, indicating severely impaired pulmonary structure and function. Thus, the above observed persistent RV dysfunction could not simply be attributed to direct myocardial injury. Preservation in cardiac consequence has been reported (10, 21–23). The study of Catena et al. reported no structural and functional sequelae in the heart of survivors of COVID-19 more than 1 month after recovery from illness (10). Daher et al. also demonstrated no echocardiographic impairments in 33 patients with severe illness after 6 weeks following discharge (23). However, these studies were limited by their short time periods at follow-up, leaving long-term

cardiovascular consequences of COVID-19 poorly understood. In the present prospective study, COVID-19 survivors were evaluated after a relatively long time period with a median interval of 327 days after diagnosis, and no elevation of cTnI and NT-proBNP were detected nor echocardiographic structural and functional abnormalities were found when compared with healthy control and risk factor-matched control, including those with myocardial injury in the acute phase. Our finding was consistent with previously published longer period follow-up studies. After a median interval of 6 months, echocardiographic measurements in COVID-19 survivors were not different between patients with and without myocardial injury during the acute COVID-19 phase (24). Combining our findings and previous follow-up results, it is suggested that myocardial injury and echocardiographic structural and functional abnormalities observed in the acute phase of COVID-19 infection might be reversible. The resolution of CMR abnormalities in COVID-19 athletes seems to be an example of this reversibility. In a consecutive follow-up study on athletes, CMR imaging revealed elevated T1, elevated T2, and late gadolinium enhancement in 2.3% of patients after a short interval (10–77 days) from diagnosis. However, a repeated CMR 4–14 weeks later from the first follow-up demonstrated resolution of T2 elevation in 100% and late gadolinium enhancement in 41% of patients (13). Thus, the cardiac abnormalities observed in COVID-19 survivors in previous studies (9, 12, 13) might be due to the short follow-up period and they might resolve in the long run. Another possible explanation for those observed persistent cardiac abnormalities in survivors could be the effect of pre-existing conditions in COVID-19 patients, such as hypertension, coronary artery disease, diabetes which are usually seen in the seniors. These patients tend to suffer more severe pneumonia (3), which further heavies the burden of the heart with mechanical ventilation. To avoid such confounders, COVID-19 survivors in our study were compared with a group of risk-factor matched control, with no significant cardiac abnormalities being found in the COVID-19 survivor group. Taken together, COVID-19 *per se* does not appear to cause long-term cardiac sequelae after recovery from acute illness.

The proposed mechanism of myocardial injury and dysfunction in patients with COVID-19 infection include cytokine-mediated damage, oxygen supply-demand imbalance, ischemic injury from microvascular thrombi formation, a direct viral infection of the myocardium, and pulmonary hypertension-induced RV dysfunction (4, 25, 26). The oxygen saturation was quite normal in COVID-19 survivors on the day of echocardiographic examination, lowering the possibility of oxygen supply-demand imbalance. Pulmonary artery systolic pressure in the COVID-19 survivors was also not different from that in healthy control. Previous studies have demonstrated that the cardiac structural and functional abnormalities caused by ischemic injury resolved after successful revascularization (27, 28). Longitudinal studies have demonstrated gradual declines of serum concentration of inflammatory biomarkers including IL-6, IL-8, tumor necrosis factor-α, and high-sensitivity C-reactive protein (hs-CRP) at the late stage of illness in COVID-19 survivors (29). Another study reported slight increased CRP levels in 16% of COVID-19 patients 2 months after symptom onset (30). Fulminant myocarditis is an inflammatory disease of the myocardium most often caused by a viral infection with severe impairment of LV systolic function in the acute phase. Previous reports showed that LV ejection fraction recovered at follow-up in survivors with fulminant myocarditis (31, 32). It is speculated that when the underlying pathogenic conditions were eliminated, the myocardial dysfunction would be reversed. Those findings in inflammatory biomarkers, oxygen saturation, and pulmonary artery systolic pressure in our study and previous studies (27, 28, 31, 32) support the observations in the present study that no significant differences exist in cTnI concentration, and echocardiographic structural and functional parameters among COVID-19 survivors, healthy control, and risk factor-matched control 327 days after diagnosis of COVID-19 infection.

Some limitations existed in our study. First, the quantitative echocardiographic data were unavailable at the onset of COVID-19 in isolation wards, which makes the longitudinal comparison of echocardiographic parameters impossible. Second, we did not perform segmental strain comparisons among groups. A previous study (33) has shown basal longitudinal strain

dysfunction in COVID-19 patients in the acute phase of illness. Nevertheless, this study also showed decreased global longitudinal strain. Global longitudinal strain was calculated by averaging peak strains in 17 segments in our study. If one or several segment(s) has or have significantly decreased strain, the global longitudinal strain would be decreased concomitantly. Since no significant differences in global longitudinal strain were found in our study, we did not do further analysis in the segmental strain. Third, our study was based on a small sampling of survivors, thus, multicenter study with a larger population and longer follow-up period would be needed to provide more valuable information on the long-term cardiac consequences of COVID-19 infection.

CONCLUSIONS

This study showed that COVID-19 survivors, including those with significantly elevated cTnI at admission and those with the severe and critical types of illness, did not have evident echocardiographic proof of cardiac structural and functional abnormalities 327 days after diagnosis.

AUTHOR CONTRIBUTIONS

Y-BD, Y-NL, X-JB, H-YL, and YZ conceived and designed the study. Y-PG, WZ, P-NH, X-QC, R-YS, Y-NL, and Y-BD collected clinical and ultrasound data. Y-PG, WZ, LL, Q-YT, JZ, and JS analyzed data and performed the statistical analysis. Y-BD, Y-NL, Y-PG, and WZ drafted the manuscript. All authors approved the manuscript.

ACKNOWLEDGMENTS

We appreciate the support of the clinical staff of the Department of Laboratory Medicine, Tongji Hospital, Huazhong University of Science and Technology, including Zi-Yong Sun, MD, Li Liu, and Jin Wang. We are also very grateful to our colleagues at Tongji Hospital for their dedicated efforts to treat patients with COVID-19. Contributors were not compensated for their work.

REFERENCES

1. Fauci AS, Lane HC, Redfield RR. COVID-19 - navigating the uncharted. N Engl J Med. (2020) 382:1268–9. doi: 10.1056/NEJMe2002387
2. Shi S, Qin M, Shen B, Cai Y, Liu T, Yang F, et al. Association of cardiac injury with mortality in hospitalized patients with COVID-19 in Wuhan, China. J Am Med Assoc Cardiol. (2020) 5:802–10. doi: 10.1001/jamacardio.2020.0950
3. Zhou F, Yu T, Du R, Fan G, Liu Y, Liu Z, et al. Clinical course and risk factors for mortality of adult inpatients with COVID-19 in Wuhan, China: a retrospective cohort study. Lancet. (2020) 395:1054–62. doi: 10.1016/S0140-6736(20)30566-3
4. Giustino G, Croft LB, Stefanini GG, Bragato R, Silbiger JJ, Vicenzi M, et al. Characterization of myocardial injury in patients with COVID-19. J Am Coll Cardiol. (2020) 76:2043–55. doi: 10.1016/j.jacc.2020.08.069
5. Lala A, Johnson KW, Januzzi JL, Russak AJ, Paranjpe I, Richter F, et al. Prevalence and impact of myocardial injury in patients hospitalized with COVID-19 infection. J Am Coll Cardiol. (2020) 76:533–46. doi: 10.1016/j.jacc.2020.06.007
6. Skaarup KG, Lassen MCH, Lind JN, Alhakak AS, Sengelov M, Nielsen AB, et al. Myocardial impairment and acute respiratory distress syndrome in hospitalized patients with COVID-19: The ECHOVID-19 study. JACC Cardiovasc Imaging. (2020) 13:2474–6. doi: 10.1016/j.jcmg.2020.08.005
7. Rothschild E, Baruch G, Szekely Y, Lichter Y, Kaplan A, Taieb P, et al. The predictive role of left and right ventricular speckle-tracking echocardiography in COVID-19. JACC Cardiovasc Imaging. (2020) 13:2471–4. doi: 10.1016/j.jcmg.2020.07.026
8. Kim J, Volodarskiy A, Sultana R, Pollie MP, Yum B, Nambiar L, et al. Prognostic utility of right ventricular remodeling over conventional risk stratification in patients with COVID-19. J Am Coll Cardiol. (2020) 76:1965–77. doi: 10.1016/j.jacc.2020.08.066
9. Moody WE, Liu B, Mahmoud-Elsayed HM, Senior J, Lalla SS, Khan-Kheil AM, et al. Persisting adverse ventricular remodeling in COVID-19 survivors: a longitudinal echocardiographic study. J Am Soc Echocardiogr. (2021) 34:562–6. doi: 10.1016/j.echo.2021.01.020
10. Catena C, Colussi G, Bulfone L, Da Porto A, Tascini C, Sechi LA. Echocardiographic comparison of COVID-19 patients with or without prior

biochemical evidence of cardiac injury after recovery. *J Am Soc Echocardiogr.* (2021) 34:193–5. doi: 10.1016/j.echo.2020.10.009

11. Brito D, Meester S, Yanamala N, Patel HB, Balcik BJ, Casaclang-Verzosa G, et al. High prevalence of pericardial involvement in college student athletes recovering from COVID-19. *JACC Cardiovasc Imaging.* (2021) 14:541–55. doi: 10.1016/j.jcmg.2020.10.023

12. Puntmann VO, Carerj ML, Wieters I, Fahim M, Arendt C, Hoffmann J, et al. Outcomes of cardiovascular magnetic resonance imaging in patients recently recovered from coronavirus disease 2019 (COVID-19). *J Am Med Assoc Cardiol.* (2020) 5:1265–73. doi: 10.1001/jamacardio.2020.3557

13. Daniels CJ, Rajpal S, Greenshields JT, Rosenthal GL, Chung EH, Terrin M, et al. Prevalence of clinical and subclinical myocarditis in competitive athletes with recent SARS-CoV-2 infection: results from the Big Ten COVID-19 cardiac registry. *J Am Med Assoc Cardiol.* (2021) 6:1078–87. doi: 10.1001/jamacardio.2021.2065

14. Lang RM, Badano LP, Mor-Avi V, Afilalo J, Armstrong A, Ernande L, et al. Recommendations for cardiac chamber quantification by echocardiography in adults: an update from the American Society of Echocardiography and the European Association of Cardiovascular Imaging. *J Am Soc Echocardiogr.* (2015) 28:1–39 e14. doi: 10.1016/j.echo.2014.10.003

15. Mor-Avi V, Lang RM, Badano LP, Belohlavek M, Cardim NM, Derumeaux G, et al. Current and evolving echocardiographic techniques for the quantitative evaluation of cardiac mechanics: ASE/EAE consensus statement on methodology and indications endorsed by the Japanese Society of Echocardiography. *Eur J Echocardiogr.* (2011) 12:167–205. doi: 10.1093/ejechocard/jer021

16. Esposito A, Palmisano A, Natale L, Ligabue G, Peretto G, Lovato L, et al. Cardiac magnetic resonance characterization of myocarditis-like acute cardiac syndrome in covid-19. *JACC Cardiovasc Imaging.* (2020) 13:2462–5. doi: 10.1016/j.jcmg.2020.06.003

17. Clark DE, Parikh A, Dendy JM, Diamond AB, George-Durrett K, Fish FA, et al. Covid-19 myocardial pathology evaluation in athletes with cardiac magnetic resonance (compete cmr). *Circulation.* (2021) 143:609–12. doi: 10.1161/CIRCULATIONAHA.120.052573

18. Kotecha T, Knight DS, Razvi Y, Kumar K, Vimalesvaran K, Thornton G, et al. Patterns of myocardial injury in recovered troponin-positive covid-19 patients assessed by cardiovascular magnetic resonance. *Eur Heart J.* (2021) 42:1866–78. doi: 10.1093/eurheartj/ehab075

19. Starekova J, Bluemke DA, Bradham WS, Eckhardt LL, Grist TM, Kusmirek JE, et al. Evaluation for myocarditis in competitive student athletes recovering from coronavirus disease 2019 with cardiac magnetic resonance imaging. *J Am Med Assoc Cardiol.* (2021) 6:945–50. doi: 10.1001/jamacardio.2020.7444

20. Zhou M, Wong CK, Un KC, Lau YM, Lee JC, Tam FC, et al. Cardiovascular sequalae in uncomplicated covid-19 survivors. *PLoS ONE.* (2021) 16:e0246732. doi: 10.1371/journal.pone.0246732

21. Sechi LA, Colussi G, Bulfone L, Brosolo G, Da Porto A, Peghin M, et al. Short-term cardiac outcome in survivors of COVID-19: a systematic study after hospital discharge. *Clin Res Cardiol.* (2021) 110:1063–72. doi: 10.1007/s00392-020-01800-z

22. de Graaf MA, Antoni ML, Ter Kuile MM, Arbous MS, Duinisveld AJF, Feltkamp MCW, et al. Short-term outpatient follow-up of COVID-19 patients: a multidisciplinary approach. *EClinicalMedicine.* (2021) 32:100731. doi: 10.1016/j.eclinm.2021.100731

23. Daher A, Balfanz P, Cornelissen C, Muller A, Bergs I, Marx N, et al. Follow up of patients with severe coronavirus disease 2019 (COVID-19): pulmonary and extrapulmonary disease sequelae. *Respir Med.* (2020) 174:106197. doi: 10.1016/j.rmed.2020.106197

24. Fayol A, Livrozet M, Boutouyrie P, Khettab H, Betton M, Tea V, et al. Cardiac performance in patients hospitalized with covid-19: a 6 month follow-up study. *ESC Heart Fail.* (2021) 8:2232–9. doi: 10.1002/ehf2.13315

25. Bavishi C, Bonow RO, Trivedi V, Abbott JD, Messerli FH, Bhatt DL. Special article - acute myocardial injury in patients hospitalized with COVID-19 infection: a review. *Prog Cardiovasc Dis.* (2020) 63:682–9. doi: 10.1016/j.pcad.2020.05.013

26. Lippi G, Lavie CJ, Sanchis-Gomar F. Cardiac troponin i in patients with coronavirus disease 2019 (COVID-19): evidence from a meta-analysis. *Prog Cardiovasc Dis.* (2020) 63:390–1. doi: 10.1016/j.pcad.2020.03.001

27. Bansal M, Jeffriess L, Leano R, Mundy J, Marwick TH. Assessment of myocardial viability at dobutamine echocardiography by deformation analysis using tissue velocity and speckle-tracking. *JACC Cardiovasc Imaging.* (2010) 3:121–31. doi: 10.1016/j.jcmg.2009.09.025

28. Allman KC, Shaw LJ, Hachamovitch R, Udelson JE. Myocardial viability testing and impact of revascularization on prognosis in patients with coronary artery disease and left ventricular dysfunction: a meta-analysis. *J Am Coll Cardiol.* (2002) 39:1151–8. doi: 10.1016/S0735-1097(02)01726-6

29. Zeng Z, Yu H, Chen H, Qi W, Chen L, Chen G, et al. Longitudinal changes of inflammatory parameters and their correlation with disease severity and outcomes in patients with COVID-19 from Wuhan, China. *Crit Care.* (2020) 24:525. doi: 10.1186/s13054-020-03255-0

30. Sonnweber T, Boehm A, Sahanic S, Pizzini A, Aichner M, Sonnweber B, et al. Persisting alterations of iron homeostasis in COVID-19 are associated with non-resolving lung pathologies and poor patients' performance: a prospective observational cohort study. *Respir Res.* (2020) 21:276. doi: 10.1186/s12931-020-01546-2

31. Ishida K, Wada H, Sakakura K, Kubo N, Ikeda N, Sugawara Y, et al. Long-term follow-up on cardiac function following fulminant myocarditis requiring percutaneous extracorporeal cardiopulmonary support. *Heart Vessels.* (2013) 28:86–90. doi: 10.1007/s00380-011-0211-8

32. Ammirati E, Cipriani M, Lilliu M, Sormani P, Varrenti M, Raineri C, et al. Survival and left ventricular function changes in fulminant versus nonfulminant acute myocarditis. *Circulation.* (2017) 136:529–45. doi: 10.1161/CIRCULATIONAHA.117.026386

33. Goerlich E, Gilotra NA, Minhas AS, Bavaro N, Hays AG, Cingolani OH. Prominent longitudinal strain reduction of basal left ventricular segments in patients with coronavirus disease-19. *J Card Fail.* (2021) 27:100–4. doi: 10.1016/j.cardfail.2020.09.469

7

Sacubitril/Valsartan: Potential Impact of ARNi "Beyond the Wall" of ACE2 on Treatment and Prognosis of Heart Failure Patients with Coronavirus Disease-19

Speranza Rubattu [1,2]*, Giovanna Gallo [1] and Massimo Volpe [1,2]

[1] Cardiology Unit, Department of Clinical and Molecular Medicine, School of Medicine and Psychology, Sant'Andrea Hospital, Sapienza University of Rome, Rome, Italy, [2] Istituto di Ricovero e Cura a Carattere Scientifico Neuromed, Pozzilli, Italy

*Correspondence:
Speranza Rubattu
rubattu.speranza@neuromed.it

Keywords: COVID-19, natriuretic peptide, ARNi, cardiovascular diseases, HFrEF—heart failure with reduced ejection fraction

INTRODUCTION

From the beginning of the SARS-CoV-2 pandemia, the type 2 angiotensin-converting enzyme (ACE2), probably the most "unloved and neglected" member of the renin-angiotensin-aldosterone (RAAS) family, has attracted increasing attention since it has been shown as the cell receptor through which the virus enters into the cells (1).

The physiological action of ACE2, a membrane protein expressed in the heart, lungs, kidneys, liver, and intestine, consists in degrading angiotensin II (Ang II) to angiotensin (1-7), a heptapeptide with a potent vasodilator function through the Mas receptor able to counterbalance the Ang II effects on vasoconstriction, sodium retention, and fibrosis (1). Previous studies have shown that Ang II type 1 receptor (AT1R) blockers (ARBs), ACE inhibitors (ACEI), and mineralocorticoid receptor antagonists (MRA) may up-regulate the expression of ACE2 both in acute and chronic settings of cardiovascular diseases (CVDs), such as hypertension, heart failure (HF) and myocardial infarction (1). These data have generated concern during the early phases of the pandemia, since it has been speculated that the increase in ACE2 level may have contributed to disease virulence and to adverse outcomes particularly in subjects affected by chronic coexisting conditions, namely hypertension, coronary artery disease, HF, and diabetes, who commonly received treatment with RAAS inhibitors and who were characterized by a worse clinical course (2).

On the other hand, it has been observed that the binding between coronavirus and ACE2 leads to ACE2 downregulation, resulting in an unopposed production of Ang II by ACE, contributing to lung damage as a consequence of AT1R mediated inflammation, fibrosis, thrombosis, vasoconstriction, and increased vascular permeability. According to these findings, RAAS inhibitors and, in particular, ARBs may even protect against COVID-19 acute lung injury (1). As a matter of fact, epidemiological studies conducted in large populations of COVID-19 patients demonstrated that ARBs or ACE inhibitors had no association with a severe or fatal course of the disease (3–5).

EVIDENCE SUPPORTING THE POTENTIAL BENEFICIAL ROLE OF ARNi IN HF PATIENTS WITH COVID-19

Natriuretic peptides (NPs), which include atrial natriuretic peptide (ANP), brain natriuretic peptide (BNP), and C-type natriuretic peptide (CNP), along with their N-terminal counterparts, may play an important protective role in COVID-19 disease. NPs are released as a consequence of increased volume overload and myocytes stress and, through their vasorelaxant, diuretic, and effects, are able to counterbalance RAAS and sympathetic nervous system actions, ultimately regulating blood pressure, electrolytes, and water homeostasis (6). At the vascular level, NPs reduce cellular growth and proliferation, preserving endothelial function and integrity as well as vascular tone, and they oppose blood clotting, inflammation, angiogenesis, and atherosclerosis progression (6). Apart from their well-described systemic hemodynamic and autocrine/paracrine functions within the cardiovascular system, NPs also play an important protective role in the lungs. In fact, ANP reduces lung endothelial permeability caused by inflammation and oxidative stress, avoiding the development of acute respiratory distress syndrome and improving arterial oxygenation during mechanical ventilation (7). According to this evidence, it has been proposed that COVID-19 patients with deficiencies in the NP system, mainly obese subjects and black people, may have an increased risk of developing severe lung complications.

Of interest, a bidirectional interaction between NPs, particularly ANP, and ACE2 has been demonstrated in experimental models. ANP, through cyclic guanosine monophosphate (cGMP) production, inhibited the Ang II-mediated activation of the extracellular signal regulated kinase (ERK1/ERK2) pathway and upregulated the mitogen-activated protein kinase phosphatase (MKP1), finally preventing the decrease in ACE2 mRNA synthesis (8). On the other hand, Ang-(1-7), the product of ACE2 activity, stimulated ANP secretion through the Mas receptor/phosphatidylinositol 3-kinase/protein kinase B (Mas/PI3K/Akt) pathway, thus reducing cardiac hypertrophy and fibrosis and potentially avoiding COVID-19 pulmonary damage (8).

Furthermore, consistently with the well-known prognostic role of NPs, it has been demonstrated that NT-proBNP level represents an independent risk factor of in-hospital death in patients with severe COVID-19, its levels being significantly higher among those patients who experienced severe clinical conditions, and increasing further during hospitalization in subjects who died, without significant changes among survivors (9).

Apart from the known pathogenetic, diagnostic, and prognostic implications in the cardiovascular system (10), NPs have relevant therapeutic properties. In this context, a field of great interest may be represented by the potential impact on the clinical course of the COVID-19 disease

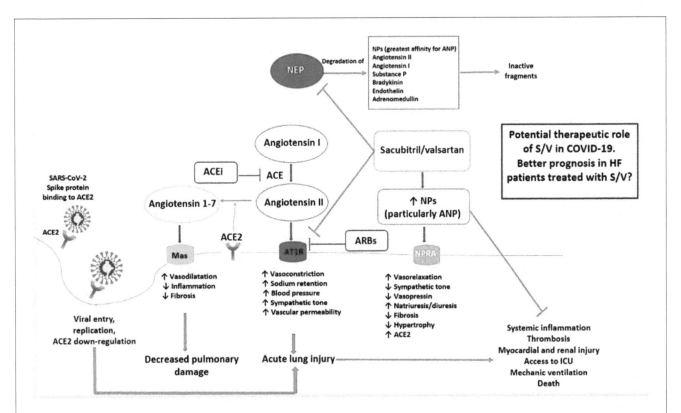

FIGURE 1 | Mechanisms underlying the potential beneficial effects of sacubitril/valsartan in HF patients with COVID-19. Ang 1-7, produced by ACE2 from Ang II, and NPs, particularly ANP, may protect from acute lung injury, systemic inflammation, and adverse outcomes during SARS-CoV-2 infection. On the other hand, local activation of the RAAS system may mediate injury responses to viral insults. S/V inhibits both the AT1R and neprilysin, which degrades NPs. As a consequence, S/V may exert an important protective function from adverse clinical course, mediated by an increase of ANP and by AT1R blockade, in HF patients with COVID-19. ACE, angiotensin converting enzyme; ACE2, type 2 angiotensin converting enzyme; ACE-i, ACE inhibitor; ANP, atrial natriuretic peptide; ARB, angiotensin type I receptor blocker; AT1R, angiotensin type I receptor; HF, heart failure; ICU, intensive care unit; NEP, neprilysin; NPs, natriuretic peptides; NPR-A, natriuretic peptide receptor A; S/V, sacubitril/valsartan.

and on its outcome of a treatment with sacubitril/valsartan (S/V), a member of the new pharmacological class of AT1R/neprilysin inhibitors (ARNi). S/V is now recognized as a cornerstone of the therapeutic management of HF with reduced ejection fraction (HFrEF) due to the impressive benefits on cardiovascular death and HF hospitalization (11).

The beneficial effects of S/V in HFrEF were confirmed in recent real-life clinical studies showing a significant reduction of cardiac death and HF rehospitalization, an improvement of echocardiographic parameters, such as left ventricular EF, systolic volume, and systolic pulmonary arterial pressure, of renal function and of quality of life (12–14). Moreover, S/V treatment can be safely started during hospitalization in daily clinical practice with no evidence of increased risk of hypotension, worsening of renal function and hyperkalaemia (15).

With regard to the trend of different NPs levels after the initiation of S/V, NT-proBNP level decreases as a consequence of the improvement of cardiac function and haemodynamic status, representing a useful biomarker of treatment response; BNP level slightly increases due to its relatively low affinity to neprilysin, whereas ANP level consistently and substantially increases both in human studies and in experimental models, mediating most of the benefits of neprilysin inhibition (16, 17).

According to these evidences, an approach based on early administration of S/V has been proposed in the therapeutic management of all COVID-19 hospitalized patients to avoid an adverse clinical course (18).

PERSPECTIVES

Based on the ability of S/V to increase ANP level while antagonizing the Ang II/AT1R effects, we propose a major protective role of this class of drugs in HFrEF patients, the only current indication for the use of ARNi, when affected by COVID-19 disease (**Figure 1**). In order to test the expected beneficial role of S/V in COVID-19, a retrospective analysis of existing registries of hospitalized COVID-19 patients could help to find out whether, among subjects affected by HFrEF, those who were already treated with S/V presented a lower disease incidence, better prognosis, and clinical course (particularly in terms of intensive care unit access, mechanical ventilation, and death), compared to patients who received other medications, including ACEI/ARBs. Furthermore, a call to action is requested to test the potential benefits of S/V in HFrEF patients affected by COVID-19 through new prospective randomized clinical trials.

AUTHOR CONTRIBUTIONS

SR, GG, and MV contributed to the conception and design, acquisition of data, or analysis and interpretation of data, drafted the article, and approved the final version to be published. All authors contributed to the article and approved the submitted version.

ACKNOWLEDGMENTS

This manuscript has been released as a pre-print at Authorea 2020 (19).

REFERENCES

1. Battistoni A, Volpe M. Might renin-angiotensin system blockers play a role in the COVID-19 pandemic? *Eur Heart J Cardiovasc Pharmacother.* (2020) 6:248–51. doi: 10.1093/ehjcvp/pvaa030
2. Volpe M, Battistoni A, the board of the Italian Society of Cardiovascular Prevention, Bellotti P, Bellone S, Bertolotti M, et al. Recommendations for cardiovascular prevention during the Sars-Cov-2 pandemic: an executive document by the board of the Italian society of cardiovascular prevention. *High Blood Press Cardiovasc Prev.* (2020) 30:1–5. doi: 10.1007/s40292-020-00401-1
3. Mancia G, Rea F, Ludergnani M, Apolone G, Corrao G. Renin-angiotensin-aldosterone system blockers and the risk of Covid-19. *N Engl J Med.* (2020) 382:2431–40. doi: 10.1056/NEJMoa2006923
4. Iaccarino G, Grassi G, Borghi C, Ferri C, Salvetti M, Volpe M, et al. Age and multimorbidity predict death among COVID-19 patients: results of the SARS-RAS study of the Italian society of hypertension. *Hypertension.* (2020) 76:366–72. doi: 10.1161/HYPERTENSIONAHA.120.15324
5. Volpe M, Battistoni A. Systematic review of the role of renin-angiotensin system inhibitors in late studies on Covid-19: a new challenge overcome? *Int J Cardiol.* (2020) 321:150–4. doi: 10.1016/j.ijcard.2020.07.041
6. Volpe M, Rubattu S, Burnett J Jr. Natriuretic peptides in cardiovascular diseases: current use and perspectives. *Eur Heart J.* (2014) 35:419–25. doi: 10.1093/eurheartj/eht466
7. Mitaka C, Hirata Y, Nagura T, Tsunoda Y, Amaha K. Beneficial effect of atrial natriuretic peptide on pulmonary gas exchange in patients with acute lung injury. *Chest.* (1998) 114:223–28. doi: 10.1378/chest.114.1.223

8. Gallagher PE, Ferrario CM, Tallant EA. Regulation of ACE2 in cardiac myocytes and fibroblasts. *Am J Physiol Heart Circ Physiol.* (2008) 295:2373–9. doi: 10.1152/ajpheart.00426.2008
9. Gao L, Jiang D, Wen XS, Cheng XC, Sun M, He B, et al. Prognostic value of NT-proBNP in patients with severe COVID-19. *Respir Res.* (2020) 21:83. doi: 10.1186/s12931-020-01352-w
10. Rubattu S, Volpe M. Natriuretic peptides in the cardiovascular system: multifaceted roles in physiology, pathology and therapeutics. *Int J Mol Sci.* (2019) 20:E3991. doi: 10.3390/ijms20163991
11. McMurray JJ, Packer M, Desai AS, Gong J, Lefkowitz MP, Rizkala AR, et al. Angiotensin-neprilysin inhibition versus enalapril in heart failure. *N Engl J Med.* (2014) 371:993–1004. doi: 10.1056/NEJMoa1409077
12. Polito MV, Silverio A, Rispoli A, Vitulano G, Auria F, De Angelis E, et al. Clinical and echocardiographic benefit of sacubitril/valsartan in a real-world population with HF with reduced ejection fraction. *Sci Rep.* (2020) 10:6665. doi: 10.1038/s41598-020-63801-2
13. Mentz RJ, Xu H, O'Brien EC, Thomas L, Alexy T, Gupta B, et al. PROVIDE-HF primary results: patient-reported outcomes investigation following initiation of drug therapy with entresto (sacubitril/valsartan) in heart failure. *Am Heart J.* (2020) 230:35–43. doi: 10.1016/j.ahj.2020.09.012
14. Spannella F, Marini M, Giulietti F, Rosettani G, Francioni M, Perna GP, et al. Renal effects of sacubitril/valsartan in heart failure with reduced ejection fraction: a real life 1-year follow-up study. *Intern Emerg Med.* (2019) 14:1287–97. doi: 10.1007/s11739-019-02111-6
15. López-Azor JC, Vicent L, Valero-Masa MJ, Esteban-Fernández A, Gómez-Bueno M, Pérez Á, et al. Safety of sacubitril/valsartan initiated during hospitalization: data from a non-selected cohort. *ESC Heart Fail.* (2019) 6:1161–6. doi: 10.1002/ehf2.12527

16. Rubattu S, Cotugno M, Forte M, Stanzione R, Bianchi F, Madonna M, et al. Effects of dual angiotensin type 1 receptor/neprilysin inhibition vs. angiotensin type 1 receptor inhibition on target organ injury in the stroke-prone spontaneously hypertensive rat. *J Hypertens.* (2018) 36:1902–14. doi: 10.1097/HJH.0000000000001762

17. Ibrahim NE, McCarthy CP, Shrestha S, Gaggin HK, Mukai R, Szymonifka J, et al. Effect of neprilysin inhibition on various natriuretic peptide assays. *J Am Coll Cardiol.* (2019) 73:1273–84. doi: 10.1016/j.jacc.2018.12.063

18. Acanfora D, Ciccone MM, Scicchitano P, Acanfora C, Casucci G. Neprilysin inhibitor-angiotensin II receptor blocker combination (sacubitril/valsartan): rationale for adoption in SARS-CoV-2 patients. *Eur Heart J Cardiovasc Pharmacother.* (2020) 6:135–6. doi: 10.1093/ehjcvp/pvaa028

19. Rubattu S, Gallo, Volpe M. Sacubitril/valsartan: potential impact of ARNi "beyond the Wall" of ACE2 on treatment and prognosis of heart failure patients with COVID-19. *Authorea. [Preprint].* (2020). doi: 10.22541/au.160157528.86277450

ECG Utilization Patterns of Patients with Arrhythmias during COVID-19 Epidemic and Post-SARS-CoV-2 Eras in Shanghai, China

Cheng Li[1†], Mu Chen[1†], Mohan Li[1†], Haicheng Wang[1], Xiangjun Qiu[2], Xiaoliang Hu[1], Qunshan Wang[1], Jian Sun[1], Mei Yang[1], Yuling Zhu[3], Peng Liao[4], Baohong Zhou[2], Min Chen[2], Xia Liu[3], Yuelin Zhao[3], Mingzhen Shen[3], Jinkang Huang[3], Li Luo[4], Hong Wu[5] and Yi-Gang Li[1,3*]

[1] Department of Cardiology, Xinhua Hospital, School of Medicine, Shanghai Jiao Tong University, Shanghai, China, [2] Shanghai Siwei Medical Co. Ltd., Shanghai, China, [3] Medical Information Telemonitoring Center, School of Medicine, Shanghai Jiao Tong University, Shanghai, China, [4] School of Public Health, Fudan University, Shanghai, China, [5] Shanghai Health Commission, Shanghai, China

*Correspondence:
Yi-Gang Li
liyigang@xinhuamed.com.cn

[†] These authors have contributed equally to this work

Background: The COVID-19 pandemic has led to concerns around its subsequent impact on global health.

Objective: To investigate the health-seeking behavior, reflected by ECG utilization patterns, of patients with non-COVID-19 diseases during and after COVID-19 epidemic.

Methods: Taking advantage of the remote ECG system covering 278 medical institutions throughout Shanghai, the numbers of medical visits with ECG examinations during the lockdown (between January 23 and April 7, 2020), post-lockdown (between April 8 and December 31, 2020) and post-SARS-CoV-2 (between January 23 and April 7, 2021) periods were analyzed and compared against those during the same periods of the preceding years (2018 and 2019).

Results: Compared with the same period during pre-COVID years, the number of medical visits decreased during the lockdown (a 38% reduction), followed by a rebound post-lockdown (a 17% increase) and a fall to the baseline level in post-SARS-CoV-2 period. The number of new COVID-19 cases announced on a given day significantly correlated negatively with the numbers of medical visits during the following 7 days. Medical visit dynamics differed for various arrhythmias. Whereas medical visits for sinus bradycardia exhibited a typical decrease-rebound-fallback pattern, medical visits for atrial fibrillation did not fall during the lockdown but did exhibit a subsequent increase during the post-lockdown period. By comparison, the volume for ventricular tachycardia remained constant throughout this entire period.

Conclusion: The ECG utilization patterns of patients with arrhythmias exhibited a decrease-rebound-fallback pattern following the COVID-19 lockdowns. Medical visits for diseases with more severe symptoms were less influenced by the lockdowns, showing a resilient demand for healthcare.

Keywords: epidemic, COVID-19, health-seeking behavior, arrhythmias, atrial fibrillation

INTRODUCTION

The Coronavirus disease 2019 (COVID-19) is a highly contagious viral infection and has spread around the world by multiple transmission modes. (1) The outbreak of COVID-19, caused by SARS-CoV-2, led to an unprecedented global public health crisis, and resulted in a large death-toll and long-term side effects for the survivors of the disease. The Chinese government imposed lockdown measures in Wuhan, the epicenter of the outbreak, from January 23 to April 7, 2020, to fight against SARS-CoV-2 in China. Since March 11, 2020, the daily number of new confirmed cases of COVID-19 has decreased significantly in China. (2) With the epidemic under control, China's prevention and control strategy were gradually adjusted to facilitate the recovery of normal economic production and life in China (3–5).

Not only did patients with COVID-19 suffer serious health damage during epidemic, but the shortage of medical resources and the strict preventive measures necessary to deal with the outbreak have also posed challenges to the routine management of non-COVID-19 diseases such as cardiovascular diseases (6–8), which has been reported in a Danish Nationwide Cohort Study regarding all-cause mortality and location of death in patients with established cardiovascular disease in COVID-19 epidemic. (9) Previous studies, mostly based on large medical centers (10), showed that the number of hospital visits decreased during the lockdowns, but research on the health-seeking behavior of populations at large have been less reported. One study from Israel showed a decrease in hospital admissions for myocardial infarction during the early stage of the pandemic, as well as a rebounding increase as the first wave of the pandemic faded (11). This research focused, however, on one specific disease and does not reflect the health-seeking dynamics of other cardiovascular diseases. The current evidence focusing on the association between COVID-19 and cardiovascular diseases is based on small, disease-specific studies and lacks quantitative backing, which highlights the importance of our study regarding the health-seeking dynamics associated with various cardiovascular diseases during and following the epidemic.

As a widely adopted routine examination characterized by its easy access and low cost, electrocardiograms (ECG) act as the diagnostic method for various types of cardiac arrhythmias. Therefore, changes to the number of medical visits with ECG examinations might reflect changes in the medical-seeking behavior of patients with cardiac arrhythmias. Taking advantage of the largest remote ECG platform in China, we were able to glimpse how COVID-19 affected the health-seeking behavior of patients with various arrhythmias during and after the epidemic.

METHODS

Study Population

This study was approved by the ethics committee at Xinhua Hospital Affiliated to Shanghai Jiao Tong University School of Medicine. All data used for this research were derived from the Siwei (Shanghai Siwei Medical, Shanghai, China) remote ECG diagnosis system. (12) As the largest ECG diagnostic system in China, the platform collected ECG data from 1,320 medical institutions across 13 provinces in China, with a volume of more than one million medical visits involving ECGs per year (**Figure 1A**). As approximately 85% of this ECG data was collected from Shanghai (**Supplementary Table 1**), which covered 278 medical institutions from almost all administrative districts (**Figure 1B** and **Supplementary Table 2**), the present study analyzes ECG data in Shanghai between January 1, 2018 and April 7, 2021.

Research Design

The numbers of medical visits with ECG examinations (ECG visits) during the lockdown (between January 23 and April 7, 2020), post-lockdown (between April 8 and December 31, 2020) and post-SARS-CoV-2 (between January 23 and April 7, 2021) periods were compared with those of the same periods during the two years prior to the COVID-19 outbreak (averages taken from 2018 and 2019). Subgroup analyses were then performed according to sex (male or female), age ($\leq$ 59 years old, 60–79 years old or $\geq$ 80 years old) and the tier of medical institution (academic hospitals or community clinics).

The number of new COVID-19 cases, new deaths, new discharged cases and existing confirmed cases in the Chinese mainland were then analyzed based on daily updates from China's Center of Disease Control (CDC) between January 11, 2020, and April 7, 2021. (2, 13) Spearman's rank correlation was analyzed for the COVID-19 data and the number of medical visits concerning various arrhythmias.

ECG-Based Diagnoses of Arrhythmias

ECG diagnoses, derived from a combination of artificial intelligence (AI) assistance and clinician diagnosis (details in **Supplementary Methods**), were adopted for the following diseases: sinus bradycardia, sinus tachycardia, atrial extrasystole, atrial tachycardia, atrial flutter, atrial fibrillation, ventricular extrasystole, ventricular tachycardia, paroxysmal supraventricular tachycardia(SVT), first-degree AV block (AVB), severe AVB (including second-degree type 2, high-degree and third-degree AVB), right bundle branch block (RBBB), left bundle branch block (LBBB) and left anterior fascicular block. Other abnormal ECG readings, such as myocardial infarction and ST segment depression, were not analyzed specifically for the inaccuracy of diagnosis due to lack of sufficient medical information.

Statistical Analysis

The numbers of daily medical visits involving ECG examinations were regarded as continuous variables, and the Mann-Whitney non-parametric test was used to compare the changes in the number of ECG visits between the different time periods or subgroups. Chi-square tests were used to compare the differences in the proportions of various arrhythmias between academic hospitals and community clinics. Spearman correlation analyses were used to reveal the correlations between the number of COVID-19 cases and the number of medical visits on following days. Statistical analyses were performed using IBM SPSS Statistics 24 (SPSS Inc., Chicago, IL). A two-sided p value of < 0.05 was considered significant.

RESULTS

Medical Visits During the Pre-COVID-19 Years (2018 and 2019)

The number of medical visits with ECG examinations remained stable during the two consecutive years preceding the COVID-19 pandemic. ECG visits in Shanghai were 696,800 and 702,989 in 2018 and 2019, respectively. Averages from 2018 and 2019 were taken as a pre-COVID baseline for subsequent comparison in this study.

The number of the ECG examinations were lower in the Jan-Feb and higher in May and June (**Figure 2**), different from the common sense that the cardiac disease patients are more prevalent in the Winter, the underlying reason remains unclear, and we checked the data from previous years. This pattern could also be observed in 2016, 2017, 2018, and 2019 (**Supplementary Figure 1**), future analysis is needed to clarify this issue.

Medical Visits During and After the Epidemic

Table 1 shows that the number of medical visits with ECG examinations decreased from 86,232 to 53,246 (a 38% reduction) during the lockdowns, after which it then increased from 591,661 to 657,774 (an 11% increase) during the post-lockdown period. Finally, this figure returned to its baseline level during the post-SARS-CoV-2 period (87,178 compared to the baseline of 86,232). When compared with the same periods during pre-COVID years, there were fewer monthly medical visits between February and June 2020, an equal number in July 2020, and higher-than-baseline levels between August and December 2020 (**Figure 2** and **Supplementary Tables 3, 4**). In addition, the yearly peak in the volume of medical visits occurred in May or June between 2016 and 2019, while in 2020, this peak was postponed to July (**Supplementary Figure 1**).

Relationship Between Medical Visits in Shanghai and Prevalence of COVID-19 in China

We analyzed the relationship between the number of new confirmed cases per day during the lockdowns in Chinese mainland and the number of medical visits in Shanghai. During the lockdowns, the number of new confirmed cases per day was negatively correlated with the number of medical visits during the following three days (r = −0.765, p < 0.001), seven days (r = −0.873, $p < 0.001$), 14 days (r = −0.804, p < 0.001), 21 days (r = −0.693, $p < 0.001$), 28 days (r = −0.615, p < 0.001), 35 days (r = −0.544, p < 0.001) and 42 days (r = −0.506, $p < 0.001$) in Shanghai (**Figure 3**, **Supplementary Figure 2** and **Supplementary Table 5**). This correlation coefficient exhibited a U-shaped curve, with a nadir at 7 days. Similarly, negative correlations with a U-shaped correlation coefficient curve were detected between the number of new COVID-related deaths in China and the number of medical visits in Shanghai during the lockdowns (**Figure 3**, **Supplementary Figure 2** and **Supplementary Table 5**). Such a correlation was not detected between the number of new discharged cases or existing confirmed cases and medical visits in Shanghai during the lockdown (**Supplementary Table 6**). No correlations between medical visit in Shanghai and COVID-19 prevalence in China were detected during the post-lockdown and post-SARS-CoV-2 periods (**Supplementary Table 5** and **Supplementary Figure 3**).

We further analyzed the relationship between medical visits in Shanghai and COVID-19 prevalence before and after the Spring Festival to exclude the impact of migration during the Spring Festival (January 23 and February 2, 2020). A similar negative correlation was observed even after factoring in for the Spring Festival migration (**Supplementary Table 7**).

Subgroup Analyses of Medical Visits in Shanghai

The impact of COVID-19 on health-seeking behavior related to cardiac arrhythmias varied by tier of medical institution (**Figure 4**). Compared with the same period during pre-COVID years, the number of medical visits to academic hospitals did not decrease during the lockdowns but increased during the post-lockdown (a 58% increase) and post-SARS-CoV-2 periods (a 30% increase). ECG visits to community clinics, however, decreased drastically during the lockdowns (a 51% reduction) followed by rebounding growth post-lockdowns and a subsequent recovery to the baseline level during the post-SARS-CoV-2 period.

In addition, medical visits from different sexes and above the age of 60 years generally followed the same decrease-rebound-fallback pattern, which was most prominent in patients between 60 and 79 years old. Medical visits by patients under 60 years of age, however, remained at a relatively constant level throughout the entire period (**Table 1**, **Supplementary Tables 3, 4** and **Supplementary Figures 4, 5**).

Similar to the results for the entire population, subgroup analyses based on age, sex and tier of medical institution revealed negative correlations between daily new cases or deaths with medical visits during the following 21 days during the lockdowns but not during the post-lockdown and post-SARS-CoV-2 periods (**Supplementary Tables 5, 6**).

Disease-Specific Medical Visits During and Following the Epidemic

The number of medical visits were further analyzed according to different arrhythmias during the lockdown, post-lockdown, and post-SARS-CoV-2 periods. During the lockdowns, the number of medical visits related to arrhythmias with severe symptoms, such as atrial flutter ($p = 0.230$), atrial fibrillation ($p = 0.172$) and severe AVB ($p = 0.816$) were comparatively similar with those from the same period during the pre-COVID years, revealing a high degree of rigidity in health seeking demand. By comparison, medical visits for diseases with little to no symptoms, such as sinus bradycardia ($p = 0.002$), ventricular extrasystole ($p = 0.004$) and RBBB ($p = 0.001$) significantly fell during the lockdown period. No matter the diagnosis, the number of medical visits exceeded baseline levels during the post-lockdown period, followed by a gradual fall to baseline levels during the post-SARS-CoV-2 period. Medical

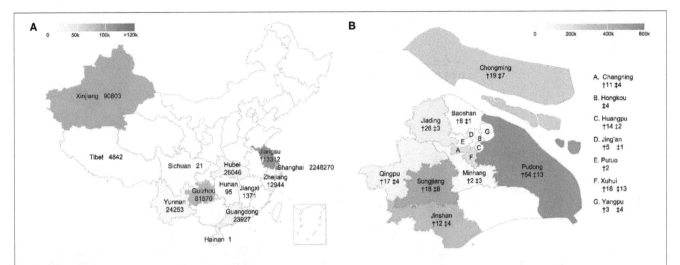

FIGURE 1 | Medical institutions covered by the ECG platform in China and Shanghai. (A) Regions covered by the remote ECG platform in China. The number following the province name shows the number of medical visits with ECG examinations in that province between Jan 1, 2018 and Apr 7, 2021. (B) Number of medical institutions covered by the ECG platform in Shanghai. † and ‡ indicate the number of community clinics and academic hospitals in that district.

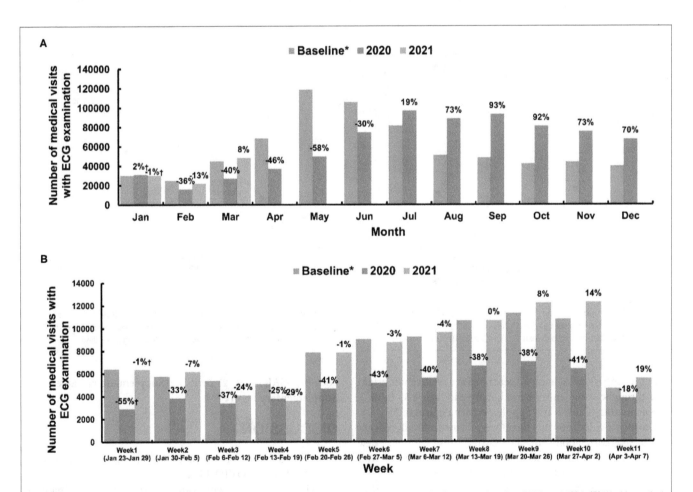

FIGURE 2 | Medical visits with ECG examination in Shanghai. (A) Monthly medical visits with ECG examinations of the baseline, 2020, and 2021. (B) Weekly medical visits during the lockdown (between January 23 and April 7, 2020) and the same period from the preceding years (baseline) and 2021. *Average number taken from 2018 and 2019. [†] The percentage difference compared with the baseline.

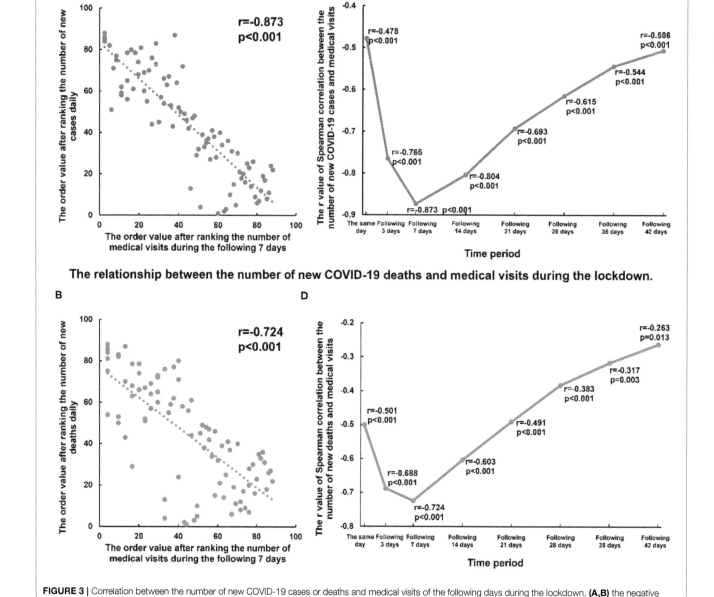

FIGURE 3 | Correlation between the number of new COVID-19 cases or deaths and medical visits of the following days during the lockdown. **(A,B)** the negative correlation between the new COVID-19 cases or deaths and the number of medical visits with ECG examination of the following 7 days during the lockdown. **(C,D)** the correlation coefficient (r) between the new COVID-19 cases or deaths and the number of medical visits of the same day and the following 3–42 days.

visits for ventricular tachycardia remained at a relatively constant level throughout the entire period analyzed (**Figure 5**, **Table 2**, **Supplementary Table 8** and **Supplementary Figures 6, 7**).

During the lockdowns, there were statistically significant but weak correlations or no correlations between new COVID-19 cases and medical visits related to diseases with severe symptoms, such as severe AVB (r = −0.495, $p <$ 0.001) and ventricular tachycardia (r = −0.055, $p = 0.614$). Negative correlations became prominent in diseases with mild symptoms, such as ventricular extrasystole (r = −0.816, $p <$ 0.001) and sinus bradycardia (r = −0.877, $p <$ 0.001). But these correlations disappeared during the post-lockdown

and post-SARS-CoV-2 periods (**Supplementary Table 9** and **Supplementary Figure 8**).

DISCUSSION

Based on a large volume of ECG data, we investigated the impact of the COVID-19 epidemic on the health-seeking behavior of patients with cardiac arrhythmias in Shanghai, China. The main findings of this study are as follows. First, the health-seeking behavior of patients with suspected cardiac arrhythmias, reflected by medical visits with ECG examinations, exhibited a decrease-rebound-fallback pattern during the period

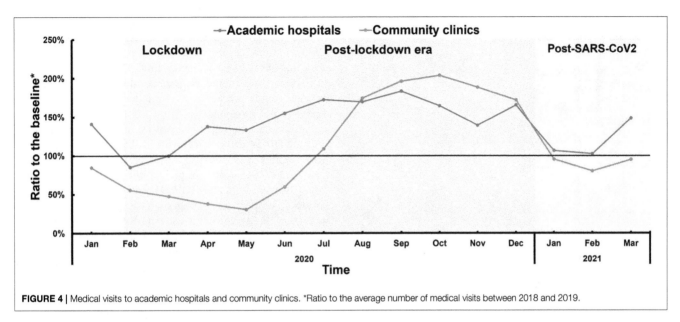

FIGURE 4 | Medical visits to academic hospitals and community clinics. *Ratio to the average number of medical visits between 2018 and 2019.

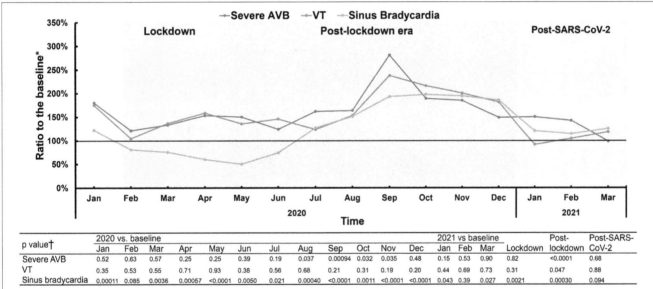

p value†	2020 vs. baseline												2021 vs baseline			Lockdown	Post-lockdown	Post-SARS-CoV-2
	Jan	Feb	Mar	Apr	May	Jun	Jul	Aug	Sep	Oct	Nov	Dec	Jan	Feb	Mar			
Severe AVB	0.52	0.63	0.57	0.25	0.25	0.39	0.19	0.037	0.00094	0.032	0.035	0.48	0.15	0.53	0.90	0.82	<0.0001	0.68
VT	0.35	0.53	0.55	0.71	0.93	0.38	0.56	0.68	0.21	0.31	0.19	0.20	0.44	0.69	0.73	0.31	0.047	0.88
Sinus bradycardia	0.00011	0.085	0.0036	0.00057	<0.0001	0.0050	0.021	0.00040	<0.0001	0.0011	<0.0001	<0.0001	0.043	0.39	0.027	0.0021	0.00030	0.094

FIGURE 5 | Different patterns of dynamics in disease-specific medical visits, represented by severe AVB, VT and sinus bradycardia. Three patterns of disease-specific medical visits dynamics during and following the pandemic were noticed, according to the ratio to the medical visits of the pre-COVID period. Pattern 1 (stable-increase-stable pattern) is represented by severe AVB. Pattern 2 (stable-stable-stable) is represented by ventricular tachycardia. Pattern 3 (decrease-rebound-fallback) is represented by sinus bradycardia. *Baseline was determined by the average number from 2018 and 2019. †The comparisons were obtained by a Mann-Whitney test. AVB, atrioventricular block; VT, ventricular tachycardia. The severe AVB includes second-degree type 2, high-degree and third-degree AVB.

starting from the COVID-19 lockdowns. This decrease in visits during the lockdown period was largely attributed to reduced patient volume at community clinics, whereas visits to academic hospitals were less affected. Second, a negative correlation was found between the number of new COVID-19 cases or deaths and medical visits on the same day as well as during the following six weeks during the lockdowns; these correlations were most prominent within the seven days after the report of new COVID-19 cases or deaths. Third, the impact of COVID-19 on health-seeking behavior varied with the types of the arrhythmias, and the medical demand for arrhythmias with potentially severe symptoms was less affected by the epidemic.

Decrease-Rebound-Fallback Pattern Following COVID-19 Lockdowns

During the initial phase of the COVID-19 outbreak, in the absence of vaccines or effective treatment protocols, self-isolation, as a standard quarantine measure, proved to be the most effective non-medical means to stop the spread of the virus. As a surging number of COVID-19 patients overwhelmed

TABLE 1 | Dynamics of medical visits of subgroups during different periods.

Groups	All year round			Lockdown			Post-lockdown			Post-SARS-CoV-2	
	Baseline*, n	2020, n	Percentage change†	Baseline*, n	2020, n	Percentage change†	Baseline*, n	2020, n	Percentage change†	2021, n	Percentage change†
Groups											
Males	321669	331239	3%	38834	23305	−40%	273130	295456	8%	40413	4%
Females	378226	407128	8%	47398	29941	−37%	318531	362318	14%	46765	−1%
≤59y	206975	214259	4%	32354	19285	−40%	165738	184151	11%	33855	5%
60–79y	389963	420944	8%	38971	23503	−40%	341967	386286	13%	40660	4%
≥80y	102957	103164	0%	14907	10458	−30%	83957	87337	4%	12663	−15%
Academic hospitals	139083	205164	48%	23273	22231	−4%	108788	171500	58%	30157	30%
Community clinics	560812	533203	−5%	62959	31015	−51%	482874	486274	1%	57021	−9%
Total	699895	738367	5%	86232	53246	−38%	591661	657774	11%	87178	1%

*Average number of 2018 and 2019.
†Compared with baseline.

medical resources during the early stage of the epidemic, the Chinese government called for non-COVID-19 patients with mild symptoms to stay at home to reserve the capacity of medical institutions for patients with COVID-19 or for patients with severe diseases and symptoms. Medical institutions also provided online consultations with doctors to help patients identify urgent situations.

Similar to the findings of previous studies in China and other countries (10, 14–18) medical visits in Shanghai, an area outside the epidemic's epicenter, also decreased by approximately 40% during the Wuhan lockdown period. But the suppressed health-seeking demand from non-COVID-19 diseases was released after the lockdown period, forming a drastic post-lockdown surge. This fall-rebound pattern was also reported by a study from Israel in that noted a decrease in hospital admissions for myocardial infarction was observed during the early stage of the epidemic, as well as a rebounding increase upon the receding end of the first wave of the epidemic (11) Another study from Korea also showed that the number of outpatient visits in internal medicine decreased during the COVID-19 pandemic and tended to rebound during the second half of the year (19) Subsequently, medical visits gradually fell back to the baseline level of prior years, reflecting the normalization of health-seeking demand during the post-SARS-CoV-2 period in China.

New cases and deaths reported daily exerted a negative influence on the health-seeking behavior of patients over the following 6 weeks, and this trend was especially strong the first week after the report. It is also of note that this negative correlation between reported new cases or deaths with medical visits was detected based on new cases or deaths reported for the whole of China rather than just Shanghai locally (**Supplementary Table 10** and **Supplementary Figure 9**), which reflects the impact of uniform policy on the behavior pattern of patients across China. As new cases per day dropped into single digits and as Wuhan lifted outbound travel restrictions, the correlation between COVID-19 cases and medical visits weakened or even disappeared, reflecting a shift of public focus and a return to normal daily life.

In addition, the general decrease in medical visits during the lockdowns was largely attributed to the decrease in visits to community clinics rather than to academic hospitals. Considering the hierarchical medical system in China, community clinics are mainly responsible for the long-term management of chronic diseases with mild symptoms, whereas patients with critical conditions and severe symptoms are usually treated at academic hospitals. This hierarchical separation of functions at different medical institutions was supported by our data regarding medical visits concerning cardiac arrhythmias during the pre-COVID-19 years (**Supplementary Table 11**). Such health-seeking preferences regarding academic hospitals and community clinics were amplified during the COVID-19 epidemic, suggesting that urgent conditions drove patients to admit themselves to academic hospitals regardless of the suggestions to isolate at home; medical visits by arrhythmic patients with mild symptoms or chronic conditions, however, largely decreased due to concerns over nosocomial infection by COVID-19.

TABLE 2 | Dynamics of medical visits of various ECG events during different periods.

Category of ECG events	All year round			Lockdown			Post-lockdown			Post-SARS-CoV-2	
	Baseline *, n	2020, n	Percentage change †	Baseline *, n	2020, n	Percentage change †	Baseline *, n	2020, n	Percentage change †	2021, n	Percentage change †
Normal ECG	310113	317929	3%	37617	20207	−46%	263332	286963	9%	37689	2%
Sinus bradycardia	64264	69573	8%	6393	4876	−24%	58051	64796	12%	7872	23%
Sinus tachycardia	28500	29462	3%	7075	5866	−17%	20126	22821	13%	5870	−17%
Atrial extrasystole	44217	45725	3%	6822	5167	−24%	36416	39526	9%	6249	−8%
Atrial tachycardia	3574	3840	7%	681	567	−17%	2779	3130	13%	570	−16%
Atrial flutter	1527	2204	44%	279	354	27%	1193	1802	51%	303	9%
Atrial fibrillation	20387	22060	8%	3466	3367	−3%	16334	18374	12%	3093	−11%
Ventricular extrasystole	26625	28982	9%	4371	3652	−16%	21667	24812	15%	4297	−2%
Ventricular tachycardia	141	206	47%	26	32	23%	110	168	53%	31	19%
Paroxysmal SVT	1168	1391	19%	203	231	14%	940	1167	24%	216	7%
First-degree AVB	25299	29582	17%	3188	2924	−8%	21664	26068	20%	3707	16%
Severe AVB	348	495	42%	61	78	28%	282	413	47%	72	18%
RBBB	36882	40705	10%	4890	4023	−18%	31337	35997	15%	5181	6%
LBBB	3309	3810	15%	476	427	−10%	2800	3324	19%	486	2%
Left anterior fascicular block	6863	6452	−6%	1000	692	−31%	5741	5656	−1%	904	−10%

*Average number of 2018 and 2019.
†Compared with baseline.
SVT, supraventricular tachycardia; atrioventricular junctional tachycardia; AVB, atrioventricular block; RBBB, right bundle branch block; LBBB, left bundle branch block.
The severe AVB includes second-degree type 2, high-degree and third-degree AVB.

Behavioral Differences Exhibited Among Various Arrhythmias

Health-seeking behavior differed among various arrhythmias regarding the number of medical visits during and following the COVID-19 epidemic. Three patterns were detected. Pattern 1 was named the "stable-increase-stable" pattern and is represented by diseases such as severe AVB and atrial fibrillation (**Supplementary Figure 6**). The number of such medical visits remained stable during the lockdowns, followed by a post-lockdown increase and a return to baseline levels during the post-SARS-CoV-2 period. No prominent cosine-like curve in medical visits was observed. Patients with diseases conforming to Pattern 1 often manifested with severe symptoms and urgent conditions, and they tended to seek health services regardless of their concerns about nosocomial infection with COVID-19, thus reflecting a rigid medical demand. Pattern 2 was named the "stable-stable-stable" pattern and is represented by VT. This pattern corresponded to a relatively constant level of medical visits during and following the epidemic. As the ECG diagnostic system did not differentiate between non-sustained VT as short as three beats and sustained VT, which can cause hemodynamic disorders, it is possible that this "stable" level represents the mixed effects of situations of different clinical severities. Pattern 3 was named the "decrease-rebound-fallback" pattern, i.e., a cosine-like curve, and is represented by sinus bradycardia and the conditions in **Supplementary Figure 7**. In this pattern, patients with arrhythmias exhibiting mild symptoms tended to follow home isolation suggestions during the lockdowns. Medical demand, however, was not suppressed after the lockdown, as a rebound in medical visits occurred. As COVID-19 was further controlled in China, health-seeking behavior returned to the rational levels of prior years. Taken together, these health-seeking behaviors during and following the epidemic were not uniform for different diseases. A rigid medical demand for some diseases, such as severe AVB and VT, was revealed by unchanging or increased medical visits during the epidemic. Our results thus highlight the importance of medical institutions coping with non-COVID-19 -but nonetheless severe - diseases during the epidemic, as well as the importance of preparing for a surge in medical visits for various arrhythmias during the post-SARS-CoV-2 period.

Implications

China's anti-COVID-19 measures included city-wide lockdowns, transportation freezes or controls in hard-hit areas, the timely release of COVID-19 information, the prevention of social gatherings and infections, thorough community screening, the quarantining of suspected individuals, the early admission and treatment of confirmed cases, extensive epidemiological investigations and a tremendous number of other efforts aimed at controlling the epidemic, such as the manufacture of sufficient medical products and vaccine research and development (20–25) As COVID-19 exerted negative effects on non-COVID diseases (7, 10) the early control of COVID-19 was also of great significance in improving the prognoses of patients with cardiac arrhythmias.

Considering that COVID-19 is still prevalent around the world and that China is now facing a new wave of Omicron

variants recently, the results of our research may have important implications for China and other countries in planning the allocation of medical resources during these new epidemic and post-SARS-CoV-2 periods. Our results show that the number of medical visits will exhibit a post-SARS-CoV-2 surge that might last for nearly half a year. As an economically developed area in China, Shanghai properly handled the prior post-SARS-CoV-2 surge in medical demand. There might be an imbalance between medical supply and demand, however, during another post-SARS-CoV-2 period in less-developed regions and rural areas with fewer medical resources. Given the rapidly expanding vaccination process, the COVID-19 pandemic is expected to be taken under control around the world in the near future. Governments and medical institutions should pay great attention to preemptively coping with post-COVID surges in medical demand among patients with cardiac arrhythmias. In addition, this might also be true for patients with other diseases.

Limitations

As the corresponding clinical, laboratory and imaging data were lacking, diagnoses made by ECG alone will result in a certain number of misdiagnoses and missed diagnoses, as well as conditions beyond arrhythmias. However, the diagnoses of cardiac arrhythmias highly relied on ECG. Second, a 30-second ECG is not able to discriminate between subtypes or between the severity of symptoms of specific arrhythmias, such as non-sustained and sustained VT, and atrial fibrillation with a fast or normal range of ventricular rate. Sinus bradycardia in this system follows the ECG criteria in which the sinus rate must be slower than 60 beats per minute. But according to new clinical guidelines, sinus bradycardia is now defined by a heart rate of <50 beats per minute (26) Also, ECG examination could be avoided to prevent contact-related infection after COVID-19, especially during the lockdown periods, which might be more prominent in community clinics and in patients with mild symptoms. These factors might bias the findings of our study.

CONCLUSIONS

The number of medical visits related to cardiac arrhythmias exhibited a decrease-rebound-fallback pattern during the period starting from the COVID-19 lockdown in Shanghai. During this lockdown period, the severity of the epidemic, reflected by daily new cases or deaths, exerted a negative 6-week impact on the patients' behaviors in their seeking of medical services, and this impact was most prominent during the week following the daily report of new cases or deaths. Medical visits for arrhythmias with potentially severe symptoms, such as severe AVB and VT, were not negatively affected by the epidemic, reflecting the rigid medical demand of these patients.

AUTHOR CONTRIBUTIONS

CL, MuC, and ML reviewed literature, analyzed the data, drafted, revised the manuscript, and designed or coded the figures and tables. HWa and XH collected the data, conducted a literature review, and interpreted the data. YZhu, BZ, and XQ developed and maintained the platform for the remote ECG diagnosis system. QW, JS, and MY critically revised the diagnosis of ECG for further analyses MiC, XL, YZha, MS, and JH provided critical feedback on

data sources. LL and PL provided guidance and support for statistical methods. HWu provided support for the development of the ECG platform. YG-L designed the study, acquired funding and managed the project. All authors had final responsibility for the decision to submit this paper for publication.

REFERENCES

1. Mehraeen E, Salehi M, Behnezhad F, Moghaddam H, SeyedAlinaghi S. Transmission modes of COVID-19: a systematic review. *Infect Disord Drug Targets*. (2021) 21:e170721187995. doi: 10.2174/1871526520666201116095934

2. CDC C. *Distribution of COVID-19 in China*. Available online at: http://2019ncov.chinacdc.cn/2019-nCoV/index.html (accessed on May 20, 2021).

3. Ren L, Wang Y, Wu Z, Xiang Z, Guo L, Xu T, et al. Identification of a novel coronavirus causing severe pneumonia in human: a descriptive study. *Chin Med J*. (2020) 133:1015–24.

4. WHO. *Report of the WHO-China Joint Mission on Coronavirus Disease 2019 (COVID-19)*. (2020). Available online at: https://www.who.int/docs/default-source/coronaviruse/who-china-joint-mission-on-covid-19-final-report.pdf (accessed on Jun 30, 2021)

5. Li Z, Chen Q, Feng L, Rodewald L, Xia Y, Yu H, et al. Active case finding with case management: the key to tackling the COVID-19 pandemic. *Lancet (London, England)*. (2020) 396:63–70. doi: 10.1016/S0140-6736(20)31278-2

6. Jeffery M, D'Onofrio G, Paek H, Platts-Mills T, Soares W, Hoppe J, et al. Trends in emergency department visits and hospital admissions in health care systems in 5 states in the first months of the COVID-19 pandemic in the US. *Jama Intern Med*. (2020) 180:1328–1333.

7. Einstein A, Shaw L, Hirschfeld C, Williams M, Villines T, Better N, et al. International impact of COVID-19 on the diagnosis of heart disease. *J Am Coll Cardiol*. (2021) 77:173–85. doi: 10.1016/j.jacc.2020.10.054

8. Schmidt A, Bakouny Z, Bhalla S, Steinharter J, Tremblay D, Awad M, et al. Cancer care disparities during the COVID-19 pandemic: COVID-19 and cancer outcomes study. *Cancer Cell*. (2020) 38:769–70. doi: 10.1016/j.ccell.2020.10.023

9. Butt J, Fosbøl E, Gerds T, Andersson C, Kragholm K, Biering-Sørensen T, et al. All-cause mortality and location of death in patients with established cardiovascular disease before, during, and after the COVID-19 lockdown: a Danish nationwide cohort study. *European Heart J*. (2021) 42:1516–23. doi: 10.1093/eurheartj/ehab028

10. Ranganathan P, Sengar M, Chinnaswamy G, Agrawal G, Arumugham R, Bhatt R, et al. Impact of COVID-19 on cancer care in India: a cohort study. *Lancet Oncology*. (2021) 970–6. doi: 10.1016/S1470-2045(21)00240-0

11. Fardman A, Oren D, Berkovitch A, Segev A, Levy Y, Beigel R, et al. Post COVID-19 acute myocardial infarction rebound. *Can J Cardiol*. (2020) 36:1832.e15–1832.e16. doi: 10.1016/j.cjca.2020.08.016

12. Yang M, Zhou R, Qiu X, Feng X, Sun J, Wang Q, et al. Artificial intelligence-assisted analysis on the association between exposure to ambient fine particulate matter and incidence of arrhythmias in outpatients of Shanghai community hospitals. *Environ Int*. (2020) 139:105745. doi: 10.1016/j.envint.2020.105745

13. Sina. *Real-Time Tracking of the COVID-19 Epidemic*. (2020). Available online at: https://news.sina.cn/zt_d/yiqing0121 (accessed on May 20, 2021)

14. Sato Y, Fujiwara Y, Fukuda N, Hayama B, Ito Y, Ohno S and Takahashi S. Changes in treatment behavior during the COVID-19 pandemic among patients at a cancer hospital. *Cancer Cell*. (2021) 39:130–31. doi: 10.1016/j.ccell.2021.01.002

15. Baum A, Kaboli P and Schwartz M. Reduced in-person and increased telehealth outpatient visits during the COVID-19 pandemic. *Ann Intern Med*. (2021) 174:129–31. doi: 10.7326/M20-3026

16. Shepherd J, Moore S, Long A, Mercer Kollar, Sumner S. Association between COVID-19 lockdown measures and emergency department visits for violence-related injuries in cardiff, wales. *JAMA*. (2021) 325:885–7. doi: 10.1001/jama.2020.25511

17. Holt A, Gislason G, Schou M, Zareini B, Biering-Sørensen T, Phelps M, et al. New-onset atrial fibrillation: incidence, characteristics, and related events following a national COVID-19 lockdown of 5.6 million people. *European Heart J*. (2020) 41:3072–79. doi: 10.1093/eurheartj/ehaa494

18. Law R, Wolkin A, Patel N, Alic A, Yuan K, Ahmed K, et al. Injury-Related emergency Department Visits During the COVID-19 Pandemic. *Am J Prev Med*. (2022) 1–8.

19. Byun H, Kang D, Go S, Kim H, Hahm J and Kim R. The impact of the COVID-19 pandemic on outpatients of internal medicine and pediatrics: a descriptive study. *Medicine*. (2022) 101:e28884. doi: 10.1097/MD.0000000000028884

20. Pan A, Liu L, Wang C, Guo H, Hao X, Wang Q, et al. Association of public health interventions with the epidemiology of the COVID-19 outbreak in Wuhan, China. *JAMA*. (2020) 323:1915–23. doi: 10.1001/jama.2020.6130

21. Maier B, Brockmann D. Effective containment explains subexponential growth in recent confirmed COVID-19 cases in China. *Science*. (2020) 368:742–6. doi: 10.1126/science.abb4557

22. Kraemer M, Yang C, Gutierrez B, Wu C, Klein B, Pigott D, et al. The effect of human mobility and control measures on the COVID-19 epidemic in China. *Science*. (2020) 368:493–7. doi: 10.1126/science.abb4218

23. Lai S, Ruktanonchai N, Zhou L, Prosper O, Luo W, Floyd J, et al. Effect of non-pharmaceutical interventions to contain COVID-19 in China. *Nature*. (2020) 585:410–13. doi: 10.1038/s41586-020-2293-x

24. Chinazzi M, Davis J, Ajelli M, Gioannini C, Litvinova M, Merler S, et al. The effect of travel restrictions on the spread of the 2019 novel coronavirus (COVID-19) outbreak. *Science*. (2020) 368:395–400. doi: 10.1126/science.aba9757

25. Tian H, Liu Y, Li Y, Wu C, Chen B, Kraemer M, et al. An investigation of transmission control measures during the first 50 days of the COVID-19 epidemic in China. *Science*. (2020) 368:638–42. doi: 10.1126/science.abb6105

26. Kusumoto F, Schoenfeld M, Barrett C, Edgerton J, Ellenbogen K, Gold M, et al. 2018 ACC/AHA/HRS Guideline on the evaluation and management of patients with bradycardia and cardiac conduction delay: a report of the american college of cardiology/american heart association task force on clinical practice guidelines and the heart rhythm society. *Circulation*. (2019) 140:e382–482. doi: 10.1161/CIR.0000000000000628

9

Hyperbilirubinemia in Gilbert Syndrome Attenuates Covid-19-Induced Metabolic Disturbances

Hayder M. Al-kuraishy[1], Ali I. Al-Gareeb[1], Saleh M. Abdullah[2], Natália Cruz-Martins[3,4,5*] and Gaber El-Saber Batiha[6*]

[1] Department of Clinical Pharmacology and Medicine, College of Medicine, Al-Mustansiriya University, Baghdad, Iraq,
[2] Department of Medical Laboratory Technology, Faculty of Applied Medical Sciences, Jazan University, Jazan, Saudi Arabia,
[3] Faculty of Medicine, University of Porto, Porto, Portugal, [4] Department of Metabolism, Nutrition and Endocrinology, Institute for Research and Innovation in Health (i3S), University of Porto, Porto, Portugal, [5] Laboratory of Neuropsychophysiology, Faculty of Psychology and Education Sciences, University of Porto, Porto, Portugal, [6] Department of Pharmacology and Therapeutics, Faculty of Veterinary Medicine, Damanhour University, Damanhour, Egypt

*Correspondence:
Natália Cruz-Martins
ncmartins@med.up.pt
Gaber El-Saber Batiha
gaberbatiha@gmail.com

Gilbert syndrome (GS) is a liver disorder characterized by non-hemolytic unconjugated hyperbilirubinemia. On the other hand, Coronavirus disease 2019 (Covid-19) is a recent viral infectious disease presented as clusters of pneumonia, triggered by the severe acute respiratory syndrome-coronavirus 2 (SARS-CoV-2). Little is known on the association between SARS-CoV-2 and GS, despite different studies have recently stated a link between hyperbilirubinemia and SARS-CoV-2 severity. In this case-report study we described a 47-year-old man, a known case of GS since the age of 4, presented to the emergency department with fever (39.8°C), dry cough, dyspnea, headache, myalgia, sweating and jaundice diagnosed with Covid-19-induced pneumonia. Interestingly, GS patient exhibited a rapid clinical recovery and short hospital stay compared to other SARS-CoV-2 positive patient, seeming that hyperbilirubinemia may exert a protective effect of against Covid-19 induced-cardiometabolic disturbances. Data obtained here underlines that the higher resistance against Covid-19 evidenced by the GS patient seems to be due to the antioxidant, anti-inflammatory, and antiviral effects of unconjugated bilirubin.

Keywords: gilbert syndrome, SARS-CoV-2, hyperbilirubinemia, COVID-19, metabolic disease

INTRODUCTION

Gilbert syndrome (GS) is a chronic liver disorder characterized by non-hemolytic unconjugated hyperbilirubinemia due to defect in the hepatic uptake of unconjugated bilirubin, which was first described by Augustin Gilbert in 1901 (1). GS is also called simple familial jaundice or icterus intermittent juvenilis, affects 5–10% of general population, being most common in male (2). Clinically, GS is presented with mild recurrent jaundice, fatigue and abdominal pain provoked by stress, infection, and menstruation. GS results from reduction in bilirubin uridine diphosphate glucuronyltransferase enzyme activity due to mutation in the UGT1A1 gene. There are more than 100 variants of UGT1A1 gene associated with GS phenotype, and generally, there is no effective treatment for GS, despite phenobarbital may be used in severe cases (3). Previously,

Maruhashi et al. (4) reported that hyperbilirubinemia in GS is associated with a cardioprotective effect attributed to the antioxidant and vasodilator effects of bilirubin.

On the other hand, coronavirus disease 2019 (Covid-19), a recent viral infectious disease presented as clusters of pneumonia and caused by the severe acute respiratory syndrome coronavirus-2 (SARS-CoV-2), has triggered a huge attention among both medical and scientific communities with the intent of discovering an effective therapeutic agent (5). The clinical spectrum of Covid-19 is asymptomatic or mild flu-like illness in around 85%, mainly in young adults; however, 10% of cases develop a severe disease with risk of development of acute respiratory distress syndrome (ARDS) (6). However, in severe cases, Covid-19 may leads to extra-pulmonary manifestations, like acute cardiac injury, arrhythmias, acute kidney injury, acute brain injury, endocrine failure, multiple organ failure, metabolic disturbances, and even death (7). In this sense, as Covid-19 pandemic has full-grown public health issues, here we present a case-report study of a patient with GS who gets infected by the SARS-CoV-2. This case is particularly relevant regarding the ameliorative role of hyperbilirubinemia in GS patients during Covid-19 pneumonia.

CASE REPORT

Presenting Concerns

A 47-year-old man, a known case of GS since age of 4-year, presented to the emergency department with fever, dry cough, dyspnea, headache, myalgia, sweating, jaundice, and generalized poor health condition without response to the empiric antibiotics and analgesics for about 3 days. Besides, a 53-years-old man presented with fever (38.9°C), cough, headache, malaise and sweating diagnosed as Covid-19 pneumonia was regarded as a control. Informed verbal consent was attained from both patients, and this study was approved (MRT 7 August 2020) by the Scientific Editorial Board in College of Medicine, Al-Mustansiriyia University, Baghdad, Iraq.

Clinical and Laboratory Findings

General physical examination showed a conscious and febrile patient (39.8°C), with jaundice and poor health status. His blood pressure was 140/90 mmHg, heart rate was 110 beats/min and body mass index (BMI) of 33.73 kg/m^2 and hypoxemia (SaO$_2$ 91%). Chest X-ray and chest computed tomography (CT) scan illustrated bilateral prominent bronchovascular marking and ground-glass opacities, respectively, suggestive of Covid-19-induced pneumonia (**Figure 1**). Radiological score was used to determine the radiological severity according to Wasilewski et al. (8).

Anti-SARS-CoV-2 antibody (IgM) was positive (2.9 U/mL) for Covid-19 patient with GS compared with (2.89 U/mL) for Covid-19 patient only, suggesting an acute SARS-CoV-2 infection in both. Complete blood count (CBC), fasting blood glucose (FBG), glycated hemoglobin (HbA1c), blood urea, serum creatinine, C-reactive protein (CRP), D-dimer, serum lactate dehydrogenase (LDH), and serum ferritin were done at the laboratory unit. Preliminary investigations showed high FBG (165 mg/dL),

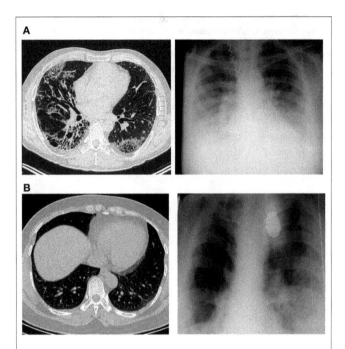

FIGURE 1 | Chest X-ray and CT scan imaging showed bilateral ground-glass appearance; **(A)** Covid-19 patients only, **(B)** Covid-19 patients with Gilbert syndrome.

HbA1c (5.5%), total serum bilirubin (6.8 mg/dL), unconjugated bilirubin (6 mg/dL), conjugated bilirubin (0.8 mg mg/dL), and high white cell counts (16.073/µL) with lymphopenia (9.12 µ/L). Similarly, the inflammatory biomarkers were increased in regard to reference ranges. D-dimer (14.000 ng/mL), CRP (243 mg/L), ferritin (654 ng/mL), and LDH (674U/L).

Liver function test and ultrasonography imaging were done to exclude liver injury. Taken together, clinical findings, radiological examinations and laboratory findings of this GS patient with Covid-19 were compared with a matched COVID-19 patient without GS at time of hospitalization (**Table 1**).

Both patients were treated with the analgesic acetaminophen (500 mg/day), azithromycin (500 mg/day) for the first 5 days, ivermectin (12 mg/day), famotidine (40 mg/day), soluble insulin (10 units) 3 times/day, and montelukast (10 mg/day). Besides oxygen therapy by high flow nasal cannula for 10 days, patients also received subcutaneous enoxaparin (60 mg/day) during the hospitalization period as a prophylaxis against venous thromboembolism.

Follow-Up and Outcomes

Following 3 weeks of management, all laboratory investigations, radiological, and clinical findings return to normal except of unconjugated bilirubin (**Table 2**) and the patient was discharged to home. Particularly, the GS patient showed a rapid clinical improvement as compared to the Covid-19 patient without GS during the hospitalization period.

An outpatient follow-up through mobile dial-up within 2 weeks following discharge disclosed a complete recovery and the GS patient returned to his prior physical fitness and normal daily activities.

TABLE 1 | Cardiometabolic and inflammatory profiles of GS patient COVID-19 positive compared to a control patient at time of admission.

Variables	Reference range	COVID-19 patient with GS	COVID-19 patient	% Difference
BMI (kg/m^2)	20–25	33.73	34.71	2.86
SBP (mmHg)	110–120	140	153	8.87
DBP (mmHg)	70–90	90	92	2.19
Covid-19 IgM (U/mL)	0.9–1.1	2.9	2.89	0.34
Covid-19 IgG (U/mL)	0.9–1.1	0.00	0.00	0.00
SaO$_2$%	95–99	91	89	1.11
TSB (mg/dL)	0.2–1.0	6.8	0.8	157.89
Conjugated bilirubin (mg/dL)	0.1–0.3	0.8	0.7	13.33
Un-conjugated bilirubin (mg/dL)	0.1–0.7	6.0	0.1	193.44
FBG (mg/dL)	70–90	165	199	18.68
HbA1c (%)	4.5–5.5	5.5	5.9	7.01
Blood urea	20–40	41	39.7	3.22
Serum creatinine	0.5–1.5	1.2	1.1	8.69
CRP (mg/L)	0.5–200	243	422	53.83
D-dimer (ng/mL)	50–10.000	14.000	22.000	44.44
Ferritin (ng/mL)	20–250	654	907.84	32.50
LDH (U/L)	230–460	674	795.21	16.50
Hb (g/dL)	12–14	13.8	14.36	3.97
WBC (μ/L)	4,000–11,000	16.073	15.74	2.09
Lymphocytes %	20–40	9.12	7.53	19.09
Neutophils %	40–80	85.31	89.45	4.73
Radiological score	1–5	4	5	22.22

Data presented as number and %, BMI, body mass index; SBP, systolic blood pressure; DBP, diastolic blood pressure; TSB, total serum bilirubin; FBG, fasting blood glucose; HbA1c, glycated hemoglobin.

TABLE 2 | Cardiometabolic and inflammatory profiles of GS patient COVID-19 positive compared to a control patient at time of discharge.

Variables	Reference range	Covid-19 with GS	Covid-19 patient	% Difference
BMI (kg/m^2)	20–25	32.65	34.71	6.11
SBP (mmHg)	110–120	119	143	18.32
DBP (mmHg)	70–90	79	82	3.72
Covid-19 IgM (U/mL)	0.9–1.1	0.9	0.89	1.11
Covid-19 IgG (U/mL)	0.9–1.1	7.84	6.01	26.42
SaO$_2$%	95–99	98	95	3.10
TSB (mg/dL)	0.2–1.0	3.4	0.8	123.81
Conjugated bilirubin (mg/dL)	0.1–0.3	0.4	0.7	54.54
Un-conjugated bilirubin (mg/dL)	0.1–0.7	3.0	0.1	187.09
FBG (mg/dL)	70–90	95	179	61.31
HbA1c (%)	4.5–5.5	5.5	5.9	7.01
Blood urea	20–40	33	34.7	5.02
Serum creatinine	0.5–1.5	1.3	1.2	8
CRP (mg/L)	0.5–200	22	122	138.88
D-dimer (ng/mL)	50–10.000	452	631.71	33.16
Ferritin (ng/mL)	20–250	105	207.84	65.74
LDH (U/L)	230–460	321	395.21	20.72
Hb (g/dL)	12–14	13.8	14.36	3.97
WBC (μ/L)	4,000–11,000	8.832	9.44	6.65
Lymphocytes %	20–40	33.7	22.53	39.72
Neutrophils %	40–80	72.88	80.45	9.87
Radiological score	1–5	1	2	66.66

Data presented as number and %, BMI, body mass index; SBP, systolic blood pressure; DBP, diastolic blood pressure; TSB, total serum bilirubin; FBG, fasting blood glucose; HbA1c, glycated hemoglobin.

CLINICAL COURSE SUMMARY

At time of hospitalization, both Covid-19 patients with or without GS presented comparable clinical presentations, like fever, headache, sweating, dry cough, fatigue, and generalized poor health status. However, these clinical features were less severe in Covid-19 patient with GS compared with Covid-19 patient only. In addition to high serum levels of unconjugated bilirubin in Covid-19 patient with GS, both laboratory and radiological findings were better as compared with Covid-19 patient only. In the management period, patients received the same course of supportive therapy, antibiotics, anticoagulants, and other drugs. During hospitalization period, the fasting blood glucose (FBG) was elevated in both Covid-19 patients (FBG = 165 mg/dL in GS, 199 mg/dL in Covid-19 control), managed through using soluble insulin subcutaneously 10 IU/day with frequent monitoring of FBG. In particular, Covid-19 patient with GS presented with a less needed for oxygen therapy compared with control Covid-19 patients who was more dependent on oxygen therapy. Near the end of hospitalization period, Covid-19 patient with GS showed a rapid clinical

improvement as compared to the Covid-19 patient without GS. At the third week of disease management, clinical, radiological and laboratory findings were re-evaluated. All investigations and clinical findings return to normal with exception of unconjugated bilirubin, which remained higher in Covid-19 patient with GS (3 mg/dL) as compared with that in control Covid-19 patient (1 mg/dL). Both patients were discharged to home with complete recovery and returned to normal daily activities.

DISCUSSION

To our knowledge, this is the first reported case study of Covid-19 in a patient with GS. The GS patient with Covid-19 showed a rapid clinical improvement and short hospital stay as compared with a Covid-19 patient. Indeed, it has been proven that bilirubin exerts potent antioxidant effects which might alleviates Covid-19 induced-oxidative stress (9). Also, it has been reported that bilirubin has cardioprotective effects, improves endothelial function and provokes the nitric oxide (NO) release (10), thus, preventing from endothelial dysfunction and cardiovascular complications in COVID-19 (11), as evident of hypertension in Covid-19 case compared to GS patient with Covid-19. Unfortunately, oxidative stress profile and endogenous antioxidant capacity were not measured in the present study to confirm the antioxidant potential of unconjugated bilirubin in Covid-19.

Liu et al. (12) found that SARS-CoV-2 infection leads to down-regulation of angiotensin converting enzyme 2 (ACE2) causing a reduction in the vasodilator angiotensins (Ang 1–7 and Ang 1–9) and augmenting of vasoconstrictor angiotensin II (AngII). These changes *per se* lead to acute lung injury (ALI), cardiovascular and metabolic disturbances in Covid-19 patients. Recently, Novák et al. (13) reported that high bilirubin levels attenuate the metabolic disorders through inhibition and attenuation of renin-angiotensin system (RAS). Besides, bilirubin has a protective effect against experimental ALI through inhibition of ischemic-reperfusion injury and exerting anti-proliferative effects (14). Therefore, high serum bilirubin level in patients with GS may lessen ALI and the development of ARDS through attenuation of AngII induced-pulmonary vasoconstriction and hyper-inflammation (15). These findings might explain a lower CT score 4 in Covid-19 with GS as compared with control Covid-19 score 5.

Lin et al. (16) also illustrated that bilirubin inhibits the nod-like receptor pyrin3 (NLRP3) inflammasomes over-activation through myeloperoxidase inhibition and subsequent reduction of inflammatory cytokines release. Thereby, high serum bilirubin levels in patients with GS may attenuate the development of cytokine storm during Covid-19 progression via inhibiting the release of interleukin (IL)-6, tumor necrosis factor (TNF)-α and IL-1β (17). These findings might explain the low rate of inflammatory biomarkers in GS patient with Covid-19 compared to the Covid-19 patient without GS. These protective effects of high bilirubin in GS are lacking in patients with Covid-19 pneumonia without GS. It has been shown that uncontrolled high pro-inflammatory cytokines, oxidative stress and unrestrained activation of NLRP3 inflammasomes contribute for development of ALI and progression of Covid-19 severity (18, 19).

Interestingly, fasting blood glucose (FBG) was increased at time of admission due to SARS-CoV-2 induced insulin resistance and transient pancreatic β-cells dysfunction. (20). However, FBG seem to be lower in Covid-19 patient with GS, since high unconjugated bilirubin in GS improves FBG and hyperinsulinemia through activation of peroxisome proliferative activated receptor alpha (PPAR-α) (21).

On the other hand, Santangelo et al. (22) disclosed that endogenous bilirubin has antiviral property against human herpes simplex virus type 1 (HSV-1), hepatitis C virus and enterovirus EV71 via up-regulation of mitogen activated protein kinase (MAPK) and c-Jun N-terminal (JNK). Both of MAPK and JNK are involved in the replication and pathogenesis of SARS-CoV-2 and other coronaviruses (23). Therefore, bilirubin may be the future endogenous agent against SARS-CoV-2. Nonetheless, Liu et al. (24) found that serum bilirubin levels are correlated with Covid-19 induced-liver injury and hemolysis, but the author ignored the antioxidant and anti-inflammatory properties of bilirubin.

The present case-report study had some limitations, including genetic sequence genotype and genetic information of family of patient with GS was not evaluated, relevant past interventions were not recorded, and antioxidant profile was not estimated. Even though this study is regarded as a baseline for future clinical trials and large-scale prospective to confirm the protective effect of unconjugated bilirubin against Covid-19.

CONCLUSION

Taken together, data obtained in this case report study shed light on the new modality for COVID-19 therapy through modulation of bilirubin metabolism. As well, high bilirubin levels in the GS patient with COVID-19 conferred a protective effect against COVID-19-derived cardiometabolic disturbances. In fact, the GS patient revealed higher resistance against COVID-19 associated cardiometabolic disturbances compared to the other COVID-19 patient without GS, directly linked to the antioxidant, anti-inflammatory and antiviral effects of unconjugated bilirubin. However, we cannot sketch any definitive conclusion from our observation; thus prospective, randomized, controlled studies are recommended in this regard.

AUTHOR CONTRIBUTIONS

All authors listed have made a substantial, direct and intellectual contribution to the work, and approved it for publication.

ACKNOWLEDGMENTS

To all members in College of Medicine, Al-Mustansiyria University. NC-M acknowledges the Portuguese Foundation for Science and Technology under the Horizon 2020 Program (PTDC/PSI-GER/28076/2017).

REFERENCES

1. Fretzayas A, Moustaki M, Liapi O, Karpathios T. Gilbert syndrome. *Eur J. Pediatrics*. (2012) 171:11. doi: 10.1007/s00431-011-1641-0

2. Aiso M, Yagi M, Tanaka A, Miura K, Miura R, Arizumi T, et al. Gilbert syndrome with concomitant hereditary spherocytosis presenting with moderate unconjugated hyperbilirubinemia. *Int Med*. (2017) 56:661–4. doi: 10.2169/internalmedicine.56.7362

3. Ha VH, Jupp J, Tsang RY. Oncology drug dosing in gilbert syndrome associated with UGT 1A1: a summary of the literature. *Pharmacotherapy*. (2017) 37:956–72. doi: 10.1002/phar.1946

4. Maruhashi T, Soga J, Fujimura N, Idei N, Mikami S, Iwamoto Y, et al. Hyperbilirubinemia, augmentation of endothelial function, and decrease in oxidative stress in Gilbert syndrome. *Circulation*. (2012) 126:598–603. doi: 10.1161/CIRCULATIONAHA.112.105775

5. Al-Kuraishy HM, Hussien NR, Al-Naimi MS, Al-Buhadily AK, Al-Gareeb AI, Lungnier C. Is ivermectin–azithromycin combination the next step for COVID-19? *Biomed Biotechnol Res J*. (2020) 4:101. doi: 10.4103/bbrj.bbrj_103_20

6. García LF. Immune response, inflammation, and the clinical spectrum of COVID-19. *Front Immunol*. (2020) 11:1441. doi: 10.3389/fimmu.2020.01441

7. Johnson KD, Harris C, Cain JK, Hummer C, Goyal H, Perisetti A. Pulmonary and extra-pulmonary clinical manifestations of COVID-19. *Front Med*. (2020) 7:526. doi: 10.3389/fmed.2020.00526

8. Wasilewski PG, Mruk B, Mazur S, Półtorak-Szymczak G, Sklinda K, Walecki J. COVID-19 severity scoring systems in radiological imaging–a review. *Polish J Radiol*. (2020) 85:e361. doi: 10.5114/pjr.2020.98009

9. Luckring EJ, Parker PD, Hani H, Grace MH, Lila MA, Pierce JG, et al. *In vitro* evaluation of a novel synthetic bilirubin analog as an antioxidant and cytoprotective agent for pancreatic islet transplantation. *Cell Transplant*. (2020) 29:0963689720906417. doi: 10.1177/0963689720906417

10. Bakrania B, Du Toit EF, Ashton KJ, Wagner KH, Headrick JP, Bulmer AC. Chronically elevated bilirubin protects from cardiac reperfusion injury in the male Gunn rat. *Acta Physiol*. (2017) 220:461–70. doi: 10.1111/apha.12858

11. Long B, Brady WJ, Koyfman A, Gottlieb M. Cardiovascular complications in COVID-19. *Am J Emerg Med.?* (2020) 38:1504–7. doi: 10.1016/j.ajem.2020.04.048

12. Liu N, Hong Y, Chen RG, Zhu HM. High rate of increased level of plasma Angiotensin II and its gender difference in COVID-19: an analysis of 55 hospitalized patients with COVID-19 in a single hospital, Wuhan, China. *medRxiv [Preprint]*. (2020) doi: 10.21203/rs.3.rs-51770/v1

13. Novák P, Jackson AO, Zhao GJ, Yin K. Bilirubin in metabolic syndrome and associated inflammatory diseases: new perspectives. *Life Sci*. (2020) 257:118032. doi: 10.1016/j.lfs.2020.118032

14. Leem AY, Kim YS, Lee JH, Kim TH, Kim HY, Oh YM, et al. Serum bilirubin level is associated with exercise capacity and quality of life in chronic obstructive pulmonary disease. *Respir Res*. (2019) 20:279. doi: 10.1186/s12931-019-1241-5

15. Karmouty-Quintana H, Thandavarayan RA, Keller SP, Sahay S, Pandit LM, Akkanti B. Emerging mechanisms of pulmonary vasoconstriction in SARS-CoV-2-induced Acute Respiratory Distress Syndrome (ARDS) and potential therapeutic targets. *Int J Mol Sci*. (2020) 21:8081. doi: 10.3390/ijms21218081

16. Lin Y, Wang S, Yang Z, Gao L, Zhou Z, Yu P, et al. Bilirubin alleviates alum-induced peritonitis through inactivation of NLRP3 inflammasome. *Biomed Pharmacother*. (2019) 116:108973. doi: 10.1016/j.biopha.2019.108973

17. Tran DT, Jeong YY, Kim JM, Bae HB, Son SK, Kwak SH. The anti-inflammatory role of bilirubin on "Two-Hit" sepsis animal model. *Int J Mol Sci*. (2020) 21:8650. doi: 10.3390/ijms21228650

18. Ragab D, Salah Eldin H, Taeimah M, Khattab R, Salem R. The COVID-19 cytokine storm; what we know so far. *Front Immunol*. (2020) 11:1446. doi: 10.3389/fimmu.2020.01446

19. de Rivero Vaccari JC, Dietrich WD, Keane RW, de Rivero Vaccari JP. The inflammasome in times of COVID-19. *Front Immunol*. (2020) 11:2474. doi: 10.3389/fimmu.2020.583373

20. Taneera J, El-Huneidi W, Hamad M, Mohammed AK, Elaraby E, Hachim MY. Expression profile of SARS-CoV-2 host receptors in human pancreatic islets revealed upregulation of ACE2 in diabetic donors. *Biology*. (2020) 9:215. doi: 10.3390/biology9080215

21. Hinds TD Jr, Stec DE. Bilirubin, a cardiometabolic signaling molecule. *Hypertension*. (2018) 72:788–95. doi: 10.1161/HYPERTENSIONAHA.118.11130

22. Santangelo R, Mancuso C, Marchetti S, Di Stasio E, Pani G, Fadda G. Bilirubin: an endogenous molecule with antiviral activity *in vitro*. *Front Pharmacol*. (2012) 3:36. doi: 10.3389/fphar.2012.00036

23. Wehbe Z, Hammoud S, Soudani N, Zaraket H, El-Yazbi A, Eid AH. Molecular insights into SARS COV-2 interaction with cardiovascular disease: role of RAAS and MAPK signaling. *Front Pharmacol*. (2020) 11:836. doi: 10.3389/fphar.2020.00836

24. Liu Z, Li J, Long W, Zeng W, Gao R, Zeng G, et al. Bilirubin levels as potential indicators of disease severity in coronavirus disease patients: a retrospective cohort study. *Front Med*. (2020) 7:598870. doi: 10.3389/fmed.2020.598870

10

Reduction of Cardiac Autonomic Modulation and Increased Sympathetic Activity by Heart Rate Variability in Patients with Long COVID

Karina Carvalho Marques[1], Camilla Costa Silva[1], Steffany da Silva Trindade[2],
Márcio Clementino de Souza Santos[3], Rodrigo Santiago Barbosa Rocha[4],
Pedro Fernando da Costa Vasconcelos[1], Juarez Antônio Simões Quaresma[1†] and
Luiz Fábio Magno Falcão[1*†]

[1] Postgraduate Program in Parasitic Biology in the Amazon, Laboratory of Infectious and Cardiopulmonary Diseases, Long COVID Program, Centre for Biological and Health Sciences, Pará State University, Belém, Brazil, [2] Laboratory of Infectious and Cardiopulmonary Diseases, Long COVID Program, Centre for Biological and Health Sciences, Pará State University, Belém, Brazil, [3] Department of Human Movement Sciences, Centre for Biological and Health Sciences, Pará State University, Belém, Brazil, [4] Centre for Biological and Health Sciences, Pará State University, Belém, Brazil

*Correspondence:
Luiz Fábio Magno Falcão
fabiofalcao@uepa.br

[†] These authors have contributed equally to this work

Although several clinical manifestations of persistent long coronavirus disease (COVID-19) have been documented, their effects on the cardiovascular and autonomic nervous system over the long term remain unclear. Thus, we examined the presence of alterations in cardiac autonomic functioning in individuals with long-term manifestations. The study was conducted from October 2020 to May 2021, and an autonomic assessment was performed to collect heart rate data for the heart rate variability (HRV) analysis. The study participants were divided into the long COVID clinical group, the intragroup, which included patients who were hospitalized, and those who were not hospitalized and were symptomatic for different periods (≤ 3, >3, ≤ 6, and >6 months), with and without dyspnoea. The control group, the intergroup, comprised of COVID-free individuals. Our results demonstrated that the long COVID clinical group showed reduced HRV compared with the COVID-19-uninfected control group. Patients aged 23–59 years developed COVID symptoms within 30 days after infection, whose diagnosis was confirmed by serologic or reverse-transcription polymerase chain reaction (swab) tests, were included in the study. A total of 155 patients with long COVID [95 women (61.29%), mean age 43.88 ± 10.88 years and 60 men (38.71%), mean age 43.93 ± 10.11 years] and 94 controls [61 women (64.89%), mean age 40.83 ± 6.31 and 33 men (35.11%), mean age 40.69 ± 6.35 years] were included. The intragroup and intergroup comparisons revealed a reduction in global HRV, increased sympathetic modulation influence, and a decrease in parasympathetic modulation in long COVID. The intragroup showed normal sympathovagal balance, while the intergroup showed reduced sympathovagal balance. Our findings indicate that long COVID leads to sympathetic excitation influence and parasympathetic reduction. The excitation can increase the heart rate and blood pressure and predispose to cardiovascular complications. Short-term HRV analysis showed good reproducibility to verify the cardiac autonomic involvement.

Keywords: autonomic nervous system, coronavirus infection, long COVID, heart rate, heart rate variability

INTRODUCTION

Coronavirus disease (COVID-19), caused by severe acute respiratory syndrome coronavirus-2 (SARS-CoV-2), manifests numerous clinical symptoms, ranging from mild to severe (1). In Brazil, 21,478,546 confirmed cases, 598,152 accumulated deaths, and 20,462,345 recovered cases were reported as of October 4, 2021. In the state of Pará, 591,872 COVID-19 cases and 16,667 deaths were registered (2).

Some patients who do recover present with symptoms that persist longer than 3–4 weeks. According to Sher (3), this post-COVID condition may be called "post-COVID syndrome," "long COVID," or "post-acute COVID-19." The persistent symptoms of patients with long-term COVID-19 include dyspnoea, fatigue, myalgia, and joint pain (3, 4). The cardiovascular effects of prolonged COVID-19 are still under debate but they may include the lack of clinical symptoms, biomarker (high-sensitivity cardiac troponin I) abnormalities, or an increased risk of myocarditis. Coronavirus infection the potential to affect the cardiovascular system. SARS-CoV-2 is not considered a cardiotropic virus, although the virus causes non-specific cytokine-mediated cardiotoxicity (5, 6). Long COVID is found to be associated with autonomic dysfunction due to neurotropism because the systemic inflammatory state can occur acutely or chronically for up to 1 year (7). Dysautonomia can thus be assessed based on heart rate variability (HRV). A reduction in HRV is a predictor of cerebrovascular and cardiovascular events and an indicator of the risk of death (8). HRV as a non-invasive index of autonomic control may reflect both sympathetic and parasympathetic effects. The HRV indicates the variations in the duration of cardiac cycles and the RR intervals. HRV can be analyzed using linear algorithms for the time and frequency domains and also by non-linear analyses (9, 10).

Changes in cardiac autonomic modulation can occur in patients with COVID-19 and, through HRV, detect autonomic dysregulation. Patients with COVID-19 with low HRV are indicated for intensive care unit admission in the first week after hospitalization, regardless of age and chronic heart disease status (11). In this context, the aim of this study was to investigate the autonomic changes in the heart among patients with long COVID.

METHODS

Study Design and Ethics

This observational, analytical, controlled, quantitative, and descriptive study was approved by the Research Ethics Committee of the Pará State University (approval number 4.252.664). Participants consented to be included in the study by signing an informed consent form; the study was performed following the Strengthening the Reporting of Observational Studies in Epidemiology guidelines for observational studies and in accordance with the principles of the Declaration of Helsinki.

The patients were followed up at the laboratory of infectious and cardiopulmonary diseases at UEPA. The study participants were divided into a long COVID clinical group (intragroup), which comprised both patients who were hospitalized and those who were not hospitalized but were symptomatic for ≤3, >3, ≤6, and >6 months, with and without dyspnoea, as well as a control group (intergroup), which comprised COVID-free individuals. As it was a cardiopulmonary program, patients with dyspnoea and respiratory symptoms such as shortness of breath were required to adhere to the program. The following patients were included in the study: those aged between 23 and 59 years, those who underwent assessment 30 days after diagnostic confirmation and onset of COVID-19 symptoms, and those whose diagnosis was confirmed by reverse-transcriptase polymerase chain reaction (PCR) or serology tests to identify the type of antibodies [immunoglobulin (Ig) M and/or IgG]. Patients who used medication that altered the HRV (such as beta-blockers, beta-mimetics, and theophylline), those who developed chronic obstructive pulmonary disease, those who had persistent lung changes, those who showed persistent desaturation, those with anemia, and those who used pacemakers were excluded. Patients with long COVID underwent regular medical examinations.

From October 2020 to May 2021, 4,100 patients with complaints of long-term symptoms (like fatigue, breathlessness, cough, joint pain, chest pain, muscle aches, and headaches) that could not be attributed to any other cause were enrolled in the clinic's database. However, only 155 patients met the inclusion criteria.

Assessment of HRV

Study participants in both groups were instructed to refrain from consuming caffeine or caffeine derivatives, smoking, and eating heavy meals at least 24 h prior to the test. In preparation for the examination, the volunteers rested for 15 min, while the patients were placed in a supine position for 10 min to measure the heart rate (HR). The patients were instructed to avoid talking or moving to prevent interference during the test. The environment temperature was maintained between 22 and 24°C, while the air humidity was maintained between 40 and 60%. The temperature and relative humidity were measured using a thermo-hygrometer (São Paulo, Brazil).

The Heart Rate (HR) was recorded using a Polar® RS800CX (Kempele, Finland) that captured the R wave on the electrocardiogram with a sampling rate of 500 Hz. The temporal distance between two consecutive peaks of the R wave was considered the iRR (the fluctuations in the intervals between consecutive heartbeats). The data series displayed on the monitor were exported using the Polar Pro Trainer 5 software (Polar Electro Ou, Finland). Subsequently, linear and nonlinear analyses were performed using the Kubios HRV version 3.1 software (Kuopio, Finland). Variability analysis was performed within a short period of time (12) to visually check the distribution of the iRRs for erroneous and absent R waves to determine the stretch with greater stability within 5 min for 256 consecutive beats. Then, the data collected during the first 30 s and final 30 s were discarded (10).

Linear Analysis

In the linear analysis of the HRV in the time domain, the following indices were included: mean iRRs, standard deviation of all normal RR intervals (SDNN), and the square root of the mean square of the differences between adjacent normal iRRs within an interval (RMSSD). SDNN indicates the sympathetic nervous system (SNS) and parasympathetic nervous system (PNS) activities, whereas RMSSD indicates the PNS (13) activity. To obtain the indices in the frequency domain, a fast Fourier transform analysis was performed and showed the components with high frequency (HF = 0.15–0.4 Hz), low frequency (LF = 0.04–0.15 Hz), and very low frequency (VLF = 0.003–0.04 Hz), as indicated in equations 1 and 2 (13, 14).

The three frequency bands (HF, LF, and VLF) were expressed in powers (ms^2) and in normalized units (n.u), which is the relative power of the LF or HF band after subtracting the VLF power from the total power. The LF/HF ratio and LF and HF bands were also obtained (15). LF and HF in normalized units represent the balance between the two autonomic nervous systems. LF demonstrates indirect sympathetic activity, while HF demonstrates the parasympathetic influence. The LF/HF ratio was reported as a marker of sympathovagal balance (10).

$$HF\ (n.u) = 100\ x\ \frac{HF}{(full\ power - VLF)} \qquad (1)$$

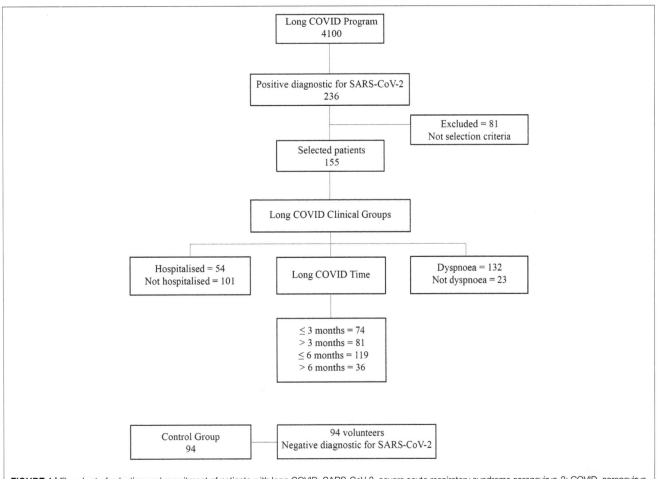

FIGURE 1 | Flowchart of selection and recruitment of patients with long COVID. SARS-CoV-2, severe acute respiratory syndrome coronavirus-2; COVID, coronavirus disease.

$$LF \ (n.u) = 100 \ x \ \frac{LF}{(\text{full power} - \text{VLF})}. \qquad (2)$$

Nonlinear Analysis

For the nonlinear analysis, geometric methods, such as the Lorenz plot or Poincaré plot, were used to obtain the HRV measurements. These were performed by measuring the dispersions of interval RRs which analyse the HRV quantitatively, by calculating the beat-to-beat standard deviation (SD). With this, the short term changes in RRs in the PNS index of the sinoatrial node control (SD1) and the long-term standard deviation of continuous iRRs (SD2), which are influenced by the PNS and SNS were measured, and the relationship between the short- term and the long-term intervals was defined as SD1/SD2 (15, 16).

In addition, other nonlinear methods based on approximate entropy (ApEn) show the degree of irregularity and complexity of the signal as the iRRs and the complexity increase (16, 17). Meanwhile, simple entropy (SampEn) shows the regularity of the selected iRR series; higher values indicate a healthy condition, while lower values indicate heart failure (10, 18).

Statistical Analysis

The information collected was stored in MS Excel 2010™ (Washington, United States) and analyzed using GraphPad Prism version 5.0™ (San Diego, United States). D'Agostino's test was used to assess the normality of the distribution to compare the measured values between the different study groups. The Student's *t*-test was used for variables with a normal distribution, whereas the Mann–Whitney *U* test was used for non-normally distributed variables. For dichotomous or nominal variables, Fisher's exact test was used. A two-tailed *P*-value of <0.05 was considered significant.

RESULTS

General Characteristics of the Study Patients

After screening 236 patients, 155 were included in the study, as shown in **Figure 1**. The demographic characteristics and comorbidities of the 155 patients with long COVID symptoms are listed in **Table 1**. Most participants were women with a mean age of over 40 years; dyspnoea was one of the most prevalent symptoms of long COVID, accounting for more than 30% of hospitalized cases.

Intragroup Comparison

Intragroup comparisons were performed between the long COVID clinical groups. The mean age of the groups was >40 years, with >40% of them admitted to the hospital for 3 months or longer, while 80% experienced dyspnoea. The demographic characteristics, comorbidities, and symptoms of the long COVID groups are shown in **Table 2**.

Regarding the HRV data, patients who experienced symptoms for >3 and >6 months had higher HRV, those who experienced symptoms for ≤3 months had reduced parasympathetic modulation and increased sympathetic modulation influence

TABLE 1 | Demographic characteristics and comorbidities of the study population and symptoms of long COVID.

Variables	Patients (n = 155)	Group control (n = 94)
Female, No (%)	95 (61.29%)	61 (64.89%)
Male, No (%)	60 (38.71%)	33 (35.11%)
Age (years), mean ± SD	43.88 ± 10.03	40.69 ± 6.35
Height (cm), mean ± SD	1.63 ± 0.08	1.64 ± 0.08
Weight (kg), mean ± SD	79.95 ± 17.84	73.73 ± 15.43
BMI, mean ± SD	30.06 ± 7.31	27.04 ± 4.30
Smoker (No, %)	3 (1.93%)	N/A
Former smoker (No, %)	28 (18.06%)	94 (100%)
Long COVID symptoms (No, %)		
Dyspnoea, No (%)	132 (85.16%)	N/A
Chest pain, No (%)	93 (60%)	N/A
Muscle weakness, No (%)	112 (72.25%)	N/A
Fatigue, No (%)	118 (76.12%)	N/A
Myalgia, No (%)	103 (66.45%)	N/A
Insomnia, No (%)	87 (56.12%)	N/A
Lower members Oedema, No (%)	58 (37.41%)	N/A
Comorbidities (No, %)		N/A
Asthma (No, %)	24 (15.48%)	N/A
DM (No, %)	13 (8.38%)	N/A
SAH (No, %)	34 (21.93%)	N/A
Obesity (No, %)	72 (46.45%)	28 (29.78%)
Hospital admission (n, %)	54 (34.83%)	
Length of hospital stay, mean ± SD	17.25 ± 15.96	N/A
≤10 days, (n, %)	19 (35.18%)	N/A
>10 days, (n, %)	35 (64.82%)	N/A
Long COVID period, mean ± SD		N/A
≤3 months, (n, %)	74 (47.74%)	N/A
>3 months, (n, %)	81 (52.26%)	N/A
≤6 months, (n, %)	119 (76.77%)	N/A
>6 months, (n, %)	36 (23.23%)	N/A
Dyspnoea	132 (85.16%)	N/A
Not dyspnoea	23 (14.84%)	N/A

BMI, body mass index; DM, diabetes mellitus; SAH, systemic arterial hypertension; SD, standard deviation.

of, and those who were hospitalized had a reduction in the sympathovagal balance (**Table 3**).

Intergroup Comparison

Major changes were observed in the intergroup comparison between the long COVID clinical groups and the control group. The clinical groups showed a reduction in global HRV (RR, SDNN, SD2, and SD1/SD2), increased the influence of sympathetic modulation (LF, LF/HF), decreased parasympathetic modulation (RMSSD, SD1, and HF), and decreased sympathovagal balance of the heart (LF/HF) in

TABLE 2 | Demographic characteristics, comorbidities, and symptoms of the study population considering the long COVID clinical group.

Variables	Hospitalised (n = 54) No, (%)	Not hospitalised (n = 101) No, (%)	P-Value	≤3 months (n = 74) No, (%)	>3 months (n = 81) No, (%)	P-Value	≤6 months (n = 119) No, (%)	>6 months (n = 36) No, (%)	P-Value	Dyspnoea (n = 132) No, (%)	Not dyspnoea (n = 23) No, (%)	P-Value
Sex												
Female	24 (44.44%)	71 (70.29%)	*0.002	38 (51.35%)	57 (70.37%)	*0.020	67 (56.30%)	28 (77.77%)	*0.020	83 (62.87%)	12 (52.17%)	0.359
Male	30 (55.56%)	30 (29.71%)		36 (48.65%)	24 (29.63%)		52 (43.70%)	8 (22.23%)		49 (37.13%)	11 (47.83%)	
Mean age (years)	44.27 ± 9.22	43.67 ± 10.47	0.837	42.17 ± 10.77	45.44 ± 9.09	0.074	43.78 ± 10.61	44.19 ± 7.90	0.940	43.43 ± 9.56	46.47 ± 12.30	0.180
Stature	1.64 ± 0.09	1.63 ± 0.08	0.441	1.64 ± 0.09	1.62 ± 0.08	0.221	1.63 ± 0.09	1.63 ± 0.08	0.739	1.63 ± 0.08	1.63 ± 0.09	0.938
Weight	86.80 ± 18.41	76.29 ± 16.49	*0.000	82.52 ± 19.21	77.60 ± 16.26	0.118	79.79 ± 17.80	80.49 ± 18.24	0.581	79.53 ± 17.78	82.35 ± 18.42	0.396
BMI	32.23 ± 7.11	28.90 ± 7.18	*0.005	30.70 ± 7.81	29.48 ± 6.82	0.361	29.94 ± 7.19	30.48 ± 7.80	0.684	29.89 ± 7.22	31.07 ± 7.88	0.422
Smoker												
Yes	0	3 (2.97%)	0.314	1 (1.35%)	2 (2.46%)	1.00	3 (2.52%)	3 (8.33%)	0.138	2 (1.51%)	1 (4.34%)	0.381
Not	54 (100%)	98 (97.03%)		73 (98.65)	79 (97.54%)		116 (97.48%)	33 (91.67%)		130 (98.49%)	22 (95.66%)	
Ex-smoker												
Yes	12 (22.22%)	6 (5.94%)	*0.006	5 (6.75%)	12 (14.81%)	0.128	10 (8.40%)	7 (19.44%)	0.123	17 (12.87%)	3 (13.04%)	0.986
Not	42 (77.78%)	95 (94.06%)		69 (93.25%)	69 (85.19%)		109 (91.6%)	29 (80.56%)		115 (87.13%)	20 (86.96%)	
Long COVID symptoms (n, %)												
Dyspnoea	47 (87.03%)	85 (84.15%)	0.813	60 (81.08%)	72 (88.88%)	0.183	97 (81.51%)	35 (97.22%)	*0.016	132 (100%)	0	0
Chest pain	31 (57.40%)	62 (61.38%)	0.731	43 (58.10%)	50 (61.72%)	*0.041	68 (57.14%)	25 (69.44%)	*0.021	78 (59.09%)	15 (65.21%)	0.649
Fatigue	40 (74.07%)	78 (77.22%)	0.695	52 (70.27%)	66 (81.48%)	0.131	86 (72.26%)	32 (88.88%)	*0.045	103 (78.03%)	15 (65.21%)	0.192
Muscle weakness	46 (85.18%)	66 (65.34%)	*0.008	55 (74.32%)	57 (70.37%)	0.595	81 (68.06%)	31 (86.11%)	*0.035	96 (72.72%)	16 (69.56%)	0.802
Myalgia	40 (74.07%)	63 (62.37%)	0.157	52 (70.27%)	51 (62.96%)	0.395	78 (65.54%)	25 (69.44%)	0.130	86 (65.15%)	17 (73.91%)	0.480
Insomnia	36 (66.66%)	51 (50.49%)	0.062	42 (56.75%)	45 (55.55%)	1.00	67 (56.30%)	20 (55.55%)	1.00	75 (56.81%)	12 (52.17%)	0.820
Lower members Oedema	28 (51.85%)	30 (29.70%)	*0.008	26 (35.13%)	32 (39.50%)	0.620	40 (33.61%)	18 (50%)	0.641	48 (36.36%)	10 (43.47%)	0.641
Comorbidities												
Asthma	3 (5.55%)	21 (20.79%)	*0.011	8 (10.81%)	16 (19.75%)	0.181	20 (16.80%)	4 (11.11%)	0.450	20 (15.15%)	4 (17.39%)	0.756
DM	7 (12.96%)	6 (5.94%)	0.221	6 (8.10%)	7 (8.64%)	1.00	11 (9.24%)	2 (5.55%)	0.733	12 (9.09%)	1 (4.34%)	0.693
SAH	11 (20.37%)	23 (22.77%)	0.839	18 (24.32%)	16 (19.75%)	0.561	28 (23.52%)	6 (16.66%)	0.492	28 (21.21%)	6 (26.08%)	0.591
Obesity	33 (61.11%)	39 (38.61%)	*0.010	37 (50%)	35 (43.20%)	0.423	53 (44.53%)	19 (52.77%)	0.447	61 (46.21%)	11 (47.82%)	1.00
Hospital admission (n, %)												
Yes	54 (100%)	0	0	32 (43.24%)	22 (27.16%)	*0.043	40 (33.61%)	14 (38.88%)	0.690	47 (35.60%)	7 (30.43%)	0.081
Not	0	101 (100%)		42 (56.76%)	59 (72.83%)		79 (66.69%)	22 (61.12%)		85 (64.40%)	16 (69.57%)	
Mean length of stay (days)												
≤10 days (n, %)	19 (35.18%)	0	0	11 (34.37%)	8 (9.87%)	1.00	15 (12.60%)	4 (28.57%)	0.747	16 (34.04%)	3 (42.85%)	0.686
>10 days (n, %)	35 (63.22%)	0		21 (65.63%)	14 (90.13%)		25 (87.4%)	10 (71.43%)		31 (65.96%)	4 (57.15%)	

BMI, body mass index; MMII, lower member; DM, diabetes mellitus; SAH, systemic arterial hypertension; SD, standard deviation.
*P significant value.

TABLE 3 | Analysis of HRV considering the long COVID clinical group.

Variables	Hospitalised (n = 54) Mean ± SD	Not hospitalised (n = 101) Mean ± SD	P-Value	≤3 months (n = 74) Mean ± SD	>3 months (n = 81) Mean ± SD	P-Value	≤6 months (n = 109) Mean ± SD	>6 months (n = 28) Mean ± SD	P-Value	Dyspnoea (n = 132) Mean ± SD	Not dyspnoea (n = 23) Mean ± SD	P-Value
RR (Ms)	794.16 ± 132.22	822.28 ± 126.72	0.228	806.93 ± 129.25	847.24 ± 138.30	*0.002	806.93 ± 129.25	830.86 ± 127.96	*0.002	812.97 ± 131.03	809.69 ± 118.88	0.925
SDNN (Ms)	28.47 ± 28.46	42.58 ± 119.92	0.171	39.84 ± 111.68	46.83 ± 133.77	0.122	39.84 ± 111.68	30.46 ± 19.96	0.571	39.81 ± 106.10	25.35 ± 20.63	0.208
RMSSD (Ms)	31.48 ± 37.22	35.05 ± 30.59	0.132	33.61 ± 34.34	38.25 ± 35.68	*0.043	33.61 ± 34.34	34.45 ± 28.44	0.529	34.57 ± 33.17	29.42 ± 32.35	0.438
SD1 (Ms)	22.29 ± 26.36	24.82 ± 21.66	0.133	23.80 ± 24.32	27.09 ± 25.27	*0.042	23.80 ± 24.32	24.40 ± 20.14	0.523	24.48 ± 23.48	20.82 ± 22.83	0.432
SD2 (Ms)	32.88 ± 31.12	35.27 ± 21.96	0.175	34.27 ± 26.80	35.93 ± 23.32	0.210	34.27 ± 26.80	35.00 ± 20.69	0.435	35.47 ± 26.30	28.52 ± 19.25	0.157
SD1/SD2	0.61 ± 0.25	0.66 ± 0.22	0.193	0.65 ± 0.24	0.69 ± 0.24	*0.011	0.65 ± 0.24	0.64 ± 0.20	0.876	0.64 ± 0.23	0.67 ± 0.23	0.604
ApEn	1.12 ± 0.15	1.14 ± 0.12	0.613	1.14 ± 0.13	1.12 ± 0.13	*0.007	1.14 ± 0.13	1.11 ± 0.15	0.176	1.14 ± 0.13	1.09 ± 0.16	0.079
SampEn	1.58 ± 0.37	1.63 ± 0.32	0.560	1.62 ± 0.34	1.59 ± 0.32	0.150	1.62 ± 0.34	1.59 ± 0.34	0.659	1.62 ± 0.33	1.55 ± 0.39	0.569
LF (n.u)	54.39 ± 21.54	48.83 ± 16.71	0.073	51.18 ± 19.26	47.29 ± 18.33	*0.014	51.18 ± 19.26	49.39 ± 16.66	0.533	50.39 ± 19.02	52.94 ± 16.60	0.572
HF (n.u)	45.54 ± 21.52	51.04 ± 16.84	0.079	48.69 ± 19.23	52.60 ± 18.33	*0.014	48.69 ± 19.23	50.56 ± 16.65	0.519	49.50 ± 18.99	46.97 ± 16.58	0.586
LF/HF	6.33 ± 30.60	1.26 ± 1.15	*0.032	1.73 ± 1.59	4.22 ± 25.06	*0.024	1.56 ± 1.56	7.90 ± 37.51	0.887	3.30 ± 19.64	1.46 ± 1.12	0.657

SD, standard deviation; RR, average of RR intervals; N.u, normalized units; SDNN, standard deviation of all normal RR intervals; SD1, rapid changes in RR intervals in parasympathetic nervous system index; SD2, long-term changes; SD1/SD2, short term ratio for long-term range variation; ApEn, approximate entropy, complexity, regularity of the RR interval series and signal complexity; SampEn, simple entropy, regularity of the RR interval series; LF, low-frequency components, ranging from 0.004 to 0.15 hertz; HF, high-frequency components, ranging from 0.15 to 0.004 hertz; LF/HF, low/high frequency components (normal range 1.5 to 2.0).
*P significant value.

relation to the control group that did not manifest COVID-19. Data are shown in **Tables 4**, **5**.

DISCUSSION

In this study, patients with long COVID had persistent symptoms of dyspnoea, fatigue, muscle weakness, and chest pain and were mostly women. Long COVID clinical groups with increased sympathetic activity influence of, less parasympathetic activity, and reduced sympathovagal balance were compared. When the participants in the clinical groups with long COVID were compared with the COVID-19-uninfected control group, they demonstrated a decreased sympathovagal balance in the heart. When linear and nonlinear analyses were performed, this population showed changes in HRV, thus suggesting changes in the autonomic control of cardiac function.

The HRV changes observed in the long-term COVID population suggest the need for non-invasive assessments and the early detection of possible changes. The study by Mol et al. (11) demonstrated that higher HRV might predict greater chances of survival in older patients with COVID-19, independent of prognostic factors. Moreover, low HRV predicted ICU admission in the first week after hospitalization. Therefore, HRV measurements may be useful not only for monitoring patients with COVID-19 but also in the early identification of patients with long COVID at risk of clinical deterioration.

The majority of the people infected with SARS-CoV-2 (mild, moderate, or severe) demonstrated chronic signs and symptoms for weeks or months after the infection, lasting 12 weeks or more (19, 20). These signs of potential chronicity were observed in our study of patients who had chronic symptoms for 12 weeks or more.

Carfi et al. (20) reported the occurrence of persistent symptoms (37%) in 179 patients (53 women) for an average of 60 days after the onset of symptoms. Fatigue (53.1%) and dyspnoea (43.4%) persistently occurred in 87.54% of patients with COVID-19. The proportion of females and the prevalence of symptoms were similar to those in our study.

The prevalence of fatigue amongst women in the present study was also confirmed in a study by Kamal et al. (21), which analyzed 287 patients (64.1% women) and reported several persistent manifestations of long COVID and a higher prevalence of fatigue in women (72.8%).

In the present study, those with persistent symptoms were closer to the beginning of COVID-19 recovery, that is, ≤3–6 months of recovery. Al-Aly et al. (22) studied patients with COVID-19, who recovered at least 30 days after their diagnosis for 6 months. This is because the first 30 days or more of the illness after the diagnosis is associated with an increased risk of death; this results from the occurrence of several respiratory, neurological, and cardiovascular disorders, as well as malaise; fatigue; and musculoskeletal pain.

Persistent post-COVID-19 symptoms within 3–6 months after "recovery" from COVID-19 were also described by González-Hermosillo et al. (23), who analyzed 130 patients. Of these, 91.5% reported at least one symptom prior to the onset of infection. The

TABLE 4 | Analysis of HRV duration of long COVID and dyspnoea in the hospitalization groups based on the control group.

Variable	Hospitalised (n=54) Mean ± DP	Control group (n=94) Mean ± DP	P-Value	Not hospitalised (n=101) Mean ± SD	Control group (n=94) Mean ± SD	P-Value	≤3 months (n=74) Mean ± SD	Control group (n=94) Mean ± SD	P-Value	>3 months (n=81) Mean ± SD	Control group (n=94) Mean ± SD	P-Value
RR (Ms)	794.16 ± 132.22	865 ± 121	*0.001	822.28 ± 126.72	865 ± 121	*0.010	806.93 ± 129.25	865 ± 121	*<0.0001	847.24 ± 138.30	865 ± 121	0.366
SDNN (Ms)	28.47 ± 28.46	46.50 ± 29.20	*<0.0001	42.58 ± 119.92	46.50 ± 29.20	*<0.0001	39.84 ± 111.68	46.50 ± 29.20	*<0.0001	46.83 ± 133.77	46.50 ± 29.20	*<0.0001
RMSSD (Ms)	31.48 ± 37.22	54.90 ± 40.64	*<0.0001	35.05 ± 30.59	54.90 ± 40.64	*<0.0001	33.61 ± 34.34	54.90 ± 40.64	*<0.0001	38.25 ± 35.68	54.90 ± 40.64	*0.000
SD1 (Ms)	22.29 ± 26.36	39.89 ± 28.39	*<0.0001	24.82 ± 21.66	39.89 ± 28.39	*<0.0001	23.80 ± 24.32	39.89 ± 28.39	*<0.0001	27.09 ± 25.27	39.89 ± 28.39	*0.000
SD2 (Ms)	32.88 ± 31.12	51.52 ± 31.79	*<0.0001	35.27 ± 21.96	51.52 ± 31.79	*<0.0001	34.27 ± 26.80	51.52 ± 31.79	*<0.0001	35.93 ± 23.32	51.52 ± 31.79	*<0.0001
SD1/SD2	0.61 ± 0.25	0.76 ± 0.324	*0.002	0.66 ± 0.22	0.76 ± 0.324	*0.028	0.65 ± 0.24	0.76 ± 0.324	*0.000	0.69 ± 0.24	0.76 ± 0.324	0.160
ApEn	1.12 ± 0.15	1.07 ± 0.130	*0.023	1.14 ± 0.12	1.07 ± 0.130	*0.000	1.14 ± 0.13	1.07 ± 0.130	*<0.0001	1.12 ± 0.13	1.07 ± 0.130	*0.046
SampEn	1.58 ± 0.37	1.47 ± 0.383	0.066	1.63 ± 0.32	1.47 ± 0.383	*0.003	1.62 ± 0.34	1.47 ± 0.383	*0.002	1.59 ± 0.32	1.47 ± 0.383	0.059
LF (n.u)	54.39 ± 21.54	44.65 ± 20.71	*0.007	48.83 ± 16.71	44.65 ± 20.71	*0.006	51.18 ± 19.26	44.65 ± 20.71	*0.001	47.29 ± 18.33	44.65 ± 20.71	0.377
HF (n.u)	45.54 ± 21.52	55.28 ± 20.69	*0.007	51.04 ± 16.84	55.28 ± 20.69	*0.006	48.69 ± 19.23	55.28 ± 20.69	*0.001	52.60 ± 18.33	55.28 ± 20.69	0.370
LF/HF	6.33 ± 30.60	1.26 ± 1.42	*0.002	1.26 ± 1.15	1.26 ± 1.42	0.099	1.56 ± 1.56	1.26 ± 1.42	*0.001	4.22 ± 25.06	1.26 ± 1.42	0.235

SD, standard deviation; RR, average of RR intervals; N.u, normalized units; SDNN, standard deviation of all normal RR intervals in a time interval; SD1, rapid changes in RR intervals is an SNP index; SD2, long-term changes; SD1/SD2, short-term ratio for long-term range variation; ApEn complexity, approximate entropy, regularity of the RR interval series and signal complexity; SampEn, simple entropy, regularity of the RR interval series; LF, low-frequency components, ranging from 0.04 to 0.15Hz; HF, high-frequency components, ranging from 0.15 to 0.4Hz; LF/HF, low/high frequency components (normal range 1.5 to 2.0).
*P significant value.

TABLE 5 | Analysis of HRV considering the duration of long COVID-19 and dyspnoea in the control group.

Variables	≤6 months (n=119) Mean ± DP	Control group (n=94) Mean ± DP	P-Value	>6 months (n=36) Mean ± DP	Control group (n=94) Mean ± DP	P-Value	Dyspnoea (n=132) Mean ± DP	Control group (n=94) Mean ± DP	P-Value	Not dyspnoea (n=23) Mean ± DP	Control group (n=94) Mean ± DP	P-Value
RR (Ms)	806.93 ± 129.25	865 ± 121	*0.001	830.86 ± 127.96	865 ± 121	0.159	812.97 ± 131.03	865 ± 121	*0.002	809.69 ± 118.88	865 ± 121	0.051
SDNN (Ms)	39.84 ± 111.68	46.50 ± 29.20	*<0.0001	30.46 ± 19.96	46.50 ± 29.20	*0.000	39.81 ± 106.10	46.50 ± 29.20	*<0.0001	25.35 ± 20.63	46.50 ± 29.20	*<0.0001
RMSSD (Ms)	33.61 ± 34.34	54.90 ± 40.64	*<0.0001	34.45 ± 28.44	54.90 ± 40.64	*0.002	34.57 ± 33.17	54.90 ± 40.64	*<0.0001	29.42 ± 32.35	54.90 ± 40.64	*0.000
SD1 (Ms)	23.80 ± 24.32	39.89 ± 28.39	*<0.0001	24.40 ± 20.14	39.89 ± 28.39	*0.001	24.48 ± 23.48	39.89 ± 28.39	*<0.0001	20.82 ± 22.83	39.89 ± 28.39	*<0.0001
SD2 (Ms)	34.27 ± 26.80	51.52 ± 31.79	*<0.0001	35.00 ± 20.69	51.52 ± 31.79	*0.001	35.47 ± 26.30	51.52 ± 31.79	*<0.0001	28.52 ± 19.25	51.52 ± 31.79	*<0.0001
SD1/SD2	0.65 ± 0.24	0.76 ± 0.324	*0.004	0.64 ± 0.20	0.76 ± 0.324	*0.050	0.64 ± 0.23	0.76 ± 0.324	*0.002	0.67 ± 0.23	0.76 ± 0.324	0.211
ApEn	1.14 ± 0.13	1.07 ± 0.130	*<0.0001	1.11 ± 0.15	1.07 ± 0.130	0.213	1.14 ± 0.13	1.07 ± 0.130	*<0.0001	1.09 ± 0.16	1.07 ± 0.130	0.501
SampEn	1.62 ± 0.34	1.47 ± 0.383	*0.003	1.59 ± 0.34	1.47 ± 0.383	0.111	1.62 ± 0.33	1.47 ± 0.383	*0.002	1.55 ± 0.39	1.47 ± 0.383	0.294
LF (n.u)	51.18 ± 19.26	44.65 ± 20.71	*0.016	49.39 ± 16.66	44.65 ± 20.71	0.221	50.39 ± 19.02	44.65 ± 20.71	*0.031	52.94 ± 16.60	44.65 ± 20.71	0.077
HF (n.u)	48.69 ± 19.23	55.28 ± 20.69	*0.015	50.56 ± 16.65	55.28 ± 20.69	0.222	49.50 ± 18.99	55.28 ± 20.69	*0.029	46.97 ± 16.58	55.28 ± 20.69	0.076
LF/HF	1.56 ± 1.56	1.26 ± 1.42	*0.017	7.90 ± 37.51	1.26 ± 1.42	0.063	3.30 ± 19.64	1.26 ± 1.42	*0.022	1.46 ± 1.12	1.26 ± 1.42	*0.033

SD, standard deviation; RR, average of RR intervals; N.u, normalized units; SDNN, standard deviation of all normal RR intervals in a time interval; SD1, rapid changes in RR intervals is an SNP index; SD2, long-term changes; SD1/SD2, short-term ratio for long-term range variation; ApEn, Approximate entropy, regularity of the RR interval series and signal complexity; SampEn, simple entropy, regularity of the RR interval series; LF, low-frequency components, ranging from 0.04 to 0.15Hz; HF, high-frequency components, ranging from 0.15 to 0.4Hz; LF/HF, low/high frequency components (normal range 1.5 to 2.0).
*P significant value.

symptom of fatigue persisted among those aged between 40 and 50 years who had long COVID for 3–6 months. As in our study, in the same age group, women were more likely to experience long-term symptoms.

The mechanism of COVID-19 development, immune system response, and Autonomic Nervous System (ANS) are complex subjects. SARS-CoV-2 can activate the innate and adaptive immune responses, generating inflammatory responses that can lead to local and systemic damage (24). Autonomic dysfunction may be mediated by the virus itself. However, during the cytokine storm, vagal stimulation induces an anti-inflammatory response, while sympathetic activation induces the release of pro-inflammatory cytokines. Some studies reported the association between autonomic dysfunction and the short and long-term neurotropism of SARS-CoV-2 (25, 26).

Increase in the influence of sympathetic activity at rest, which can generate an increase in premature deaths, remains of great concern (27). This alteration may increase the HR, while the emergence of cardiovascular diseases predisposes the patient to systemic arterial hypertension and incorrect adaptations of the ANS in response to this (28), thus impairing cardiac regulation.

Heart rate variability has been used to diagnose autonomic regulation, and sympathetic and parasympathetic imbalance occurs in dysautonomia. It is unclear, how dysautonomia with HRV dysregulation occurs in patients with COVID-19 and long COVID. This could be due to neurotropism, hypoxia, and inflammation caused by the autonomic-virus pathway or immune-mediated processes after viral exposure (29). Cardiovascular dysautonomia frequently occurs in patients who recover from COVID-19. There is a reduction in the HRV components (rMSSD and SDNN) when compared with that in uninfected individuals. Despite the scarcity of HRV data, some researchers have been investigating autonomic dysfunction in patients with long COVID to improve disease management and prognosis and limit the progression of the disease (30). Further, the adverse effects of viral infection can generate an increase the sympathetic tone influence, thus preventing the balance in parasympathetic modulation in patients with long COVID.

We reported an increase influence of in the resting sympathetic tone, a decrease in parasympathetic tone, and significant changes in RMSSD and SDNN in long COVID clinical groups compared with those in long-term COVID groups and reduced LF/HF compared with that in the COVID-19-uninfected control group. A previous cross-sectional study conducted by Kaliyaperumal et al. (31) analyzed 106 patients treated for COVID-19 (asymptomatic or mildly to moderately symptomatic). Of these, 63 (59.4%) had COVID-19, while 43 (40.6%) were healthy. The authors demonstrated high rates of autonomic imbalance in patients with COVID-19. Parasympathetic modulation (rMSSD and SDNN) increased in the patients with COVID-19 independent of age, sex, and comorbidities, while the HRV components in LF and HF potencies decreased in COVID-19 patients, when compared with the healthy uninfected individuals.

The parasympathetic activity (RMSSD, SD1, and HF) decreased in long COVID clinical groups; this finding suggests that parasympathetic changes may be associated with mediation of the inflammatory process. However, in a meta-analysis of 159 studies by Williams et al. (32), a negative association was found between HRV and vagal indices (e.g. HF), SDNN, and inflammation markers. SDNN was strongly associated with inflammatory markers and had greater effects in women than in men.

Other decreases in parasympathetic modulation were reported by Gifford et al. (33), who examined the autonomic function and HRV after extreme resistance exercise. They reported that healthy women have a lower sympathetic profile; an increase in HRV within 15 days after performing exercise showed better parasympathetic activity (RMSSD, SD1, and HF), increased global HRV (SD1/SD2), and increased SampEn.

In the present study, changes in ApEn and SampEn entropies were not observed in the long COVID clinical groups compared with that in the COVID-19-free control group. However, Bajic, Đajić, and Milovanović (34), when analyzing the different entropies (Apen, SampEn, binary, sample, and multiscale) of 116 patients with COVID-19 (mild to severe) and 77 healthy controls, only found significant cross-entropies in heart rate signals and systolic pressure. Most of the patients with COVID-19 had lower SampEn values compared with those in the control group. Considering that ANS dysfunctions are associated with COVID-19 severity, we believe that signal acquisition is complex; moreover, no difference was found in the entropies between patients with COVID-19 and controls.

Heart rate variability has been assessed in other studies to determine autonomic functions (35). Linear and nonlinear methods were used to analyse HRV to assess cardiac modulation (36). Our study demonstrated HRV alterations in the long COVID population with cardiac autonomic dysfunction; increased influence of sympathetic activity at rest was associated with increased HR and blood pressure levels, cardiovascular problems, poorer prognosis, and sudden death. However, this finding still needs to be extensively explored to understand the mechanisms leading to these alterations. In addition, the usefulness of this tool in clinical practice should be evaluated.

Strengths and Limitations

Heart rate variability analysis was performed using a cardiofrequency meter, which is influenced by individual and behavioral factors. The study was performed at a single center and had a small sample size. The sample was representative of the population studied; few studies described in the scientific literature used HRV analysis for assessing cardiac modulation in the long COVID population. However, further studies need to be conducted to understand the repercussions of long COVID in different body organs and on breathing controls to understand whether long COVID impacts cardiac autonomic modulation. The results collected in this study will be fundamental for the initial understanding of cardiac autonomic alterations in patients with long COVID.

CONCLUSIONS

Our results demonstrated that the long COVID clinical groups showed reduced HRV compared with the COVID-19-uninfected control group. Short-term linear and nonlinear methods demonstrated good precision in this population. Therefore, changes in long COVID should be monitored to understand its involvement in cardiac autonomic modulation and detect possible cardiovascular changes for short- or long-term prevention. In particular, increased influence of sympathetic activity may be linked with cardiovascular imbalances, chronic disease, and sudden death. Hence, further tests and clinical trials should be conducted to understand the after-effects of long COVID on cardiac autonomous modulation. Although changes in the ANS were observed, it is unclear, whether the changes were caused directly or indirectly by infection or systemic inflammatory state in patients who recovered from COVID-19.

AUTHOR CONTRIBUTIONS

JQ and LF: project administration, support, supervision, review, and scientific collaboration. MS and RR: support, review, and edition. CS and ST: investigation, data collection, and written. KM: investigation, data collection, written, and edition and review. All authors read and approved the final manuscript.

REFERENCES

1. Hamid S, Mir MY, Rohela GK. Novel coronavirus disease (COVID-19): a pandemic (epidemiology, pathogenesis and potential therapeutics). *New Microbes New.* (2020) 35:100679. doi: 10.1016/j.nmni.2020.100679

2. Ministry of Health (BR). *Special Epidemiological Bulletin. Coronavirus Panel-Covid-19.* (2021). https://covid.saude.gov.br/. Accessed October 4, 2021.

3. Sher L. Post-COVID syndrome and suicide risk. *QJM.* (2021) 114:95–8. doi: 10.1093/qjmed/hcab007

4. Kingstone T, Taylor AK, O'donnel CA, Atherton H, Blane DN, Chew-Graham CA. Finding the 'right' GP: a qualitative study of the experiences of people with long-COVID. *BJGP Open.* (2020) 4:1–12. doi: 10.3399/bjgpopen20X101143

5. Mascia G, Pescetelli F, Baldari A, Gatto P, Seitun S, Sartori P et al. Interpretation of elevated high-sensitivity cardiac troponin I in elite soccer players previously infected by severe acute respiratory syndrome coronavirus 2. *Int J Cardiol.* (2021) 326:248–51. doi: 10.1016/j.ijcard.2020.11.039

6. Li DL, Davogustto G, Soslow JH, Wassenaar JW, Parikh AP, Chew JD et al. Characteristics of COVID-19 myocarditis with and without multisystem inflammatory syndrome. *Am J Cardiol.* (2022) 168:135–41. doi: 10.1016/j.amjcard.2021.12.031

7. Becker RC. Autonomic dysfunction in SARS-COV-2 infection acute and long-term implications COVID-19 editor's page series. *J Thromb Thombolysis.* (2021) 17:1–16. doi: 10.1007/s11239-021-02549-6

8. Berger M, Raffin J, Pichot V, Hupin D, Garet M, Labeix P et al. Effect of exercise training on heart rate variability in patients with obstructive sleep apnea: a randomized controlled trial. *Scand J Med Sci Sports.* (2019) 29:1254–62. doi: 10.1111/sms.13447

9. Francesco B, Grazia BM, Emanuele G, Valentina F, Sara C, Chiara F et al. Linear and nonlinear heart rate variability indexes in clinical practice. *Comput Math Methods Med.* (2012) 2012:1–5. doi: 10.1155/2012/219080

10. Task Force of the European Society of Cardiology and the North American Society of Pacing and Electrophysiology. *Eur Heart J.* (1996) 17: 354–381.

11. Mol MBA, Strouss MTA, Osch FHMV, Vogelaar FJ, Barten DG, Farchi M, et al. Heart-rate-variability (HRV), predicts outcomes in COVID-19. *PLoS ONE.* (2021) 16:e0258841. doi: 10.1371/journal.pone.0258841

12. Arêas GPT, Caruso FCR, Simões RP, Simões VC, Jaenisch RB, Sato TO, et al. Ultra-short-term heart rate variability during resistance exercise in the elderly. *Braz J Med Biol Res.* (2018) 51:e6962. doi: 10.1590/1414-431x20186962

13. Burr RL. Interpretation of normalized spectral heart rate variability indices in sleep research: a critical review. *Sleep-New York Then Westchester.* (2007) 30:913–9. doi: 10.1093/sleep/30.7.913

14. Vanderlei LC, Pastre CM, Hoshi RA, Carvalho TD, Godoy MF. Noções Básicas de variabilidade da frequência cardíaca e sua aplicabilidade clínica. *Rev Bras Cir Cardiovasc.* (2009) 24:205–17. doi: 10.1590/S0102-76382009000200018

15. Martin J, Schneider F, Kowalewskij A, Jordan D, Hapfelmeier A, Kochs EF, et al. Linear and non-linear heart rate metrics for the assessment of anaesthetists workload during general anaesthesia. *Br J Anaesth.* (2016) 117:767–74. doi: 10.1093/bja/aew342

16. Hoshi RA, Pastre CM, Vanderlei LC, Godoy MF. Poincaré plot indexes of heart rate variability: Relationships with other nonlinear variables. *Auton Neurosc.* (2013) 177:271–4. doi: 10.1016/j.autneu.2013.05.004

17. Pincus S. Approximate entropy (ApEn) as a complexity measure. *Chaos.* (1995) 5:110–7. doi: 10.1063/1.166092

18. Thu TNP, Hérnandez AL, Costet N, Patural H, Pichot V, Carrault G et al. Improving methodology in hearth rate variability analysis for the premature infants: impact of the time length. *PLoS ONE.* (2019) 14:1–14. doi: 10.1371/journal.pone.0220692

19. Carod-Artal FJ. [Post-COVID-19 syndrome: epidemiology, diagnostic criteria and pathogenic mechanisms involved]. *Rev Neurol.* (2021) 72:384–96. doi: 10.33588/rn.7211.2021230

20. Carfi A, Bernabei R, Landi F. Persistent symptoms in patients after acute COVID-19. *JAMA.* (2020) 324:603–5. doi: 10.1001/jama.2020.12603

21. Kamal M, Omirah MA, Hussein A, Saeed H. Assessment and characterization of Post-COVID-19 manifestations. *Int J Clin Pract.* (2021) 75:e13746. doi: 10.1111/ijcp.13746

22. Al-Aly Z, Xie Y, Bowe B. High-dimensional characterization of post-acute sequelae of COVID-19. *Nature.* (2021) 594:259–64. doi: 10.1038/s41586-021-03553-9

23. González-Hermosillo JA, Martínez-López JP, Carrillo-Lampón SA, Ruiz-Ojeda D, Herrera-Ramírez S, Amezcua-Guerra LM, et al. Post-acute COVID-19 symptoms, a potential link with myalgic encephalomyelitis/chronic fatigue syndrome: a 6-month survey in a Mexican cohort. *Brain Sci.* (2021) 11:1–13. doi: 10.3390/brainsci11060760

24. Anka AU, Tahir MI, Abubakar SD, Alsabbagh M, Zian Z, Hamedifar H, et al. Coronavirus disease 2019 (COVID-19): an overview of the immunopathology, serological diagnosis and management. *Scand J Immunol.* (2020) 93:e12998. doi: 10.1111/sji.12998

25. Dani M, Dirksen A, Taraborreli P, Torocastro M, Panagopoulos D, Sutton R, et al. Autonomic dysfunction in 'long COVID': rationale, physiology and management strategies. *Clin Med.* (2021) 21:e63–7. doi: 10.7861/clinmed.2020-0896

26. Hu J, Jolkkoken J, Zhao C. Neurotropism of SARS-CoV-2 and its neuropathological alterations: similarities with other coronaviruses. *Neurosci Biobehav Rev.* (2020) 119:184–93. doi: 10.1016/j.neubiorev.2020.10.012

27. Notarius CF, Millar PJ, Floras JS. Muscle sympathetic activity in resting and exercising humans with and without heart failure. *Appl Physiol Nutr Metab.* (2015) 40:1107–15. doi: 10.1139/apnm-2015-0289

28. Júnior JRZ, Viana AO. de Melo Gel, de Angelis K. The impact of sedentarism on heart rate variability (HRV) at rest and in response to mental stress in young women. *Physiol Rep.* (2018) 6:1–8. doi: 10.14814/phy2.13873

29. Barizien N, Guen ML, Russel S, Touche P, Huang F. Vallée. Clinical characterization of dysautonomia in long COVID-19 patients. *Sci Rep.* (2021) 11:14042. doi: 10.1038/s41598-021-93546-5

30. Shah B, Kunal S, Bansal A, Jain J, Poundrik S, Shetty MK, et al. Heart rate variability as a marker of cardiovascular dysautonomia in post-COVID-19 syndrome using artificial intelligence. *Indian Pacing Electrophysiol J.* (2022) 22:70–6. doi: 10.1016/j.ipej.2022.01.004

31. Kaliyaperumal D. Karthikeyan Rk, Alagesan M, Ramalingam S. Characterization of cardiac autonomic function in COVID-19 using heart rate variability: a hospital based preliminar observational study. *J Basic Clin Physiol Pharmacol.* (2021) 32:247–53. doi: 10.1515/jbcpp-20 20-0378

32. Williams DP, Koening J, Carnevali L, Sgoifo A, Jarcok MN, Sternberg EM Thayer JF. Heart rate variability and inflammation: a meta-analysis of human studies. *Brain Behav Immun.* (2019) 80:219–26. doi: 10.1016/j.bbi.2019.03.009

33. Gifford RM, Boos CJ, Reynolds RM, Woods DR. Recovery time and heart rate variability following extreme endurance exercise in healthy women. *Physiol Rep.* (2018) 6:e13905. doi: 10.14814/phy2.13905

34. Bajić D, ðajić V, Milovanović B. Entropy analysis of COVID-19 cardiovascular signals. *Entropy.* (2021) 23:87. doi: 10.3390/e23010087

35. Hayano J, Yuda E. Pitfalls of assessment of autonomic function by heart rate variability. *J Physiol Anthopol.* (2019) 38:1–8. doi: 10.1186/s40101-019-0193-2

36. Hoshi RA, Andrea RY, Santos IS, Dantas EM, Mill JG, Lotufo PA, et al. Linear and nonlinear analyses of heart rate variability following orthostatism in subclinical hypothyroidism. *Medicine.* (2019) 98:1–7. doi: 10.1097/MD.0000000000014140

11

Acute Coronary Syndromes and SARS-CoV-2 Infection: Results from an Observational Multicenter Registry during the Second Pandemic Spread in Lombardy

Marco Ferlini[1], Diego Castini[2], Giulia Ferrante[3], Giancarlo Marenzi[4],
Matteo Montorfano[5], Stefano Savonitto[6], Maurizio D'Urbano[7], Corrado Lettieri[8],
Claudio Cuccia[9], Marcello Marino[10], Luigi Oltrona Visconti[1] and Stefano Carugo[3]*

[1] Division of Cardiology, Fondazione IRCCS Policlinico San Matteo, Pavia, Italy, [2] Cardiology Department, ASST Santi Paolo e Carlo, Milan, Italy, [3] Department of Clinical Sciences and Community Health, Division of Cardiology, University of Milan, Fondazione IRCCS Cà Granda Ospedale Maggiore Policlinico, Milan, Italy, [4] IRCCS Centro Cardiologico Monzino, University of Milan, Milan, Italy, [5] Interventional Cardiology Unit, IRCCS San Raffaele, Milan, Italy, [6] Cardiology Department, Manzoni Hospital, Lecco, Italy, [7] Cardiology Department, Legnano Hospital, ASST Ovest Milanese, Legnano, Italy, [8] Cardiology Department, Carlo Poma Hospital, ASST Mantova, Mantua, Italy, [9] Cardiology Department, Poliambulanza Hospital, Brescia, Italy, [10] Cardiology Department, Ospedale Maggiore di Crema, ASST Crema, Crema, Italy

*Correspondence:
Stefano Carugo
stefano.carugo@unimi.it

Background: COVID-19 had an adverse impact on the management and outcome of acute coronary syndromes (ACS), but most available data refer to March-April 2020.

Aim: This study aims to investigate the clinical characteristics, time of treatment, and clinical outcome of patients at hospitals serving as macro-hubs during the second pandemic wave of SARS-CoV-2 (November 2020-January 2021).

Methods and Results: Nine out of thirteen "macro-hubs" agreed to participate in the registry with a total of 941 patients included. The median age was 67 years (IQR 58-77) and ST-elevation myocardial infarction (STEMI) was the clinical presentation in 54% of cases. Almost all patients (97%) underwent coronary angiography, with more than 60% of patients transported to a macro-hub by the Emergency Medical Service (EMS). In the whole population of STEMI patients, the median time from symptom onset to First Medical Contact (FMC) was 64 min (IQR 30-180). The median time from FMC to CathLab was 69 min (IQR 39-105). A total of 59 patients (6.3%) presented a concomitant confirmed SARS-CoV-2 infection, and pneumonia was present in 42.4% of these cases. No significant differences were found between STEMI patients with and without SARS-CoV-2 infection in treatment time intervals. Patients with concomitant SARS-CoV-2 infection had a significantly higher in-hospital mortality compared to those without (16.9% vs. 3.6%, $P < 0.0001$). However, post-discharge mortality was similar to 6-month mortality (4.2% vs. 4.1%, $P = 0.98$). In the multivariate analysis, SARS-CoV-2 infection did not show an independent association with in-hospital mortality, whereas pneumonia had higher mortality (OR 5.65, $P = 0.05$).

Conclusion: During the second wave of SARS-CoV-2 infection, almost all patients with ACS received coronary angiography for STEMI with an acceptable time delay. Patients with concomitant infection presented a lower in-hospital survival with no difference in post-discharge mortality; infection by itself was not an independent predictor of mortality but pneumonia was.

Keywords: acute coronary syndrome, COVID-19, coronary angiography, hub, STEMI (myocardial infarction)

INTRODUCTION

From the beginning of 2020, the world has had to face the COVID-19 pandemic caused by Severe Acute Respiratory Syndrome Coronavirus-2 (SARS-CoV-2) infection. Italy has been one of the most affected countries in Europe with more than seven million infections and over one hundred thousand deaths (1). In addition to mortality directly caused by severe acute respiratory syndrome and viral interstitial pneumonia, the COVID-19 pandemic played an indirect adverse effect on overall mortality excess, mainly by the necessity to divert resources from the optimal treatment of time-dependent medical and surgical emergencies to COVID-19 cases as a consequence of the dramatic surge in hospital admissions due to SARS-CoV-2 infection (2). An excess in cardiovascular deaths has been observed during 2020 compared to 2019 (3), which could be related to several factors, including reduction of acute coronary syndrome (ACS) hospitalizations, delay in ST-elevation myocardial infarction (STEMI) hospital presentation, an increase of out-of-hospital cardiac arrests, reduction of coronary revascularization procedures, and reduction of outpatient surveillance (4–7). Moreover, direct cardiac involvement has been reported in patients with COVID-19, and patients with ACS and concomitant infection had the worst outcome compared to patients without (8–12). Most of the available data refer to the first spread of the SARS-CoV-2 pandemic that occurred during the first months of 2020, while a second wave of the pandemic was observed worldwide between the end of 2020 and the beginning of 2021.

Lombardy, the most densely populated region in Italy, has been dramatically affected both during the first and the second wave of infection. To guarantee an optimal time of treatment for clinical emergencies, the regional healthcare authorities applied, during the first spread, a model of centralization called "macro-hubs" that was organized according to the estimated patient transportation time and the geographical features of the region. A detailed description of this model has been previously described and a retrospective analysis of its application, during the first wave, found an acceptable time delay in the ACS treatment (13, 14) of patients. This centralization model was, hence, further adopted during the second pandemic wave.

In the present study, we aimed to investigate the clinical characteristics, time to treatment, and clinical outcome of patients hospitalized at the macro-hub centers identified by the healthcare authorities of Lombardy during the second pandemic wave of SARS-CoV-2, from November 2020 to January 2021.

Moreover, we performed an exploratory assessment of the GRACE score predictive performance in the present pandemic context.

MATERIALS AND METHODS

This study presents a retrospective analysis of prospectively collected data from a multicenter observational registry of consecutive patients with diagnoses of ACS hospitalized during the second SARS-CoV-2 pandemic spread. The macro-hubs involved in the registry and the duration of data collection (from 2 November 2020 to 31 January 2021) were based on the application of the decrees by Lombardy health authorities. The decrees defining a macro-hub were: (a) to perform primary percutaneous coronary intervention (PPCI) to all incoming STEMI on a 24/7 basis; (b) to guarantee a PPCI team was available 24/7 in the hospital (rather than on-call); (c) to provide separate pathways for patients with ACS and suspected/diagnosed COVID-19 from triage to catheterization laboratory and isolated care unit to avoid the risk of cross-infections.

At each participating hospital, a principal investigator was responsible for data collection in a custom electronic database provided by the coordinating center (Cardiology Department, University of Milan, ASST Santi Paolo e Carlo, Milan, Italy). At the end of data collection, the completed databases were submitted to the coordinating center for data analysis.

The study complies with the Declaration of Helsinki and was approved by the local institutional review board of each participating center. Patients gave their informed consent at admission for data collection and future publications in anonymous studies.

Study Population

Eligible patients were included in the registry if they received a diagnosis of ACS during hospitalization. STEMI was defined as typical symptoms lasting at least 20 min and persistent ST-elevation of ≥ 2 mm in at least two contiguous leads or new or presumed new left bundle-branch block. NSTEMI was defined as new onset or worsening angina (or equivalent) and elevated biomarkers of myocardial necrosis (troponin I or T above the upper limits of normal at each study site) with or without associated electrocardiographic signs of ischemia (ST-depression, transient ST-elevation, or T-wave inversion). Unstable angina (UA) was defined by the absence of troponin elevation.

The diagnosis of SARS-CoV-2 infection was based on the positive nasopharyngeal swab, bronchoalveolar lavage, and a pulmonary TAC diagnostic for interstitial pneumonia, as a single test or in combination.

Patients with either STEMI or high-risk non-ST-elevation ACS (NSTE-ACS) (presence of hemodynamic and/or electrical instability, recurrent or ongoing chest pain refractory to medical treatments, and/or relevant ST-T wave changes) were directly transferred to the catheterization laboratory with the execution of a nasopharyngeal swab. Patients with low- or intermediate-risk NSTE-ACS were evaluated in the emergency department (ED) and underwent nasopharyngeal swab immediately, deferring percutaneous coronary intervention (PCI) decision after swab results and clinical conditions. All patients, regardless of the immediate treatment decision, were admitted to different wards according to their molecular nasopharyngeal swab results.

Data Collection

For each patient, the following data were collected: demographic characteristics, cardiovascular risk factors, prior cardiac events or procedures, presence of cardiogenic shock, pulmonary edema or cardiac arrest on or before admission, site of STEMI at ECG, and echocardiographic left ventricular ejection fraction (LVEF). Moreover, blood hemoglobin, white blood cells, estimated glomerular filtration rate (eGFR) (CKD-EPI formula), and troponins values at admission were collected. Finally, the Global Registry of Acute Coronary Events (GRACE) score at admission was calculated (15). Data about in-hospital pharmacological treatments and interventional procedures had to be reported for all included patients.

For patients with STEMI, we analyzed the critical time intervals: "symptom-onset to first medical contact (FMC) (defined as the diagnosis by 12-lead electrocardiogram) and "FMC to arrival at catheterization laboratory (CathLab)."

As clinical adverse events, we considered the in-hospital occurrence of all-cause death, acute pulmonary edema, shock, cardiac arrest, acute kidney injury (AKI), major bleedings, pneumonia, and need for invasive and/or non-invasive ventilation. AKI was defined according to Kidney Disease Improving Global Outcomes (KDIGO) guidelines (16) and bleeding events were appraised according to Bleeding Academic Research Consortium (BARC) definitions (17). Total mortality was also collected at a 6-month follow-up.

Statistical Analysis

Categorical data are reported as absolute values and percentages and compared using the chi-square test; continuous variables are described as the median and interquartile range (IQR) and compared using the Mann–Whitney test. The associations between clinical variables and clinical events were investigated using univariate and multivariate logistic regression analysis. The GRACE score predictive performance for in-hospital and post-discharge mortality was assessed using the C-statistic and receiver operating characteristic curves. The software used for statistical analysis was MedCalc Statistical Software version 16.2.0 (MedCalc Software bvba, Ostend, Belgium) and the cut-off adopted for statistical significance was $P < 0.05$.

RESULTS

Nine out of thirteen "macro-hubs" of the Lombardy region agreed to participate in the registry during the second pandemic wave and a total of 941 consecutive patients were included.

The baseline demographic and clinical characteristics and in-hospital treatments of the overall population are summarized in **Table 1**. The median age was 67 years (IQR 58-77), 30% were ≥ 75 years old, and 26% were females. STEMI

TABLE 1 | Baseline characteristics of the overall population.

VARIABLE	N = 941
Age, years, median (IQR)	67 (58–77)
Age ≥ 75 years, n (%)	284 (30)
Females, n (%)	242 (26)
Arterial hypertension, n (%)	625 (66.4)
Diabetes mellitus, n (%)	225 (24)
Hyperlipidemia, n (%)	477 (51)
Active smoking, n (%)	237 (25)
Previous MI, n (%)	195 (20.7)
Previous PCI, n (%)	212 (22.5)
Previous CABG, n (%)	54 (5.7)
Clinical presentation	
STEMI, n (%)	507 (54)
NSTE-ACS, n (%)	434 (46)
LVEF,%, median (IQR)	50 (40–55)
GRACE score, median (IQR)	121 (100–143)
Acute pulmonary edema, n (%)	55 (5.8)
Shock, n (%)	37 (3.9)
Cardiac arrest, n (%)	40 (4.3)
SARS-CoV-2 infection, n (%)	59 (6.3)
Blood samples	
Hemoglobin at admission, gr/dl, median (IQR)	14 (13–15)
White blood cells at admission, n/mcl, median (IQR)	9.8 (7.6–12)
Troponin at admission, ng/dl, medin (IQR)	0.25 (0.04–1.75)
eGFR at admission, ml/min/1.73 mq, median (IQR)	79.9 (59–92.6)
Coronary angiography and revascularization	
Coronary angiography, n (%)	914 (97)
STEMI, n (%)	494 (97.4)
NSTE-ACS, n (%)	420 (96.8)
Radial artery access, n (%)	809 (88.5)
PCI, n (%)	762 (83.4)
CABG, n (%)	60 (6.5)
Complete revascularization, n (%)	574 (60)
IABP, n (%)	56 (6)
PMCS, n (%)	7 (0.7)
Drug therapy	
Aspirin, n (%)	857 (91)
P2Y12 inhibitors, n (%)	778 (82.6)
Glycoprotein IIb/IIIa inhibitors, n (%)	125 (13.3)
Inotropic drugs, n (%)	91 (9.7)

CABG, coronary artery by-pass grafting; eGFR, estimated glomerular filtration rate; IABP, intra-aortic balloon pump; LVEF, left ventricular ejection fraction; MI, myocardial infarction; NSTE-ACS, non ST elevation acute coronary syndrome; PCI, percutaneous coronary intervention; PMCS, percutaneous mechanic circulatory support; STEMI, ST elevation myocardial infarction.

was the clinical presentation in 54% of the cases (anterior site in 52%). The GRACE score at admission was 121 (IQR 100-143). Overall, 97% of the patients underwent coronary angiography (97.4% of STEMI and 96.8% of NSTE-ACS patients). Multivessel coronary artery disease (CAD) was present in 51% of cases, and there was no significant angiographic CAD in 8% of cases. A PCI was performed in 83.4% of the cases (90.7% of patients with STEMI and 74.8% of patients with NSTE-ACS), and coronary artery by-pass grafting (CABG) was performed in 6.5% of cases. Complete revascularization was obtained in 60% of cases within index admission.

Sixty percent of the patients were transported to a macro-hub by the Emergency Medical Service (EMS), whereas 26% self-presented to the ED of a macro-hub and 12.8% were transferred from spoke centers; the remaining patients were already at the hospital at the time of ACS.

Patients With Concomitant SARS-CoV-2 Infection

A total of 59 patients (6.3%) had concomitant confirmed SARS-CoV-2 infection. **Table 2** shows the comparisons between demographic, baseline clinical characteristics,

TABLE 2 | Comparison between patients with and without SARS-CoV-2 infection.

VARIABLE	SARS-CoV-2 (N = 59)	No SARS-CoV-2 (N = 882)	P-value
Age, years, median (IQR)	69 (62–77)	67 (58–77)	0.29
Age ≥ 75 years, n (%)	19 (32.2)	265 (30)	0.72
Females, n (%)	11 (18.6)	231 (26.2)	0.19
Arterial hypertension, n (%)	44 (74.6)	581 (65.9)	0.17
Diabetes mellitus, n (%)	19 (32.2)	206 (23.4)	0.12
Hyperlipidemia, n (%)	27 (45.8)	450 (51)	0.43
Previous MI, n (%)	16 (27)	179 (20.3)	0.21
Previous PCI, n (%)	16 (27)	196 (22.2)	0.38
Clinical presentation			
STEMI, n (%)	33 (56)	474 (53.7)	0.74
NSTE-ACS, n (%)	26 (44)	408 (46.3)	
LVEF,%, median (IQR)	48 (38–55)	50 (40–55)	0.09
GRACE score, median (IQR)	139 (105–158)	121 (100–142)	0.02
Acute pulmonary edema, n (%)	4 (6.8)	51 (5.8)	0.75
Shock, n (%)	3 (5.1)	34 (3.9)	0.64
Cardiac arrest, n (%)	3 (5.1)	37 (4.2)	0.74
Pneumonia, n (%)	25 (42.4)	7 (0.8)	<0.0001
Blood samples			
Hemoglobin at admission, gr/dl, median (IQR)	13.9 (12.3–15.4)	14 (12.8–15.2)	0.57
White blood cells at admission, n/mcl, median (IQR)	9.04 (7.55–11.19)	9.81 (7.64–12.20)	0.18
Troponin at admission, ng/dl, median (IQR)	0.61 (0.13–2.14)	0.24 (0.04–1.67)	0.04
eGFR at admission, ml/min/1.73 mq, median (IQR)	74 (52–90)	80 (59–93)	0.27
Diagnostic and therapeutic procedures			
Coronary angiography, n (%)	58 (98)	856 (97)	0.57
No significant CAD, n (%)	6 (10.3)	67 (8)	0.25
SVD, n (%)	18 (31)	355 (41.5)	
MVD, n (%)	34 (58.6)	434 (50.7)	
PCI, n (%)	47 (81)	715 (83.5)	0.62
CABG, n (%)	4 (6.9)	56 (6.5)	0.90
Complete revascularization, n (%)	29 (49)	545 (64)	0.04
IABP, n (%)	5 (8.5)	51 (5.8)	0.39
PMCS, n (%)	0 (0)	7 (0.8)	0.78
NIV, n (%)	13 (22)	26 (2.9)	<0.0001
IMV, n (%)	1 (1.7)	13 (1.5)	0.89
Drug therapy			
Aspirin, n (%)	52 (88)	805 (91)	0.41
P2Y12 inhibitors, n (%)	47 (79.7)	731 (82.9)	0.53
Glycoprotein IIb/IIIa inhibitors, n (%)	11 (18.6)	114 (12.9)	0.21
Inotropic drugs, n (%)	6 (10.2)	85 (9.6)	0.89

CABG, coronary artery by-pass grafting; CAD, coronary artery disease; eGFR, estimated glomerula filtration rate; IABP, intra-aortic balloon pump; IMV, invasive mechanical ventilation; LVEF, left ventricular ejection fraction; MI, myocardial infarction; MVD, multivessel disease; NIV, non -invasive ventilation; NSTE-ACS, non ST elevation acute coronary syndrome; PCI, percutaneous coronary intervention; PMCS, percutaneous mechanic circulatory support; STEMI, ST elevation myocardial infarction; SVD, single vessel disease.

TABLE 3 | Time to treatment in the overall STEMI population and separately in patients with and without SARS-CoV-2 infection.

	Overall STEMI *N* = 507	SARS-Cov-2 *N* = 33	No SARS-Cov-2 *N* = 474	*P*-value
Symptom onset-FMC, median (IQR)	64 (30–180)	77 (37–240)	60 (30–180)	0.40
FMC-CathLab, median (IQR)	69 (39.5–105)	65 (37–160)	70 (40–125)	0.98

FMC, first medical contact.

TABLE 4 | Clinical outcomes in the overall population and separately in patients with and without SARS-CoV-2 infection.

	Overall population	SARS-Cov-2	No SARS-Cov-2	*P*-value
Acute pulmonary edema, n (%)	38 (4)	1 (1.7)	37 (4.2)	0.34
Shock, n (%)	49 (5.1)	7 (11.9)	42 (4.8)	0.02
In-hospital cardiac arrest, n (%)	66 (7)	6 (10.2)	60 (6.8)	0.32
Major bleedings, n (%)	37 (3.9)	3 (5.1)	34 (3.8)	0.84
AKI, n (%)	91 (9.7)	10 (16.9)	81 (9.2)	0.13
In-hospital mortality, n (%)	42 (4.5)	10 (16.9)	32 (3.6)	<0.0001
Mortality at 6 months among hospital survivors, n (%)	36 (4.1)	2 (4.2)	34 (4.1)	0.98

AKI, acute kidney injury.

and in-hospital treatments of patients with and without SARS-CoV-2 infection.

In these patients, STEMI was the clinical presentation in 56% of cases (a rate comparable to that observed in patients without SARS-CoV-2 infection). The GRACE score was 139 (IQR 105-158), significantly higher than in patients without infection. Almost all patients (about 98%) underwent coronary angiography in both groups, and no significant differences were found in CAD extension; however, patients with SARS-CoV-2 infection presented a non-significant higher rate of no significant CAD (10.3 vs. 8%). PCI was performed in 81% of cases and CABG in 6.9%. Complete revascularization was obtained in 49% of cases, a significantly lower rate compared to that observed in patients without SARS-CoV-2 infection (64%, *P* = 0.04).

Pneumonia was present in 42.4% of patients with SARS-CoV-2 infection (vs.8% in patients without SARS-CoV-2 infection, *P* < 0.0001). Significantly more patients with COVID-19 underwent non-invasive ventilation (NIV) (22 vs. 2.9%, *P* < 0.0001), whereas no significant difference was observed regarding invasive mechanical ventilation utilization (IMV) between patients with and without COVID-19.

Diagnosis and Treatment Times

Table 3 shows treatment times in the overall STEMI population and patients with and without SARS-CoV-2 infection.

In the whole population, the median time from symptoms-onset to FMC was 64 min (IQR 30-180). The median time from FMC to CathLab was 69 min (IQR 39-105). No significant differences were found between STEMI patients with and without infection in both time intervals.

Clinical Outcomes

Table 4 summarizes the clinical outcomes observed in the overall population and separately in patients with and without SARS-CoV-2 infection.

Except for cardiogenic shock, which was higher in patients with SARS-CoV-2 infection (11.9 vs. 4.8%, *P* = 0.02), no

significant differences were found in the incidence of the other adverse events. In-hospital mortality was 4.5% in the overall population and was significantly higher in patients aged ≥ 75 years (8.1 vs. 2.9%, *P* = 0.004) and in STEMI (5.9 vs. 2.8%, *P* = 0.02).

In patients with concomitant SARS-CoV-2 infection, in-hospital mortality was significantly higher than in patients without (16.9 vs. 3.6%, *P* < 0.0001). Although in the univariate logistic regression analysis the presence of infection was significantly associated with in-hospital mortality (OR 5.41, 95% CI 2.51–11.65, *P* < 0.0001), in the multivariate analysis it showed a weak and not significant association, whereas the presence of pneumonia showed an independent association but with a borderline statistical significance (**Table 5**).

Of the 899 patients discharged alive, mortality data at 6 months was available in 877 (98%). At this time point, mortality was 4.1% in the overall population and no significant difference

TABLE 5 | Regression coefficients and odds ratios from multivariate logistic regression analysis testing association between clinical variables and in-hospital mortality.

VARIABLE	Regression coefficient (SE)	*P*-value	Odds ratios (95% CI)
Age	0.046 (0.024)	0.05	1.04 (0.99–1.09)
Diabetes mellitus	0.130 (0.542)	0.79	0.87 (0.30–2.52)
STEMI	0.445 (0.550)	0.41	1.56 (0.53–4.58)
MVD	1.237 (0.359)	0.02	3.44 (1.17–10.15)
LVEF ≤ 35%	1.568 (0.526)	0.003	4.79 (1.71–13.46)
eGFR < 60 ml/min/1.73 mq	1.027 (0.530)	0.05	2.79 (0.98–7.90)
Cardiac arrest	1.327 (1.160)	0.25	0.26 (0.02–2.57)
Shock	2.537 (0.670)	0.0002	12.65 (3.39–47.10)
SARS-CoV-2 infection	1.415 (0.834)	0.08	4.11 (0.80–21.12)
Pneumonia	1.732 (0.901)	0.05	5.65 (0.96–33.06)

eGFR, estimated glomerular filtration rate; LVEF, left ventricular ejection fraction; MVD, multivessel disease; STEMI, ST elevation myocardial infarction. In the model were included all variables with P < 0.10 at the univariate analysis.

was found between patients with and without SARS-CoV-2 infection (4.2 vs. 4.1%, *P* = 0.98). Infection was not significantly associated with post-discharge mortality. In the multivariate regression analysis only age, LVEF ≤ 35% at discharge, and the diagnosis of pneumonia were independently associated with post-discharge mortality.

In order to evaluate the predictive performance of the GRACE score in the present pandemic context, with particular regard to SARS-CoV-2 patients, we tested the predictive accuracy of the GRACE score at admission both for in-hospital and post-discharge mortality. **Table 6** reports the results of the C-statistic. The score showed globally a good predictive performance for mortality, with higher C-statistic for in-hospital (0.85 95% CI.82–0.87, *p* < 0.0001) as compared to post-discharge mortality (0.75 95% CI.71–0.77, *p* < 0.0001), particularly with regard to in-hospital death in patients with concomitant SARS-CoV-2 infection (0.94 95% CI.82–0.98, *p* < 0.0001).

DISCUSSION

In the present article, we describe the presentation, time of care, and mortality data of patients with ACS managed at hospitals identified as "macro-hubs" in a specific geographical area during the second spread of SARS-CoV-2 infection with a modified network of assistance based on a model of centralization of care.

The main findings of our analysis are as follows: more than half of patients presented with STEMI and these were treated within the ESC-recommended time delay (18); patients with ACS and positive at SARS-CoV-2 had a higher baseline risk profile, as suggested by a significantly higher GRACE score, and significantly higher mortality compared to patients without infection. This excess mortality risk appears to be attributable to the presence of concomitant pneumonia.

A delay in STEMI treatment was one of the first observations reported as a consequence of the COVID-19 outbreak at the beginning of the pandemic (19); particularly, patients with STEMI and COVID-19 presented the longest time of assistance as a consequence of a prolonged time from symptom onset to hospital admission, mainly due to the lack of dedicated organization of the healthcare system and for the limited availability of EMS due to systemic overload (12).

The centralized model used in Lombardy did not show a negative impact on time to treatment; furthermore, as previously reported, the time from symptom onset to CathLab was significantly shorter during the second compared to the first spread of infection (February-May 2020) (20). In the present analysis, about 60% of STEMI were directly transported to a macro-hub by EMS. The STEMI care network available for 15 years in the Lombardy Region comprising 55 CathLabs, mostly performing 24/7 primary PCI, and a well territorially distributed EMS certainly contributed to this positive result. However, the application of standardized protocols for fast-tracking the treatment of STEMI during the pandemic was endorsed by scientific societies, (21) allowing healthcare workers to obtain results in terms of the time of reperfusion, clinical outcomes, and staff safety in line with those before pandemic (22).

Patients with concomitant infection presented a significantly higher rate of in-hospital death compared to patients without infection (16.9 vs. 3.6%), whereas post-discharge mortality was not affected (4.2 vs. 4.1%); furthermore, in the multivariate analysis, infection by itself was not an independent predictor of mortality, whereas pneumonia was, though with a borderline statistical significance. It has been previously reported that patients with ACS, particularly STEMI, and concomitant COVID-19 present worse outcomes: in the North American COVID-19 Myocardial Infarction Registry, the in-hospital mortality of these patients was 33% (11). In the present data, a significant difference between patients with and without infection was found only in the rate of pneumonia and in the need of non-invasive ventilation: therefore, it is likely that pulmonary complications continue to have an adverse prognostic impact on these patients during the acute phase, whereas for survivors no significant difference in mortality was found at mid-term follow-up. However, we have reported a higher rate of pneumonia during the first spread of COVID-19 (about 60%) in patients with ACS and concomitant infection (14) that has been reduced (but not erased!) in the second wave by early and specific treatment (e.g., steroids and ventilation strategies); furthermore, the wide availability of diagnostic tools led to the diagnosis of patients with less severe clinical infection.

Although the GRACE score is a well-established predictive tool for outcomes prediction in patients with ACS (15), to our knowledge little information exists about its usefulness during the COVID-19 pandemic. Based on this, we tried an explorative investigation on the predictive value of the GRACE score on mortality and we found a good value of C-statistic for the overall population that was even stronger for patients with SARS-CoV-2 infection. Although the GRACE score is used to predict clinical outcomes in patients with ACS beyond infections, the baseline value was higher in patients with SARS-Cov2. These observations suggest that patients with ACS and SARS-CoV-2 might have a worse baseline risk profile and that the GRACE score retains a good predictive power in these patients. In a similar study, a significant difference was not found for GRACE score between patients with and without infection but a value > 140 and the presence of COVID-19 were independent risk factors associated with higher in-hospital mortality (23).

TABLE 6 | Predictive values of the GRACE score for in-hospital and post-discharge mortality in the overall population and separately in patients with and without SARS-CoV-2 infection.

	C-statistic (95% CI)	Sens/Spec	P-value
In-hospital mortality			
Overall population	0.85 (0.82–0.87)	70/88	<0.0001
SARS-CoV-2 patients	0.94 (0.82–0.98)	100/88	<0.0001
NoSARS-CoV-2 patients	0.82 (0.79–0.85)	60/82	<0.0001
Post-discharge mortality			
Overall population	0.75 (0.71–0.77)	52/91	<0.0001
SARS-CoV-2 patients	0.82 (0.67–0.93)	100/62	<0.002
NoSARS-CoV-2 patients	0.73 (0.70–0.76)	50/90	<0.0001

Limitations

Small sample size, retrospective analysis, and lack of correction for covariates with consequent confounding bias can be considered as the main limitations of the present study. Furthermore, complete information on pharmacologic therapies was lacking. Finally, geographical differences do not allow definite conclusions and make our findings not necessarily representative of different areas in Italy or worldwide.

CONCLUSION

The main aim of our work was to offer an overall clinical picture of ACS population during the second pandemic wave of SARS-CoV-2 infection and to describe its prognosis within the macro-hub network implemented by the Lombardy region in order to cope with the COVID-19 pandemic (13). The present article adds further confirmation to what we observed previously (14, 20): a timely adequate treatment of STEMI patients was obtained and a better prognosis in overall patients with ACS, both with and without SARS-CoV-2 infection, was observed during the second pandemic wave, corroborating in our opinion the beneficial effect of the organizational strategy adopted. Moreover, patients with concomitant infection had lower in-hospital survival, whereas post-discharge mortality was similar; infection by itself was not an independent predictor of mortality, whereas pneumonia implied a higher mortality risk.

AUTHOR CONTRIBUTIONS

SC, MF, and DC contributed to the conception and design of the study. DC, MF, and GF organized the database. DC performed the statistical analysis. MF and DC wrote the first draft of the manuscript. GM, MMo, SS, MD'U, CL, CC, MMa, and LV wrote the sections of the manuscript. All authors contributed to manuscript revision, read, and approved the submitted version.

REFERENCES

1. COVID-19 Excess Mortality Collaborators. Estimating excess mortality due to the COVID-19 pandemic: a systematic analysis of COVID-19 related mortality, 2020-21. *Lancet.* (2022) 399:1513–36. doi: 10.1016/S0140-6736(21)02796-3

2. Wadhera RK, Shen C, Gondi S, Chen S, Kazi DS, Yeh RW. Cardiovascular deaths during the COVID-19 pandemic in the United States. *J Am Coll Cardiol.* (2021) 77:159–69. doi: 10.1016/j.jacc.2020.10.055

3. De Rosa S, Spaccarotella C, Basso C, Calabrò MP, Curcio A, Filardi PP, et al. Reduction of hospitalizations for myocardial infarction in Italy in the COVID-19 era. *Eur Heart J.* (2020) 41:2083–8.

4. Baldi E, Sechi G, Mare C, Canevari F, Brancaglione A, Primi R, et al. Out-of-hospital cardiac arrest during the COVID-19 outbreak in Italy. *N Engl J Med.* (2020) 382:496–8. doi: 10.1056/NEJMc2010418

5. De Luca G, Verdoia M, Cercek M, Jensen LO, Vavlukis M, Calmac L, et al. Impact of COVID-19 pandemic on mechanical reperfusion for patients with STEMI. *J Am Coll Cardiol.* (2020) 76:2321–30.

6. Quadri G, Rognoni A, Cerrato E, Baralis G, Boccuzzi G, Brscic E, et al. Catheterization laboratory activity before and during COVID-19 spread: a comparative analysis in Piedmont, Italy, by the Italian Society of Interventional Cardiology (GISE). *Int J Cardiol.* (2021) 323:288–91. doi: 10.1016/j.ijcard.2020.08.072

7. Nijjer SS, Petraco R, Sen S. Optimal management of acute coronary syndromes in the era of COVID-19. *Heart.* (2020) 106:1609–16. doi: 10.1136/heartjnl-2020-317143

8. Capone V, Cuomo V, Esposito R, Canonico ME, Ilardi F, Prastaro M, et al. Epidemiology, prognosis, and clinical manifestation of cardiovascular disease in COVID-19. *Expert Rev Cardiovasc Ther.* (2020) 18:531–9. doi: 10.1080/14779072.2020.1797491

9. Cameli M, Pastore MC, Mandoli GE, D'Ascenzi F, Focardi M, Biagioni G, et al. COVID-19 and Acute Coronary Syndromes: Current Data and Future Implications. *Front. Cardiovasc. Med.* (2021) 7:593496. doi: 10.3389/fcvm.2020.593496

10. The European Society for Cardiology. ESC guidance for the diagnosis and management of cardiovascular disease during the COVID-19 pandemic: part 2—care pathways, treatment, and follow-up. *Eur Heart J.* (2022) 43:1059–03. doi: 10.1093/eurheartj/ehab697

11. Garcia S, Dehghani P, Grines C, Davidson L, Nayak KR, Saw J, et al. Initial findings from the North American COVID-19 myocardial infarction registry. *J Am Coll Cardiol.* (2021) 77:1994–2003.

12. Kite TA, Ludman PF, Gale CP, Wu J, Caixeta A, Mansourati J, et al. International prospective registry of acute coronary syndromes in patients with COVID-19. *J Am Coll Cardiol.* (2021) 77:2466–76. doi: 10.1016/j.jacc.2021.03.309

13. Ferlini M, Andreassi A, Carugo S, Cuccia C, Bianchini B, Castiglioni B, et al. Centralization of the ST elevation myocardial infarction care network in the Lombardy region during the COVID-19 outbreak. *Int J Cardiol.* (2020) 312:24–6. doi: 10.1016/j.ijcard.2020.04.062

14. Carugo S, Ferlini M, Castini D, Andreassi A, Guagliumi G, Metra M, et al. Management of acute coronary syndromes during the COVID-19 outbreak in Lombardy: the "macro-hub" experience. *Int J Cardiol Heart Vasc.* (2020) 31:100662. doi: 10.1016/j.ijcha.2020.100662

15. Fox KA, Dabbous OH, Goldberg RJ, Pieper KS, Eagle KA, Van de Werf F, et al. Prediction of risk of death and myocardial infarction in the six months after presentation with acute coronary syndromes: prospective multinational observational stuady (GRACE). *BMJ.* (2006) 333:1091. doi: 10.1136/bmj.38985.646481.55

16. Khwaja A. KDIGO clinical practice guidelines for acute kidney injury. *Nephron Clin Pract.* (2012) 120:c179–84. doi: 10.1159/000339789

17. Mehran R, Rao SV, Bhatt DL, Gibson CM, Caixeta A, Eikelboom J, et al. Standardized bleeding definitions for cardiovascular clinical trials: a consensus from the Bleeding academic research consortium. *Circulation.* (2011) 123:2736–47. doi: 10.1161/CIRCULATIONAHA.110.009449

18. Ibanez B, James S, Agewall S, Antunes MJ, Bucciarelli-Ducci C, Bueno H, et al. 2017 ESC Guidelines for the management of acute myocardial infarction in patients presenting with ST-segment elevation. *Eur Heart J.* (2018) 39:119. doi: 10.5603/KP.2018.0041

19. Tam CF, Cheung KS, Lam S, Wong A, Yung A, Sze M, et al. Impact of Coronavirus disease 2019 (COVID-19) outbreak on ST-segment-elevation myocardial infarction care in Hong Kong, China. *Circ Cardiovasc Qual Outcomes.* (2020) 13:e006631. doi: 10.1161/CIRCOUTCOMES.120.006631

20. Ferlini M, Castini D, Oltrona Visconti L, Carugo S. Acute coronary syndromes during the first and the second wave of COVID-19. *Eur J Int Med.* (2022) 99:109–11. doi: 10.1016/j.ejim.2022.02.001

21. Chieffo A, Stefanini GG, Price S, Barbato E, Tarantini G, Karam N, et al. EAPCI position statement on invasive management of acute coronary syndromes during the COVID-19 pandemic. *Eur Heart J.* (2020) 41:1839–51.doi: 10.1093/eurheartj/ehaa381

22. Salarifar M, Ghavami M, Poorhosseini H, Masoudkabir F, Jenab Y, Amirzadegan A, et al. The impact of a dedicated coronavirus disease 2019 primary angioplasty protocol on time components related to ST-segment elevation myocardial infarction management in a 24/7 primary percutaneous coronary intervention–capable hospital. *Kardiol Pol.* (2020) 78:1227–34. doi: 10.33963/KP.15607

23. Solano-Lopez J, Luis Zamorano J, Pardo San A, Amat-Santos I, Sarnago F, Gutiérrez Ibañes E, et al. Risk factors for in-hospital mortality in patients with acute myocardial infarction during the COVID-19 outbreak. *Rev Esp Cardiol.* (2020) 73:985–93. doi: 10.1016/j.rec.2020.07.009

12

Changes of Vascular Reactivity and Arterial Stiffness in a Patient with Covid-19 Infection

Philipp Jud[1]*, Harald H. Kessler[2] and Marianne Brodmann[1]

[1] *Division of Angiology, Department of Internal Medicine, Medical University of Graz, Graz, Austria,* [2] *Diagnostic and Research Institute of Hygiene, Microbiology, and Environmental Medicine, Medical University of Graz, Graz, Austria*

*Correspondence:
Philipp Jud
philipp.jud@medunigraz.at

Covid-19 infection may be associated with a higher incidence developing cardiovascular complications, however, the underlying mechanisms contributing to cardiovascular complications are largely unknown, while endothelial cell damage may be present. We want to report a 24-year-old woman with Covid-19 infection who had undergone measurements of vascular reactivity and arterial stiffness, including flow-mediated dilation (FMD), nitroglycerin-mediated dilation (NMD), aortic pulse wave velocity (PWV), augmentation index and carotid intima-media-thickness (cIMT) at the time when Covid-19 was diagnosed. Reduced FMD of 0.0% and NMD of 15.5% were observed, while PWV (5.9 m/s), Aix (27%) and cIMT with 0.4 mm of both common carotid arteries were unremarkable. Repeated measurements of FMD, NMD, PWV, Aix, and cIMT 6 weeks after Covid-19 infection revealed persistently reduced FMD (0.0%), while NMD (17.24%), PWV (5.6 m/s) and augmentation index (13%) ameliorated. This case suggests potential impact of Covid-19 infection on endothelial function, also in young Covid-19 patients without any co-morbidity.

Keywords: Covid-19, endothelial dysfunction, vascular reactivity, arterial stiffness, vasculopathy

INTRODUCTION

Covid-19 is caused by the severe acute respiratory syndrome coronavirus 2 (SARS-CoV-2) affecting primarily the respiratory system. Patients with cardiovascular comorbidities have an increased risk of in-hospital death and Covid-19 infection may lead to a higher risk of cardiovascular complications like heart failure, venous thromboembolism or stroke (1–4). Although prior data suggested a direct viral infection of the endothelial cell and diffuse endothelial inflammation which may promote to cardiovascular changes in Covid-19, a recent study assumed that direct endothelial infection by SARS-CoV-2 *via* angiotensin-converting enzyme 2 (ACE2) receptors is unlikely as there is a lack of ACE2 in human endothelial cells (5, 6). Furthermore, other pathways have been suggested contributing also to endothelial changes in Covid-19 (7–9). We report a 24-year-old woman with Covid-19 infection who had undergone measurements of vascular reactivity and arterial stiffness on the day of proven Covid-19 infection and 6 weeks after infection.

CASE REPORT

A 24-year-old woman underwent measurements of flow-mediated dilation (FMD), nitroglycerin-mediated dilation (NMD), pulse wave velocity (PWV), and carotid intima-media-thickness (cIMT) due to a preventive medical check-up at the beginning of December 2020. She was otherwise healthy, had a body-mass-index of 23.8 kg/m² without any known atherosclerotic risk factor and worked as a secretary for a medical office in a hospital. Additionally, she was a non-smoker without a family history of cardiovascular disease and did not take any medications. Due to governmental initiated shutdown in Austria from November 3rd, 2020 to December 23rd, 2020, the patient refrained from sports activities during that shutdown, but she was active with regular sport activity of 30 min three times a week prior to that shutdown.

Measurements of FMD, NMD, cIMT, and pulse-wave analysis were performed in the morning between 7:00 a.m. and 9:00 a.m. after overnight fasting in a temperature-controlled (22–24°C) and quiet room by one trained technician. At the beginning of the FMD measurement, a blood pressure cuff was placed on the right forearm below the antecubital fossa and the baseline diameter of the right brachial artery was examined in a longitudinal plane between 2 and 7 centimeters proximal to the antecubital fossa in the patient. Three end-diastolic diameters between two intimal layers were measured ECG-gated during image acquisition in a one-centimeter-long segment of the brachial artery. Subsequently, the cuff was inflated >50 mmHg above the resting systolic pressure for 5 min, then deflated and 60 s after cuff release, the post-ischemic diameter of the brachial artery was measured. During a rest of 15 min, pulse-wave analysis including measurement of the aortic PWV and augmentation index was performed on the left arm and calculated *via* the oscillometric device Mobil-O-Graph® (I.E.M. Mobil-O-Graph, I.E.M., Cockerillstr., Stolberg, Germany) by an automated analysis. A size-adjusted cuff was placed on the patient's left upper arm about 2-4 centimeters above the antecubital fossa in supine position and subsequent pulse-wave analysis was performed, while the patient did not to speak or move over the whole pulse-wave analysis. Also, during the same rest of 15 min, the patient underwent measurement of the cIMT of both common carotid artery in supine position using a high-resolution linear array probe with 8–13 MHz (Siemens ACUSON S2000™, Siemens Healthcare Corp., Henkelstr., Erlangen, Germany). The thickness of the intimal and medial layers of the common carotid wall

was measured on frozen longitudinal images in at least one-centimeter-long segment of the artery. After that rest of 15 min, the diameter of the right brachial artery was recorded similar to the technique described for FMD before and 5 min after sublingual administration of 0.4 mg glyceryl trinitrate spray. FMD and NMD measurements were performed with an 8–13 MHz linear array transducer using a conventional ultrasound scanner (Siemens ACUSON S2000™, Siemens Healthcare Corp., Henkelstr., Erlangen, Germany). Most recommendations for the measurement of FMD and NMD were fulfilled according to recent guidelines (10). The measurements revealed a reduced FMD of 0.0% and a reduced NMD of 15.5% according to proposed reference values (11). Pulse-wave analysis revealed a PWV of 5.9 m/s and an augmentation index of 27% while ultrasonography revealed a cIMT of 0.4 mm of both common carotid arteries.

The patient was asymptomatic at the time of the respective measurements without potential symptoms of Covid-19 infection or any other infection. One hour after the respective measurements, testing for Covid-19 by polymerase chain reaction (PCR) was performed in that patient due to a routine testing for hospital staff which confirmed an acute Covid-19 infection with a cycle threshold of 22. The initial physical examination including auscultation was unremarkable with a body temperature of 36.6°C and a blood pressure of 127/88 mmHg. Measurement of oxygen level and chest x-ray were not performed as the patient was asymptomatic without respiratory symptoms. There was only a slightly elevated C-reactive protein (8.4 mg/L, reference value 0–5 mg/L) without lymphopenia and lipid parameters were also normal. The patient was subsequently home-isolated and was advised to monitor her health. During home-quarantine, the patient developed headache and myalgia within the first 3 days, which were treated by acetaminophen on demand and resolved afterwards, followed by loss of taste and smell as well as by mild dyspnea on exertion after the fifth and seventh day of home quarantine, respectively. On the tenth day of quarantine, Covid-19 PCR was performed again with a cycle threshold of 26. The patient was asymptomatic after 20 days of initial Covid-19 PCR and repeated PCR testing for Covid-19 was negative on the 21st day after initial Covid-19 PCR. A timeline

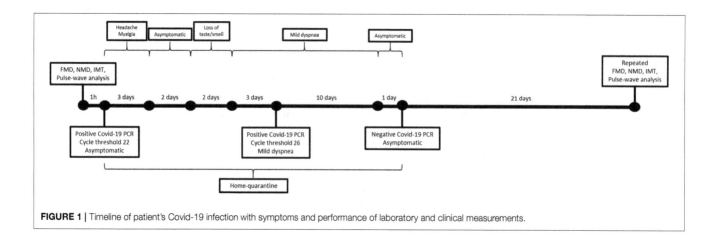

FIGURE 1 | Timeline of patient's Covid-19 infection with symptoms and performance of laboratory and clinical measurements.

of patient's Covid-19 infection with symptoms and performance of Covid-19 PCR and clinical measurements are shown in **Figure 1**.

Six weeks after initial Covid-19 testing, measurements for FMD, NMD, cIMT, and pulse-wave analysis were repeated by the same measurement methods as describes above evaluating changes of the respective parameters. FMD remained unchanged with 0.0% while NMD ameliorated to 17.24%. Furthermore, also PWV with 5.6% and augmentation index with 13% decreased while cIMT was unchanged.

DISCUSSION

We demonstrated with our case a potential impact of Covid-19 infection on endothelial dysfunction. Prior investigations of endothelial changes in Covid-19 infection have demonstrated direct viral infection of endothelial cells and endothelial inflammation with microthrombi and microangiopathy (5, 12). As the vascular endothelium is essential for the maintenance of vascular homoeostasis, dysfunction of the endothelium may result in cardiovascular changes. So far, there are only limited data about the pathophysiological mechanisms how SARS-CoV-2 contributes to endothelial dysfunction. While potential interactions of SARS-CoV-2 with ACE2 receptors have been suggested initially, recent data indicate that there is lacking evidence of ACE2 receptors expression on human endothelial cells assuming thus that direct infection of endothelial cells by SARS-CoV-2 is unlikely (5, 6, 13). Besides potential microvascular damage, also macrovascular damage may be promoted by Covid-19 infection since low values of FMD and NMD of the brachial artery were present in our patient. Additionally, amelioration of NMD, aortic PWV and Aix were observed after Covid-19 infection which indicates that Covid-19 infection may influence vascular homeostasis also in large arteries. Brachial FMD and NMD as well as aortic PWV are proven predictors of cardiovascular events and mortality and changes of those parameters are also associated cardiovascular events and mortality (14, 15). So far, data evaluating vascular reactivity or arterial stiffness in Covid-19 infection are very limited. Only one study investigated FMD and PWV in young adults 4 weeks after positive testing for SARS-CoV-2 revealing significantly lower values of FMD and higher values of PWV in the group of subjects with a suffered SARS-CoV-2 (16). However, data about vascular reactivity and arterial stiffness in acute Covid-19 infection are still lacking and follow-up changes of these parameters during a Covid-19 infection have not been investigated yet.

Underlying pathways by which SARS-CoV-2 may contribute to endothelial dysfunction are yet unknown. Our case and previous data suggest that both, direct cytotoxicity and indirect endothelial injury promote to endothelial dysfunction. Besides a potential but unlikely pathway of SARS-CoV-2 with ACE2 receptors, other pathways promoted by inflammatory mediators including interleukin-6 and prothrombotic mediators, like von Willebrand factor and neutrophil extracellular traps, may result in widespread inflammation and also in endothelial dysfunction (5–8, 13, 17, 18). As acetaminophen has only a weak anti-inflammatory effect, potential interaction of acetaminophen on inflammatory mediators which may affect endothelial dysfunction can be excluded (19). Additionally, as FMD and NMD indicates bioavailability of nitric oxide and PWV and augmentation index are parameters of arterial elasticity, we hypothesize that SARS-CoV-2 exhibits also an influence on nitric oxide metabolism and morphological changes of the arterial wall.

One limitation of our measurements was that we did not fulfill all recent recommendations for the assessment of FMD and NMD according to recent guidelines (10). Recommendations regarding subject preparation, operator-dependent factors and protocol were fulfilled, except for the recommended dose of sublingual glyceryl trinitrate. In our case, 0.4 mg glyceryl trinitrate was used instead of recommended 25 µg glyceryl trinitrate. Additionally, all other recommendations for technique and analysis were fulfilled, except for continuous measurement of velocity and diameter using simultaneous live duplex ultrasound, the use of continuous edge-detection and wall tracking software and calculating peak diameter and shear rate stimulus, since such a software was not available. Instead, offline analysis by a blinded observer was performed. Other limitations are that we conducted measurements of vascular reactivity and arterial stiffness only in one patient with Covid-19 infection and the lacking comparison of the results to a potential healthy, sex- and age-matched control subject.

Our case demonstrated that endothelial dysfunction may be present at a very early stage of Covid-19 infection and seems to be partly persistent even if SARS-CoV-2 is not detectable anymore. Our patient was asymptomatic at the time of verified Covid-19 infection when measurements of vascular reactivity and arterial stiffness were performed and symptoms occurred a few days later. It needs to be elucidated if parameters differ between asymptomatic and symptomatic patients as well as between patients with a different severity of symptoms. Furthermore, it needs to be elucidated if parameters of vascular reactivity and arterial stiffness remain altered as a long-term consequence of Covid-19 or if these changes may be present only in the acute phase of this infection. Moreover, studies evaluating parameters of vascular reactivity and arterial stiffness as potential predictors for cardiovascular events and mortality need to be performed.

In conclusion, we could demonstrate that infection by SARS-CoV-2 may alter different parameters of vascular reactivity and arterial stiffness probably by causing direct and indirectly endothelial dysfunction, which may promote to cardiovascular complications in patients with Covid-19 infection. Further studies evaluating parameters of endothelial dysfunction are urgently needed.

AUTHOR CONTRIBUTIONS

PJ and MB contributed to conception and design of the study.

HK contributed to data analysis. PJ wrote the first draft of the manuscript. All authors contributed to manuscript revision.

REFERENCES

1. Figliozzi S, Masci PG, Ahmadi N, Tondi L, Koutli E, Aimo A, et al. Predictors of adverse prognosis in COVID-19: a systematic review and meta-analysis. *Eur J Clin Invest.* (2020) 50:e13362. doi: 10.1111/eci.13362
2. Zhou F, Yu T, Du R, Fan G, Liu Y, Liu Z, et al. Clinical course and risk factors for mortality of adult inpatients with COVID-19 in Wuhan, China: a retrospective cohort study. *Lancet.* (2020) 395:1054–62. doi: 10.1016/S0140-6736(20)30566-3
3. Klok FA, Kriup MJHA, van der Meer NJM, Arbous MS, Gommers D, Kant KM, et al. Incidence of thrombotic complications in critically ill ICU patients with COVID-19. *Thromb Res.* (2020) 191:145–47. doi: 10.1016/j.thromres.2020.04.013
4. Diener HC, Berlit P, Masjuan J. COVID-19: patients with stroke or risk of stroke. *Eur Heart J Suppl.* (2020) 22(Suppl. Pt t):P25–8. doi: 10.1093/eurheartj/suaa174
5. Varga Z, Flammer AJ, Steiger P, Haberecker M, Andermatt R, Zinkernagel AS, et al. Endothelial cell infection and endotheliitis in COVID-19. *Lancet.* (2020) 395:1417–18. doi: 10.1016/S0140-6736(20)30937-5
6. McCracken IR, Saginc G, He L, Huseynov A, Daniels A, et al. Lack of evidence of angiotensin-converting enzyme 2 expression and replicative infection by SARS-CoV-2 in human endothelial cells. *Circulation.* (2021) 143:865–8. doi: 10.1101/2020.12.02.391664
7. Wang K, Gheblawi M, Oudit GY. Angiotensin converting enzyme 2: a double-edged sword. *Circulation.* (2020) 142:426–8. doi: 10.1161/CIRCULATIONAHA.120.047049
8. Panigada M, Bottino N, Tagliabue P, Grasselli G, Novembrino C, Chantarangkul V, et al. Hypercoagulability of COVID-19 patients in intensive care unit: a report of thromboelastography findings and other parameters of hemostasis. *J Thromb Haemost.* (2020) 18:1738–42. doi: 10.1111/jth.14850
9. Dou Q, Wei X, Zhou K, Yang S, Jia P. Cardiovascular manifestations and mechanisms in patients with COVID-19. *Trends Endocrinol Metab.* (2020) 31:893–904. doi: 10.1016/j.tem.2020.10.001
10. Thijssen DHJ, Bruno RM, van Mil ACCM, Holder SM, Faita F, Greyling A, et al. Expert consensus and evidence-based recommendations for the assessment of flow-mediated dilation in humans. *Eur Heart J.* (2019) 40:2534–47. doi: 10.1093/eurheartj/ehz350
11. Maruhashi T, Kajikawa M, Kishimoto S, Hashimoto H, Takaeko Y, Yamaji T, et al. Diagnostic criteria of flow-mediated vasodilation for normal endothelial function and nitroglycerin-induced vasodilation for normal vascular smooth muscle function of the brachial artery. *J Am Heart Assoc.* (2020) 9:e013915. doi: 10.1161/JAHA.119.013915
12. Ackermann M, Verleden SE, Kuehnel M, Haverich A, Welte T, Laenger F, et al. Pulmonary vascular endothelialitis, thrombosis, and angiogenesis in Covid-19. *N Engl J Med.* (2020) 383:120–8. doi: 10.1056/NEJMoa2015432
13. Gheblawi M, Wang K, Viveiros A, Nguyen Q, Zhong JC, Turner AJ, et al. Angiotensin-converting enzyme 2: SARS-CoV-2 receptor and regulator of the renin-angiotensin system: celebrating the 20th anniversary of the discovery of ACE2. *Circ Res.* (2020) 126:1456–74. doi: 10.1161/CIRCRESAHA.120.317015
14. Inaba Y, Chen JA, Bergmann SR. Prediction of future cardiovascular outcomes by flow-mediated vasodilatation of brachial artery: a meta-analysis. *Int J Cardiovasc Imaging.* (2010) 26:631–40. doi: 10.1007/s10554-010-9616-1
15. Vlachopoulos C, Aznaouridis K, Stefanadis C. Prediction of cardiovascular events and all-cause mortality with arterial stiffness: a systematic review and meta-analysis. *J Am Coll Cardiol.* (2010) 55:1318–27. doi: 10.1016/j.jacc.2009.10.061
16. Ratchford SM, Stickford JL, Province VM, Stute N, Augenreich MA, Koontz LK, et al. Vascular alterations among young adults with SARS-CoV-2. *Am J Physiol Heart Circ Physiol.* (2021) 320:H404–10. doi: 10.1152/ajpheart.00897.2020
17. Pathan N, Hemingway CA, Alizadeh AA, Stephens AC, Boldrick JC, Oragui EE, et al. Role of interleukin 6 in myocardial dysfunction of meningococcal septic shock. *Lancet.* (2004) 363:203–9. doi: 10.1016/S0140-6736(03)15326-3
18. Middleton EA, Hue XY, Denorme F, Campbell RA, Ng D, Salvatore SP, et al. Neutrophil extracellular traps contribute to immunothrombosis in COVID-19 acute respiratory distress syndrome. *Blood.* (2020) 136:1169–79. doi: 10.1182/blood.2020007008
19. Flower R, Gryglewski R, Herbaczyńska-Cedro K, Vane JR. Effects of anti-inflammatory drugs on prostaglandin biosynthesis. *Nat New Biol.* (1972) 238:104–6. doi: 10.1038/newbio238104a0

13

The Predictive Value of Myoglobin for COVID-19-Related Adverse Outcomes

Chaoqun Ma[1†], Dingyuan Tu[1†], Jiawei Gu[2†], Qiang Xu[1], Pan Hou[1], Hong Wu[1], Zhifu Guo[1], Yuan Bai[1*], Xianxian Zhao[1*] and Pan Li[1*]

[1] Department of Cardiology, Changhai Hospital, Naval Medical University, Shanghai, China, [2] Department of General Surgery, The Fifth People's Hospital of Shanghai, Fudan University, Shanghai, China

*Correspondence:
Pan Li
15021333603@163.com
Xianxian Zhao
13764924032@163.com
Yuan Bai
yuanbai@smmu.edu.cn

† These authors have contributed equally to this work

Objective: Cardiac injury is detected in numerous patients with coronavirus disease 2019 (COVID-19) and has been demonstrated to be closely related to poor outcomes. However, an optimal cardiac biomarker for predicting COVID-19 prognosis has not been identified.

Methods: The PubMed, Web of Science, and Embase databases were searched for published articles between December 1, 2019 and September 8, 2021. Eligible studies that examined the anomalies of different cardiac biomarkers in patients with COVID-19 were included. The prevalence and odds ratios (ORs) were extracted. Summary estimates and the corresponding 95% confidence intervals (95% CIs) were obtained through meta-analyses.

Results: A total of 63 studies, with 64,319 patients with COVID-19, were enrolled in this meta-analysis. The prevalence of elevated cardiac troponin I (cTnl) and myoglobin (Mb) in the general population with COVID-19 was 22.9 (19–27%) and 13.5% (10.6–16.4%), respectively. However, the presence of elevated Mb was more common than elevated cTnl in patients with severe COVID-19 [37.7 (23.3–52.1%) vs.30.7% (24.7–37.1%)]. Moreover, compared with cTnl, the elevation of Mb also demonstrated tendency of higher correlation with case-severity rate (Mb, $r = 13.9$ vs. cTnl, $r = 3.93$) and case-fatality rate (Mb, $r = 15.42$ vs. cTnl, $r = 3.04$). Notably, elevated Mb level was also associated with higher odds of severe illness [Mb, OR = 13.75 (10.2–18.54) vs. cTnl, OR = 7.06 (3.94–12.65)] and mortality [Mb, OR = 13.49 (9.3–19.58) vs. cTnl, OR = 7.75 (4.4–13.66)] than cTnl.

Conclusions: Patients with COVID-19 and elevated Mb levels are at significantly higher risk of severe disease and mortality. Elevation of Mb may serve as a marker for predicting COVID-19-related adverse outcomes.

Prospero Registration Number: https://www.crd.york.ac.uk/prospero/display_record.php?ID=CRD42020175133, CRD42020175133.

Keywords: COVID-19, myoglobin, cardiac troponin I, predictive value, severe illness, mortality

INTRODUCTION

Coronavirus disease 2019, caused by severe acute respiratory syndrome coronavirus 2 (SARS-CoV-2), was first reported in Wuhan City, Hubei province of China in December 2019 (1). The pandemic spread rapidly worldwide from China, resulting in 230 million confirmed cases and more than 4 million deaths by September 22, 2021. Clinical manifestations differ greatly among patients with coronavirus disease 2019 (COVID-19), ranging from asymptomatic infections to severe or critical disease and even death (2). Although SARS-CoV-2 was initially thought to be a respiratory tract virus, it has been widely reported that the adverse prognosis of patients with COVID-19 relates largely to the involvement of multisystem organs such as the heart, liver, kidney, brain, and the nervous system (3–5).

Cardiac injury, manifested as the elevation of cardiac biomarkers, namely, cardiac troponin I (cTnI), lactate dehydrogenase (LDH), creatine kinase (CK), CK isomer-MB (CK-MB), myoglobin (Mb), and B-type natriuretic peptide (BNP) or N-terminal pro-B type natriuretic peptide (NT-proBNP), has been detected in numerous patients with COVID-19, and is closely related to the clinical prognosis (6–9). In particular, elevation of cTnI, which was widely reported in several studies, has been identified as an independent variable associated with in-hospital mortality (10).

Nevertheless, elevation of Mb in patients with COVID-19 has been widely mentioned in several studies (11–15). More importantly, Mb presents a potential predictive value in COVID-19-related adverse outcomes. In a study reported by Qin et al., elevated Mb presented with higher frequency on admission and showed the highest overall performance for predicting the risk of COVID-19 mortality among the various cardiac biomarkers (16). However, to the best of our knowledge, a pooled analysis regarding the advantage of Mb in predicting the prognosis of COVID-19 is lacking. Therefore, we conducted a systematic review and meta-analysis to explore the predictive value of elevated Mb for adverse outcomes of patients with COVID-19.

METHODS
Study Protocol
This study was performed according to the Preferred Reporting Items for Systematic Reviews and Meta-Analyses (PRISMA) statement and Meta-analysis of Observational Studies in Epidemiology (MOOSE) reporting guidelines (17, 18). The protocol was preregistered in the International prospective register of systematic reviews (PROSPERO, CRD42020175133). The detailed definitions of laboratory-confirmed COVID-19 cases and severe illness are described in **Supplementary Method S1**.

Search Strategy and Study Selection
Two investigators (DT and JG) independently searched the PubMed, Embase, and Web of Science Core Collection (Clarivate Analytics) databases for relevant articles published between December 2019 and September 8, 2021 using the following keywords: "coronavirus," "nCoV," "HCoV," "SARS-CoV-2,"

"COVID*," "NCP*," "cardiac injury," "cardiac," "biomarker*," "myocardial," "heart," "troponin," and "myoglobin" alone and in combination. The detailed search strategies are presented in **Supplementary Methods S2**. After removing duplicate studies, three reviewers (CM, DT, and JG) were assigned to independently screen the titles and abstracts, and then examine the full texts. Any disagreement was resolved by the senior authors (YB and XZ). The inclusion criteria were as follows: (1) diagnosis of COVID-19 according to the World Health Organization interim guidance (19), (2) gives the specific number of COVID-19 patients with the elevation of cTnI and/or Mb, (3) studies in English only, and (4) sample size of ≥10 individuals. The exclusion criteria were as follows: (1) studies with data that could not be reliably extracted, and (2) editorials, comments, expert opinions, case reports.

Data Extraction and Quality Assessment
Using a predesigned spreadsheet, three authors (DT, CM, and JG) independently extracted the relevant data from the included studies. Corresponding authors were asked via email to clarify or provide additional information. Study quality assessments were performed using the Quality Assessment Forms recommended by the Agency for Healthcare Research and Quality (AHRQ) for cross-sectional studies (**Supplementary Methods S3**). Studies were defined as high quality if a score of ≥7 was attained. Any conflicts with the assessments were resolved either by consensus or by the adjudicators (XZ and PL).

Statistical Analysis
Effect estimates were presented as pooled prevalence or odds ratio (OR) with 95% confidence interval (CI) and visualized with forest plots. A fixed or random-effects model was used according to heterogeneity across studies (if I^2 ≤50%, fixed-effects model; if I^2 >50%, random-effects model) (20). We performed Egger's test and the test performed by Peters et al., and visually inspected the funnel plots to investigate publication bias (21). Sensitivity analyses were performed by systematically removing each study in turn to explore its effect on the outcome. All the analyses were performed using R (version 3.5.3), RStudio (version 1.2.1335), and Comprehensive Meta-Analysis.

Patient and Public Involvement
Patients or the public were not involved in the design, conduct, reporting, and dissemination plans of our research.

RESULTS
Literature Search and Study Characteristics
A total of 106,925 articles were initially retrieved, of which the full texts of 6,542 articles were reviewed (**Figure 1**). Finally, 63 studies were eligible for our analysis (**Table 1** and **Supplementary Tables S1, S2**), and included 64,319 confirmed patients with COVID-19 who presented to a hospital. All these studies were retrospective observational ones. Of the 63 studies, 31 were conducted in China, 18 in the United States, 5 in Italy, 4 in Spain, 2 in Turkey, and 3 in other countries (Libya, Finland,

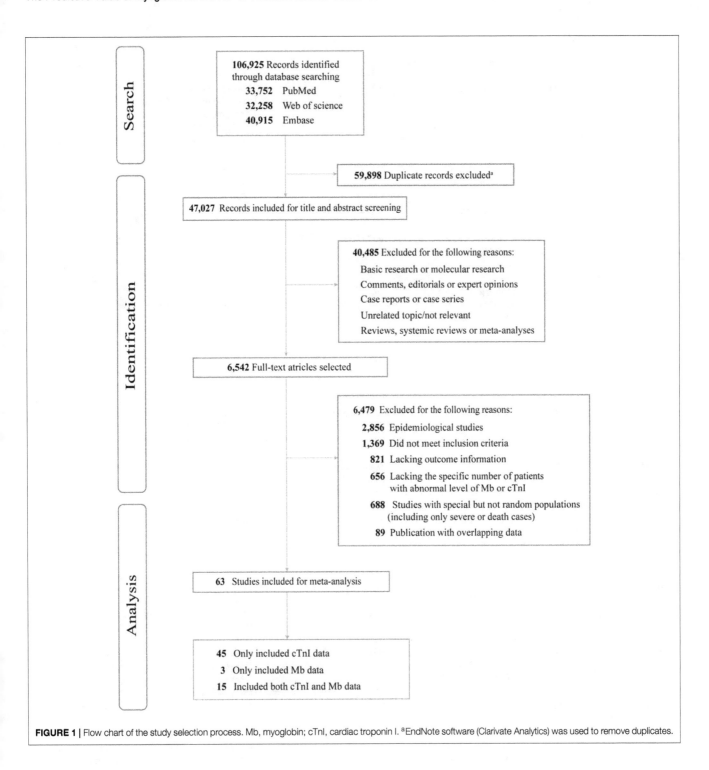

FIGURE 1 | Flow chart of the study selection process. Mb, myoglobin; cTnl, cardiac troponin I. ªEndNote software (Clarivate Analytics) was used to remove duplicates.

and Iran) (**Supplementary Table S2**). Among them, 45 studies only mentioned data of cTnI, 3 studies only mentioned Mb, and 15 studies included both Mb and cTnI. Regarding the differences in Mb or cTnI detection methods and criteria among different hospitals, we listed in **Table 1** the average level of Mb or cTnI, cut-off value of abnormal Mb or cTnI, and number of patients with elevated Mb or cTnI in each study. In addition, preexisting cardiovascular conditions, such as the prevalence of coronary

artery disease (CAD) and heart failure (HF), and the average level of BNP or NT-proBNP were also summarized (**Table 1**).

Incidence of cTnl/Mb Elevation

Among the 63 included studies, the pooled case-severity rate (CSR), case-fatality rate (CFR), and intensive-care unit (ICU)-admission rate were 31.3 (95% CI 23.2–39.4%, $I^2 = 99\%$), 12.5

TABLE 1 | Characteristics of the included studies.

Authors	No.	Cardiovascular condition	Mb	cTnI	Outcome
Arcari L et al.	111	CAD, 12 (11.0); HF, 8 (7.0)	NA	Average level of cTnI, 17 (5–47) pg/mL; cut-off value, 14 pg/ml; elevated patients, 39/103 (37.9%)	Death
Bardaji' A et al.	186	CAD, 20 (10.8); HF, 14 (7.5)	NA	Elevated patients, 41 (22.0%)	Death, admission to ICU
Bhatla A et al.	700	CAD, 76 (11.0); HF, 88 (13.0); BNP, 2,940 (7,962) pg/mL	NA	Cut-off value, 0.01 ng/mL; elevated patients, 82/373 (22.0%)	NA
Cai Q et al.	298	CAD, 25 (8.4); HF, 7 (2.3)	Average level of Mb, 37.1 (29.2–51.5) µg/L; elevated patients, 10/260 (3.8%)	NA	Death, discharge
Calvo-Fernández A et al.	872	CAD, 59 (6.83); HF, 41 (4.73)	NA	Cut-off value, 14.0 ng/L; elevated patients, 225/651 (34.6%)	Death, admission to ICU, mechanical ventilation
Cao J et al.	102	CAD, 5 (4.9); BNP, 12.2 (0–63.1) pg/mL; NT-pro BNP, 417 (132–1,800) pg/mL	NA	Average level of cTnI, 8.0 (3.0–35.7) pg/mL; cut-off value, 0.026 ng/mL; elevated patients, 15/55 (27.3%)	Discharge, death
Cao J et al.	244	NA	Average level of Mb in severe patients, 39.35 (29.21–74.19) µg/L; Cut-off value, 110 µg/L	Cut-off value, 0.04 ng/mL; elevated patients, 27/244 (11.1%)	Severe COVID-19, death, mechanic ventilation
Cao M et al.	198	CAD, 12 (6.0)	Average level of Mb, 5.9 (2.8–15.7) µg/L; cut-off value, 48.8 µg/L; elevated patients, 33/194 (17.0%)	Average level of cTnI, 0.02 (0.01–0.04) ng/ml; cut-off value, 0.04 ng/mL; elevated patients, 22/194 (11.3%)	Severe COVID-19
Chen N et al.	99	CAD, 40 (40.0)	Average level of Mb, 49.5 (32.2–99.8) µg/L; cut-off value, 146.9 µg/L; elevated patients, 15 (15.2%)	NA	Discharge, death
Chorin E et al.	204	CAD, 25 (12.0); HF, 7 (3.0)	NA	Average level of cTnI, 0.02 (0.01–0.04) ng/Ml; cut-off value, 0.05 ng/mL; elevated patients, 84 (41.2%)	Death
Cipriani A et al.	109	CAD, 18 (17.0); HF, 16 (15.0%); BNP, 90 (22–262) pg/ml	NA	Average level of cTnI, 18.0 (7.0–96.0) ng/L; cut-off value, 32 ng/L for males, 16 ng/L for females; elevated patients, 46 (42.2%)	Death, admission to ICU, discharge
Deng Q et al.	112	CAD, 15 (13.4); HF, 6 (5.4); NT-pro BNP, 430.1 (100.6–2859.3) ng/L	NA	Average level of cTnI, 0.01 (0.00–0.14) ng/ml; cut-off value, 0.04 ng/mL; elevated patients, 42 (37.5%)	Severe COVID-19, death
Elhadi M et al.	1,207	CAD, 25 (2.1)	NA	Cut-off value, 26 pg/mL; elevated patients, 90/292 (30.8%)	Death, admission to ICU
Feng Y et al.	476	CAD, 38 (8.0); BNP, 40.85 (21.64–79.37) pg/ml	Average level of Mb, 18.85 (4.8–51.48) µg/L	Elevated patients, 86/384 (22.4%)	Death, discharge, severe COVID-19
Ferguson J et al.	72	NA	NA	Cut-off value, 0.055 ng/mL; elevated patients, 2/45 (4.4%)	Death, mechanical ventilation, admission to ICU
Ferrante G et al.	332	CAD, 49 (14.5); BNP, 72.5 (34.5–198.0) pg/mL	NA	Average level of cTnI, 11.4 (4.7–37.3) mg/L; cut-off value, 0.02 ng/mL; elevated patients, 123 (37.0%)	Death, admission to ICU

(Continued)

TABLE 1 | Continued

Authors	No.	Cardiovascular condition	Mb	cTnI	Outcome
Franks C et al.	182	NA	NA	Cut-off value, 0.03 ng/mL; elevated patients, 80/143 (55.9%)	Death
García de Guadiana-Romualdo L et al.	1,280	CAD, 328 (25.6)	NA	Elevated patients, 344 (26.9%)	Death, admission to ICU
Garibaldi BT et al.	832	CAD, 266 (32.0); HF, 127 (15.0); NT-pro BNP 214 (45–960) pg/mL	NA	Elevated patients, 194/682 (28.4%)	Death, severe COVID-19
Guo T et al.	187	CAD, 21 (11.2); NT-pro BNP, 268.4 (75.3–689.1) pg/mL	Average level of Mb, 38.5 (21.0–78.0) μg/L	Elevated patients, 52 (27.8%)	Death
Han H et al.	273	NA	Cut-off value, 110 μg/L; elevated patients, 29/273 (10.6%)	Cut-off value, 0.04 ng/mL; elevated patients, 27/273 (9.9%)	Death, severe COVID-19
Harmouch F et al.	560	Vascular disease, 36 (6.4); HF, 54 (9.6)	NA	Cut-off value, 0.05 ng/mL; elevated patients, 97/482 (20.1%)	Death, mechanical ventilation, admission to ICU
He F et al.	288	CAD, 85 (29.5); BNP, 35 (13–117.5) pg/mL	Elevated patients, 8/276 (2.9%)	Cut-off value, 0.03 ng/mL; elevated patients, 22/190 (11.6%);	Death, admission to ICU
He X et al.	1,031	CAD, 83 (8.1); NT-pro BNP 124 (43–374) pg/mL	NA	Average level of cTnI, 5.3 (2.5–14.0) pg/Ml; elevated patients, 215 (20.9%)	Death
Hu L et al.	323	CAD, 41 (12.7)	NA	Cut-off value, 0.04 pg/mL; elevated patients, 68 (21.1%)	Death, severe COVID-19, mechanical ventilation
Huang C et al.	41	CAD, 6 (15.0)	NA	Average level of cTnI, 3.4 (1.1–9.1) pg/mL; cut-off value, 0.028 ng/mL; elevated patients, 5/41 (12.2%)	Death, severe COVID-19, discharge
Huang J et al.	98	CAD, 6 (6.0); BNP 119 (54–392) pg/mL	NA	Cut-off value, 0.0229 ng/Ml; elevated patients, 7 (7.1%)	Death, discharge, severe COVID-19
Huang R et al.	202	CAD, 5 (2.5)	NA	Elevated patients, 2/103 (1.9%)	Admission to ICU, mechanical ventilation, severe COVID-19
Karbalai Saleh S et al.	386	CAD, 97 (25.1)	NA	Cut-off value, 26 ng/L for males, 11 ng/L for females; elevated patients, 115 (29.8%)	Death, admission to ICU
Lala A et al.	2,736	CAD, 453 (16.6); HF, 276 (10.1)	NA	Cut-off value, 0.03 ng/mL; OR for in-hospital mortality, 1.75 (1.37–2.24); elevated patients, 985 (36.0%)	Death
Li C et al.	2,068	CAD, 182 (8.8); HF, 14 (0.7); NT-pro BNP 108 (36–370) pg/mL	Average level of Mb, 40.7 (28.4–73.8) μg/L; elevated patients, 174/1,554 (11.2%)	Average level of cTnI, 4.2 (1.9–11.0) pg/mL; elevated patients, 181 (8.8%)	Death, severe COVID-19
Li X et al.	548	CAD, 34 (6.2)	NA	Cut-off value, 15.6 pg/mL; elevated patients, 119 (21.7%)	Discharge, death, severe COVID-19
Maeda T et al.	181	CAD, 36 (19.9); HF, 24/180 (13.3)	NA	Elevated patients, 54 (29.8%)	Death
Majure D et al.	6,247	CAD, 833 (13.0); HF, 529 (9.0)	NA	Cut-off value, 0.045 ng/mL; elevated patients, 1,821 (29.1%)	Death, admission to ICU, mechanical ventilation

(Continued)

TABLE 1 | Continued

Authors	No.	Cardiovascular condition	Mb	cTnI	Outcome
Manocha KK et al.	446	CAD, 94 (21.1); HF, 38 (8.5); BNP 84 (25–300) pg/mL	NA	Average level of cTnI, 0.05 (0–0.34) ng/Ml; cut-off value, 0.34 ng/mL; elevated patients, 112 (25.1%)	Death, admission to ICU
Merugu GP et al.	217	NA	NA	Elevated patients, 34/201 (16.9%)	Death
Mikami T et al.	6,493	NA	NA	Average level of cTnI, 0.03 (0.02–0.10) ng/dl; cut-off value, 0.03 ng/dL; elevated patients, 1,312/2,526 (51.9%)	Death
Özyilmaz S et al.	105	CAD, 14 (21.1)	NA	Average level of cTnI, 2.6 (0–1774.5) pg/mL[a]; cut-off value, 7.8 ng/mL; elevated patients, 21 (20.0%)	Death
Palaiodimos L et al.	200	CAD, 33 (16.5); HF, 34 (17.0)	NA	Cut-off value, 0.01 ng/mL; elevated patients, 56 (28.0%)	Mortality, intubation, O_2 requirement, ARDS, ICU, AKI, RRT, length of stay
Peiró ÓM et al.	196	CAD, 19 (9.7); HF, 14 (7.1)	NA	Average level of cTnI, 14 (4–37) ng/L; cut-off value, 21 ng/L; elevated patients, 77 (39.3%)	Death, admission to ICU, mechanical ventilation
Price-Haywood E et al.	3,481	CAD, 139 (4.0); HF, 128 (3.7)	NA	Cut-off value, 0.06 ng/mL; elevated patients, 270/1,084 (24.9%)	Death, admission to ICU
Qin J et al.	3,219	CAD, 206 (6.4)	Elevated patients, 228/1,895 (12.0%); HR for in-hospital mortality, 6.84 (4.95–9.45) AUC for mortality, 0.83 (0.80–0.86)	Elevated patients, 95/1,462 (6.5%); HR for in-hospital mortality, 9.59 (6.36–14.47); AUC for in-hospital mortality, 0.78 (0.73–0.84)	Death
Richardson S et al.	5,700	CAD, 595 (11.1); HF, 371 (6.9); BNP, 385.5 (160–1996.8), $n = 1,818$	NA	Elevated patients, 801/3,533 (22.7%)	Admission to ICU, mechanical ventilation, kidney replacement therapy, Death
Schiavone M et al.	674	HF, 111 (16.5)	NA	Average level of cTnI, 18 (8–40) ng/L; elevated patients, 130 (19.3%)	Death, admission to ICU, mechanical ventilation
Shah P et al.	309	CAD, 28 (9.1); HF, 65 (21.0)	NA	Elevated patients, 116 (37.5%)	Death, admission to ICU, mechanical ventilation
Shen Y et al.	325	NA	Cut-off value, 48.8 µg/L; elevated patients, 28/325 (8.6%)	Cut-off value, 0.04 ng/mL; elevated patients, 80/325 (24.6%)	Death, discharge
Singh N et al.	276	Vascular disease, 49 (17.8); HF, 56 (20.3)	NA	Cut-off value, 0.017 ng/mL; elevated patients, 132/276 (47.8%) OR for in-hospital mortality, 4.43 (1.61–12.19)	Death
Stefanini G et al.	397	Prior MI, 33/395 (8.4); HF, 18/395 (4.6); BNP, 67 (30–191) pg/mL	NA	Average level of cTnI, max 10.8 (4.3–39.5) ng/L, baseline 7.8 (4.5–25.6) ng/L; elevated patients, 130 (32.7%)	Death, admission to ICU, discharge
Suleyman G et al.	463	CAD, 59 (12.7); HF, 49 (10.6)	NA	Elevated patients, 107 (23.1%)	Death, admission to ICU

(Continued)

TABLE 1 | Continued

Authors	No.	Cardiovascular condition	Mb	cTnI	Outcome
Tanboga IH et al.	14,855	CAD, 2,341 (15.3); HF, 776 (5.1)	NA	Average level of cTnI, 0.08 (0.00–0.28) ng/mL; elevated patients, 1,027 (6.9%)	Death, admission to ICU, mechanical ventilation
Tomasoni D et al.	692	CAD, 148 (21.4); HF, 90 (13.0); NT-pro BNP 303 (96–1,201) pg/mL	NA	Elevated patients, 272/605 (45.0%)	Death
Wang D et al.	138	CAD, 20 (14.5)	NA	Average level of cTnI, 6.4 (2.8–18.5) pg/mL; cut-off value, 0.0262 ng/mL; Elevated patients, 10 (7.2%)	Admission to ICU
Wang Z et al.	293	CAD, 21 (7.2)	Average level of Mb, 57.6 (30.8–116.4) μg/L; cut-off value, 110 μg/L; elevated patients, 58/213 (27.2%)	Average level of cTnI, 0.007 (0.006–0.046) ng/mL; cut-off value, 0.0796 ng/mL; elevated patients, 36/216 (16.7%)	Death
Wei J et al.	101	CAD, 5 (5.0); NT-pro BNP, 71.2 (31.6–237.5) pg/mL	NA	Average level of cTnI, 6.8 (4.3–10.1) pg/mL; cut-off value, 0.014 ng/mL; elevated patients, 16 (15.8%)	Death, severe case, admission to ICU, mechanical ventilation
Wu Y et al.	125	CAD, 11 (8.8); BNP, 65.0 (23.0–178.0) pg/mL	Average level of Mb, 35.0 (27.7–75.65) μg/L; cut-off value, 154.9 μg/L; elevated patients, 14 (11.2%)	Average level of cTnI, 3.9 (1.9–10.3) pg/ml; cut-off value, 0.0342 ng/mL; elevated patients, 10 (8.0%)	Long-term hospitalization
Xu P et al.	703	CAD, 35 (5.0)	Elevated patients, 33/181 (18.2%)	NA	Death, admission to ICU, mechanical ventilation
Zeng J et al.	416	CAD, 13 (3.1); HF, 5/57 (8.8)	Cut-off value, 100 μg/L; elevated patients, 30/174 (17.2%)	Cut-off value, 0.026 ng/mL; elevated patients, 29/345 (8.4%)	Death, discharge
Zhang G et al.	221	CAD, 22 (10.0)	NA	Average level of cTnI, 7.6 (3.6–21.5) pg/mL; cut-off value, 0.0262 ng/mL; elevated patients, 17 (7.7%)	Discharge, death, severe COVID-19
Zhang Q et al.	41	CAD, 1 (2.4)	Average level of Mb, 26.0 (19.7–118.6) μg/L; elevated patients, 11 (26.8%)	Average level of cTnI; 1.5 (0.8–5.0) ng/mL; elevated patients, 41 (100%)	Severe COVID-19
Zhang Y et al.	166	CAD, 30 (18.1); NT-proBNP, 179.0 (67.0–457.0) pg/mL	Average level of Mb, 54.8 (33.8–127.2) μg/L; cut-off value, 106 μg/L; elevated patients, 28/166 (16.9%)	Average level of cTnI, 5.0 (2.2–10.7) pg/mL; cut-off value, 0.0156 ng/mL; elevated patients, 17/166 (10.2%)	Discharge, death
Zhao M et al.	1,000	CAD, 60 (6.0)	Average level of Mb, 44.54 (28.5–85.05) μg/L; cut-off value, 110 μg/L; elevated patients, 132/754 (17.5%)	Average level of cTnI, 0.006 (0.006–0.018) ng/mL; cut-off value, 0.0796 ng/mL; elevated patients, 66/758 (8.7%)	Death, discharge
Zhao X et al.	91	HF, 14 (15.4)	NA	Cut-off value, 0.01 ng/mL; elevated patients, 3/88 (3.4%)	Death, discharge
Zhou F et al.	191	CAD, 15 (8.0); HF, 44 (23.0)	NA	Average level of cTnI, 4.1 (2.0–14.1) ng/mL; cut-off value, 28 ng/mL; elevated patients, 24/145 (16.6%)	Death, admission to ICU

No., confirmed number of patients with coronavirus disease 2019(COVID-19); Mb, myoglobin; cTnI, cardiac troponin I; CAD, coronary artery disease; HF, heart failure; BNP, B-type natriuretic peptide; NT-proBNP, N-terminal pro-B type natriuretic peptide; ICU, intensive-care unit; NA, data not available. [a]Median (range).

(95% CI 10.7–14.6%, $I^2 = 98\%$), and 20.1% (95% CI 15.3–24.9%, $I^2 = 99\%$) (**Supplementary Figure S1**). The prevalence of elevated cTnI and Mb in the general population with COVID-19 was 22.9 (95% CI 19–27%, $I^2 = 99\%$) and 13.5% (95% CI 10.6–16.4%, $I^2 = 92\%$), respectively (**Figure 2**). Furthermore, the meta-analysis showed that elevated cTnI occurred in 30.7% (24.7–37.1%, $I^2 = 86\%$) of the patients in the severe disease group, while the estimated rate of elevated Mb was 37.7% (23.3–52.1%, $I^2 = 90\%$) in patients with severe COVID-19. For the non-survivor group, the elevation rate of Mb and cTnI was 53.4 (95% CI 46.9–59.9%, $I^2 = 0\%$) and 55.5% (95% CI 47.1–64%, $I^2 = 94\%$), respectively (**Figure 3**).

Meta-regression demonstrated that both CSR and CFR were positively associated with the proportion of patients with elevated cTnI or Mb. Regarding logit CSR, the prevalence of elevated Mb showed tendency of higher regression coefficient compared with cTnI (Mb: $r = 13.9$, [95% CI 3.51–24.29, $p < 0.01$] vs. cTnI: $r = 3.93$, [95% CI 0–8.52, $p < 0.05$]). A similar trend was observed in logit CFR (Mb: $r = 15.42$, [95% CI 11.2–19.65, $p < 0.0001$] vs. cTnI: $r = 3.04$, [95% CI 1.84–4.25, $p < 0.0001$]) (**Figure 4**).

Risk of Elevated cTnI/Mb for Adverse Outcomes

The ORs of elevation of Mb/cTnI for the development of severe illness and death were further estimated. In the overall analysis, patients COVID-19 and elevated cTnI were at higher risk of severe illness (OR = 7.06, 95% CI 3.94–12.65, n = 15, $I^2 = 88\%$). Nevertheless, elevated Mb showed tendency of better predictive value for severe illness (OR = 13.75, 95% CI 10.2–18.54, $n = 6$, $I^2 = 39\%$) compared with cTnI. Regarding in-hospital mortality, elevated cTnI (OR = 7.75, 95% CI 4.4–13.66, $n = 13$, $I^2 = 95\%$) and Mb (OR = 13.49, 95% CI 9.3–19.58, $n = 3$, $I^2 = 0\%$) were associated with COVID-19-related deaths (**Figure 5**).

Sensitivity Analysis and Publication Bias

Sequential removal of each trial from the analysis revealed no meaningful differences (**Supplementary Figure S2**). We observed no evidence of publication bias by inspecting the funnel plot or with Egger's test, Begger's test or the test used by Peters et al. ($p > 0.05$; **Supplementary Figure S3**).

DISCUSSION

This systematic review and meta-analysis of 63 high-quality retrospective studies systematically investigated the predictive value of Mb for COVID-19-related severe disease or death compared with cTnI. The main findings of the study are as follows: (1) more patients with COVID-19-related severe disease showed elevated Mb compared with elevated cTnI; (2) elevated Mb presented obvious superiority over cTnI for predicting severe illness, showing 3-fold higher meta-regression coefficient and 2-fold higher OR; (3) furthermore, Mb elevation was more strongly associated with high risk of COVID-19-related death compared with cTnI.

Severe acute respiratory syndrome coronavirus 2 has been reported to be more contagious than previously discovered human coronaviruses (22), with the progression of the COVID-19 pandemic worldwide, there has been increasing concern regarding the "destructive power" of SARS-CoV-2 for multiple system organ damage, such as in the heart, liver, kidney, brain, and the nervous system (5, 23). Among them, myocardial injury is an important manifestation (6). Madjid et al. reported that up to 15% of hospitalized patients with COVID-19 exhibit myocardial injury, with some developing significant cardiac complications, such as biventricular heart failure, arrhythmias, and cardiogenic shock (9, 24). Liu et al. demonstrated that the mortality rate of patients with COVID-19 and cardiovascular disease was as high as 10.5%, which was 11.67 times higher than that of patients with COVID-19 with no preexisting conditions (25). Consistently, our analysis showed that the pooled incidence rate of cardiac injury was 22.9% in the general population, while the rate increased to 55.5% in the non-survivor group, indicating that cardiac injury was common in patients with COVID-19, especially those with poor prognosis.

Abnormal levels of cardiac biomarkers, including cTnI, CK-MB, Mb, and NT-proBNP, have been identified as indicators for COVID-19-related poor prognosis, such as severe illness (26), ICU admission and in-hospital mortality (27, 28). However, there is no consensus on the optimal biomarker for predicting COVID-19-related outcomes. cTnI elevation has been widely studied for its high prevalence in patients with COVID-19. However, in a study by Qin et al., elevated Mb presented with obviously higher frequency on admission compared with cTnI (12 vs. 6.5%) (16). Similarly, our subgroup analysis revealed that elevated Mb was more common in patients with severe COVID-19 than cTnI. Several recent studies have highlighted elevated cTnI as an important risk factor for adverse outcomes, such severe illness (29, 30), ICU admission (31, 32), and death (10, 26, 33). However, our meta-regression analysis suggested that the elevation rate of Mb presented 3-fold stronger association with CSR and 5-fold stronger association with CFR than cTnI. Notably, elevated Mb level showed higher risk of severe illness and mortality compared with cTnI. The results suggested that Mb may serve as a better biomarker for the severity of COVID-19. Accordingly, the dynamic monitoring of Mb might facilitate timely initiation of intensive care, thereby reducing the risk of other adverse events, such as COVID-19-related death.

Myoglobin is an iron and oxygen-binding protein that plays an important role in the storage of oxygen in skeletal and cardiac muscles (34). Previously, it was generally believed that Mb, while sensitive, was not specific for cardiac injury *per se*. Therefore, the prognostic value of Mb as a marker of myocardial injury in patients with COVID-19 has not been taken seriously (35). However, our meta-analysis suggested that Mb has a potential advantage over cTnI in predicting COVID-19-related adverse outcomes, such as the occurrence of severe illness and death. The mechanistic link between Mb and COVID-19 prognosis is unclear, but it may be the distribution of Mb in skeletal muscle besides myocardium, making it more sensitive to the dynamics of systemic states (36). de Andrade-Junior et al. reported that patients with severe COVID-19 are prone to develop muscle wasting and impaired muscle function (37). Moreover, Mb can be rapidly released into the blood in response

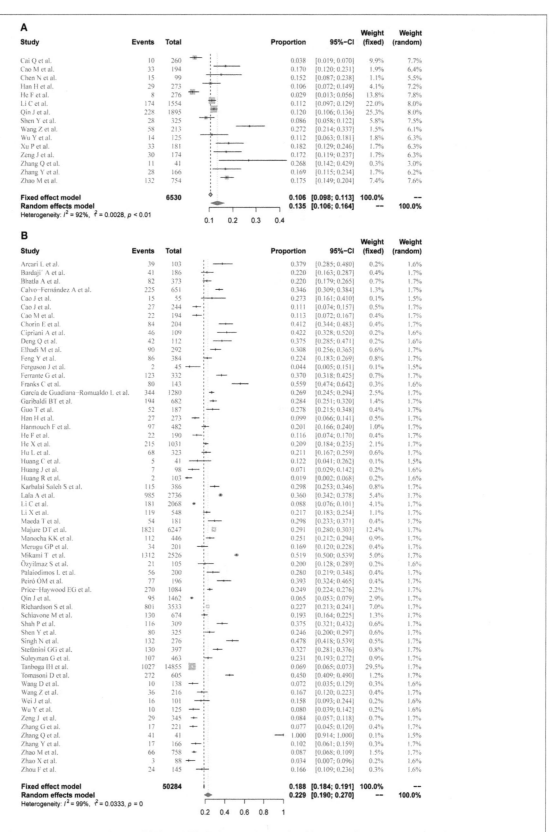

FIGURE 2 | Forest plot for the pooled prevalence of elevated **(A)** Mb and **(B)** cTnI in general population. Mb, myoglobin; cTnI, cardiac troponin I. Proportions are presented with fixed-effects when $I^2 \leq 50\%$ and random-effects otherwise.

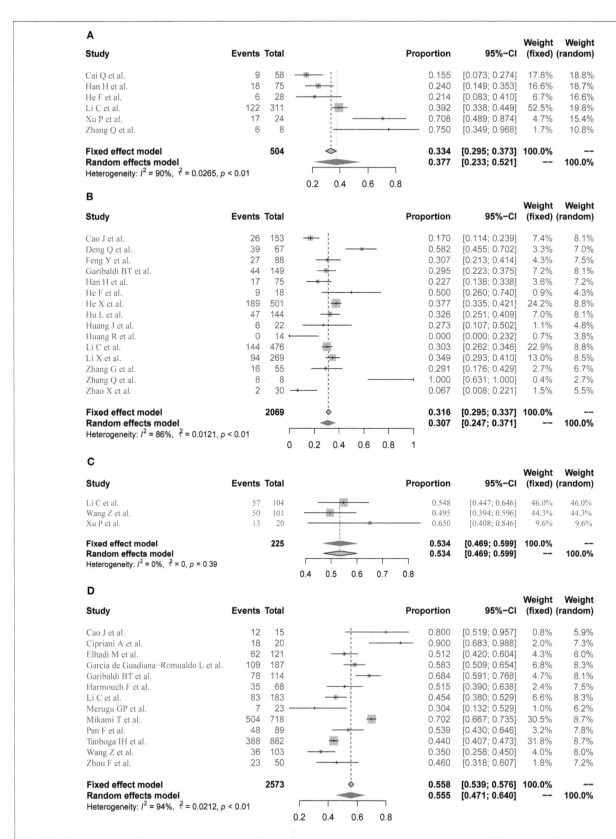

FIGURE 3 | Forest plot for the pooled prevalence of elevated Mb and cTnI in the severe disease and non-survivor groups. **(A)** Prevalence of elevated Mb in the severe disease group. **(B)** Prevalence of elevated cTnI in the severe disease group. **(C)** Prevalence of elevated Mb in the non-survivor group. **(D)** Prevalence of elevated cTnI in the non-survivor group. Mb, myoglobin; cTnI, cardiac troponin I. Proportions are presented with fixed-effects when $I^2 \leq 50\%$ and random-effects otherwise.

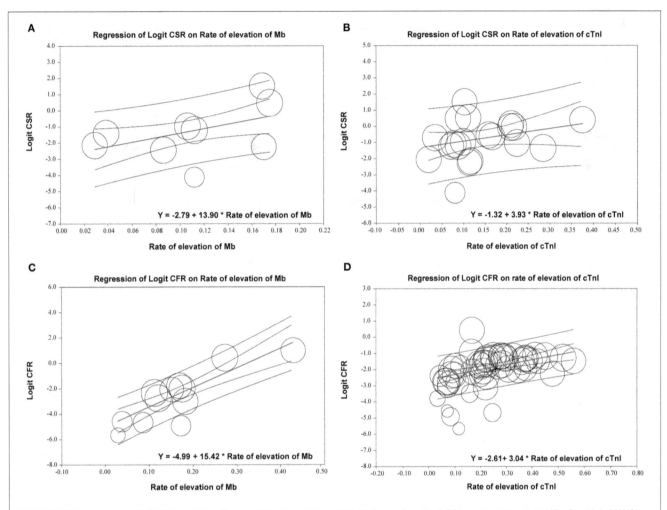

FIGURE 4 | Meta-regression of logit CSR or CFR on the rate of elevation of Mb or cTnI. **(A)** Regression of logit CSR on rate of elevation of Mb; $R = 13.9$, 95% CI 3.51–24.29, $p < 0.01$. **(B)** Regression of logit CSR on rate of elevation of cTnI; $r = 3.93$, 95% CI 0–8.52, $p < 0.05$. **(C)** Regression of logit CFR on rate of elevation of Mb; $r = 15.42$, 95% CI 11.2–19.65, $p < 0.0001$. **(D)** Regression of logit CFR on rate of elevation of cTnI; $r = 3.04$, 95% CI 1.84–4.25, $p < 0.0001$. CSR, case-severity rate; CFR, case-fatality rate; Mb, myoglobin; cTnI, cardiac troponin I. Each circle represents one study; size of the circle is proportional to the population size of each study.

to inflammatory stimuli (38). Wang et al. reported that oxidized Mb can act as a useful marker of myocardial inflammation (39). Furthermore, emerging evidence suggests that inflammatory responses, such as lymphopenia and cytokine storm, are closely associated with severe COVID-19 and high mortality (40, 41). Therefore, besides myocardial injury, the link between elevated Mb and COVID-19 prognosis may also be explained by inflammation and muscle injury. In addition to SARS-CoV-2 infection, increased Mb may also be caused by other preexisting comorbidities, such as chronic obstructive pulmonary disease (COPD), liver diseases, kidney diseases, and cardiovascular diseases, which have also been identified as risk factors for COVID-19 severity and mortality (42–45). Taken together, elevated Mb may be involved in damage directly caused by SARS-COV-2 infection and subsequent multiple organ failure, which partly explains the predictive value of Mb for adverse prognosis of COVID-19.

In the past year, the development and application of vaccines against SARS-CoV-2 brought hope to people worldwide. Notably, for the prevention of adverse outcomes of COVID-19, Chung et al. reported that two doses of mRNA COVID-19 vaccines were highly effective against symptomatic infection and severe consequences (46). Cornberg et al. demonstrated that priority vaccination for COVID-19 in patients with chronic liver diseases may be an important measure to intervene in the course of severe COVID-19 (47). However, the exact efficacy of COVID-19 vaccines against various comorbidities associated with myoglobin elevation is unknown and remains to be elucidated.

This meta-analysis had several potential limitations. First, all the studies included in this meta-analysis were retrospective, and there were relatively few studies involving both Mb and cTnI. Hence, the superiority of Mb over cTnI in predicting value should be interpreted as an observational conclusion.

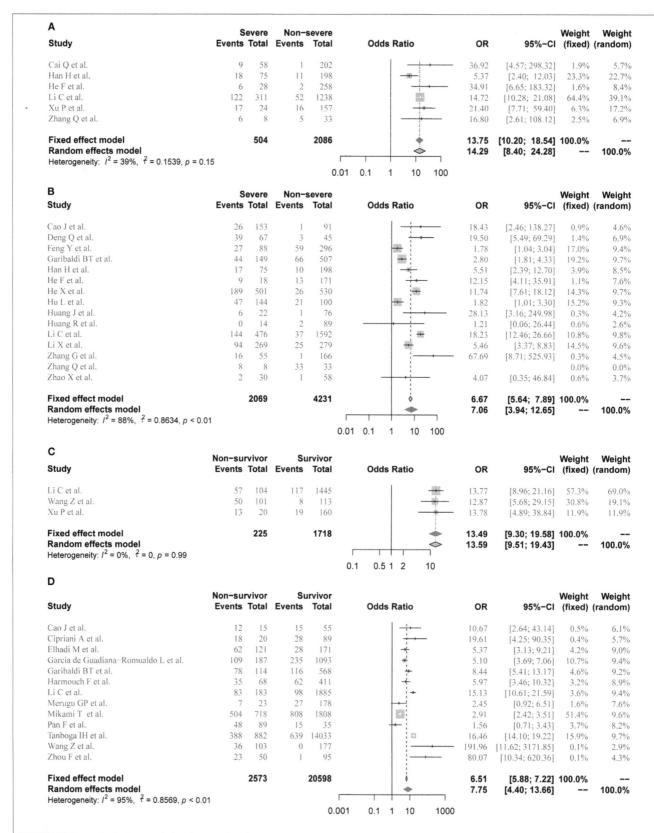

FIGURE 5 | Forest plot for the association of coronavirus disease 2019 (COVID-19)-related adverse outcomes with abnormal level of Mb or cTnl. **(A)** Severe illness and elevation of Mb. **(B)** Severe illness and elevation of cTnl. **(C)** In-hospital mortality and elevation of Mb. **(D)** In-hospital mortality and elevation of cTnl. Mb, myoglobin; cTnl, cardiac troponin I. Odds ratios (ORs) are presented with fixed-effects when I^2 ≤50% and random-effects otherwise.

Further high-quality comparative studies are needed to confirm the difference between Mb and cTnI in predicting prognosis of COVID-19. Second, because of the nature of meta-regression and high heterogeneity across the analyses, we were unable to obtain a definite causal relationship between elevated Mb and poor prognosis of COVID-19. The potential sources of heterogeneity include different cutoffs of elevated cTnI or Mb, mean ages (48, 49), and sex ratios (50) in different studies. Therefore, considering the confounding factors, our results need to be further confirmed by rigorous prospective studies and randomized controlled trials. Third, because of the limited number of included studies, this meta-analysis did not analyze the predictive value of CK-MB, NT-proBNP, LDH, and other cardiac markers except Mb and cTnI. Fourth, studies enrolled in this meta-analysis had a relatively short follow-up period. Therefore, the predictive value of Mb for long-term prognosis of COVID-19 needs to be further explored.

In summary, this meta-analysis showed that patients with COVID-19 and elevated Mb levels are at higher risk of severe disease and mortality. Hence, elevated Mb could be used as a predictor of adverse outcomes in COVID-19. However, high-quality studies are required to confirm these findings and establish the link between elevated Mb and prognosis of patients with COVID-19.

AUTHOR CONTRIBUTIONS

PL, XZ, and YB were the judicators and contributed to the conception of the study. CM, DT, JG, YB, ZG, and HW designed the protocol. CM, DT, and JG searched the databases and finished data extraction, quality assessment, and statistical analysis. CM and DT wrote the first draft of the manuscript. All authors reviewed the manuscript, provided critical revision, and have approved the final version for publication.

ACKNOWLEDGMENTS

We sincerely wish to thank all the medical staff worldwide who made great contribution to the prevention and control of the COVID-19 pandemic. In addition, we are grateful to the investigators of all the studies included in this meta-analysis for providing access to their data.

REFERENCES

1. Li Q, Guan X, Wu P, Wang X, Zhou L, Tong Y, et al. Early transmission dynamics in Wuhan, China, of novel coronavirus-infected pneumonia. *N Engl J Med.* (2020) 382:1199–207. doi: 10.1056/NEJMoa2001316

2. Zeng J, Wu W, Qu J, Wang Y, Dong C-F, Luo Y-F, et al. Cardiac manifestations of COVID-19 in Shenzhen, China. *Infection.* (2020) 48:861–70. doi: 10.1007/s15010-020-01473-w

3. Simoneau C, Ott M. Modeling multi-organ infection by SARS-CoV-2 using stem cell technology. *Cell Stem Cell.* (2020) 27:859–68. doi: 10.1016/j.stem.2020.11.012

4. Synowiec A, Szczepański A, Barreto-Duran E, Lie L, Pyrc K. Severe acute respiratory syndrome coronavirus 2 (SARS-CoV-2): a systemic infection. *Clin Microbiol Rev.* (2021) 34:e00133-20. doi: 10.1128/CMR.00133-20

5. Bae S, Kim S, Kim M, Shim W, Park S-M. Impact of cardiovascular disease and risk factors on fatal outcomes in patients with COVID-19 according to age: a systematic review and meta-analysis. *Heart.* (2021) 107:373–80. doi: 10.1136/heartjnl-2020-317901

6. Dou Q, Wei X, Zhou K, Yang S, Jia P. Cardiovascular manifestations and mechanisms in patients with COVID-19. *Trends Endocrinol Metabol.* (2020) 31:893–904. doi: 10.1016/j.tem.2020.10.001

7. Guo T, Fan Y, Chen M, Wu X, Zhang L, He T, et al. Cardiovascular implications of fatal outcomes of patients with coronavirus disease 2019 (COVID-19). *JAMA Cardiol.* (2020) 5:811–8. doi: 10.1001/jamacardio.2020.1017

8. Kawakami R, Sakamoto A, Kawai K, Gianatti A, Pellegrini D, Nasr A, et al. Pathological evidence for SARS-CoV-2 as a cause of myocarditis: JACC review topic of the week. *J Am Coll Cardiol.* (2021) 77:314–25. doi: 10.1016/j.jacc.2020.11.031

9. Li X, Guan B, Su T, Liu W, Chen M, Waleed KB, et al. Impact of cardiovascular disease and cardiac injury on in-hospital mortality in patients with COVID-19: a systematic review and meta-analysis. *Heart.* (2020) 106:1142–7. doi: 10.1136/heartjnl-2020-317062

10. Nie S, Yu M, Xie T, Yang F, Wang H-B, Wang Z-H, et al. Cardiac troponin i is an independent predictor for mortality in hospitalized patients with COVID-19. *Circulation.* (2020) 142:608–10. doi: 10.1161/CIRCULATIONAHA.120.048789

11. Han H, Xie L, Liu R, Yang J, Liu F, Wu K, et al. Analysis of heart injury laboratory parameters in 273 COVID-19 patients in one hospital in Wuhan, China. *J Med Virol.* (2020) 92:819–23. doi: 10.1002/jmv.25809

12. Xu PP, Tian RH, Luo S, Zu ZY, Fan B, Wang XM, et al. Risk factors for adverse clinical outcomes with COVID-19 in China: a multicenter, retrospective, observational study. *Theranostics.* (2020) 10:6372–83. doi: 10.7150/thno.46833

13. Chen N, Zhou M, Dong X, Qu J, Gong F, Han Y, et al. Epidemiological and clinical characteristics of 99 cases of 2019 novel coronavirus pneumonia in Wuhan, China: a descriptive study. *Lancet.* (2020) 395:507–13. doi: 10.1016/S0140-6736(20)30211-7

14. Cai Q, Huang D, Ou P, Yu H, Zhu Z, Xia Z, et al. COVID-19 in a designated infectious diseases hospital outside Hubei Province, China. *Allergy.* (2020) 75:1742–52. doi: 10.1111/all.14309

15. Zhang Q, Xu Q, Chen Y, Lou L, Che L-H, Li X-H, et al. Clinical characteristics of 41 patients with pneumonia due to 2019 novel coronavirus disease (COVID-19) in Jilin, China. *BMC Infect Dis.* (2020) 20:961. doi: 10.1186/s12879-020-05677-1

16. Qin J, Cheng X, Zhou F, Lei F, Akolkar G, Cai J, et al. Redefining cardiac biomarkers in predicting mortality of inpatients with COVID-19. *Hypertension.* (2020) 76:1104–12. doi: 10.1161/HYPERTENSIONAHA.120.15528

17. Shamseer L, Moher D, Clarke M, Ghersi D, Liberati A, Petticrew M, et al. Preferred reporting items for systematic review and meta-analysis protocols (PRISMA-P) 2015: elaboration and explanation. *BMJ.* (2015) 350:g7647. doi: 10.1136/bmj.g7647

18. Stroup D, Berlin J, Morton S, Olkin I, Williamson GD, Rennie D, et al. Meta-analysis of observational studies in epidemiology: a proposal for reporting. Meta-analysis of Observational Studies in Epidemiology (MOOSE) group. *JAMA.* (2000) 283:2008–12. doi: 10.1001/jama.283.15.2008

19. World Health Organization. *Clinical Management of Severe Acute Respiratory Infection (SARI) When COVID-19 Disease Is Suspected: Interim Guidance, 13 March 2020.* Geneva: World Health Organization (2020). doi: 10.15557/PiMR.2020.0003

20. Higgins J, Thompson S, Deeks J, Altman D. Measuring inconsistency in meta-analyses. *BMJ.* (2003) 327:557–60. doi: 10.1136/bmj.327.7414.557

21. Peters J, Sutton A, Jones D, Abrams K, Rushton L. Comparison of two methods to detect publication bias in meta-analysis. *JAMA*. (2006) 295:676–80. doi: 10.1001/jama.295.6.676

22. Zhu N, Zhang D, Wang W, Li X, Yang B, Song J, et al. A novel coronavirus from patients with pneumonia in China, 2019. *N Engl J Med*. (2020) 382:727–33. doi: 10.1056/NEJMoa2001017

23. Gupta A, Madhavan M, Sehgal K, Nair N, Mahajan S, Sehrawat TS, et al. Extrapulmonary manifestations of COVID-19. *Nat Med*. (2020) 26:1017–32. doi: 10.1038/s41591-020-0968-3

24. Madjid M, Safavi-Naeini P, Solomon S, Vardeny O. Potential effects of coronaviruses on the cardiovascular system: a review. *JAMA Cardiol*. (2020) 5:831–40. doi: 10.1001/jamacardio.2020.1286

25. Liu P, Blet A, Smyth D, Li H. The science underlying COVID-19: implications for the cardiovascular system. *Circulation*. (2020) 142:68–78. doi: 10.1161/CIRCULATIONAHA.120.047549

26. Cipriani A, Capone F, Donato F, Molinari L, Ceccato D, Saller A, et al. Cardiac injury and mortality in patients with coronavirus disease 2019 (COVID-19): insights from a mediation analysis. *Int Emerg Med*. (2021) 16:419–27. doi: 10.1007/s11739-020-02495-w

27. Metkus T, Sokoll L, Barth A, Czarny M, Hays AG, Lowenstein CJ, et al. Myocardial injury in severe COVID-19 compared to non-COVID acute respiratory distress syndrome. *Circulation*. (2020) 143:553–65. doi: 10.1161/CIRCULATIONAHA.120.050543

28. Shi S, Qin M, Shen B, Cai Y, Liu T, Yang F, et al. Association of cardiac injury with mortality in hospitalized patients with COVID-19 in Wuhan, China. *JAMA Cardiol*. (2020) 5:802–10. doi: 10.1001/jamacardio.2020.0950

29. Zhao XY, Xu XX, Yin HS, Hu QM, Xiong T, Tang Y-Y, et al. Clinical characteristics of patients with 2019 coronavirus disease in a non-Wuhan area of Hubei Province, China: a retrospective study. *BMC Infect Dis*. (2020) 20:311. doi: 10.1186/s12879-020-05010-w

30. Huang R, Zhu L, Xue L, Liu L, Yan X, Wang J, et al. Clinical findings of patients with coronavirus disease 2019 in Jiangsu province, China: a retrospective, multi-center study. *PLoS Negl Trop Dis*. (2020) 14:e0008280. doi: 10.1371/journal.pntd.0008280

31. Singh N, Anchan RK, Besser SA, Belkin MN, Cruz MD, Lee L, et al. High sensitivity troponin-T for prediction of adverse events in patients with COVID-19. *Biomarkers*. (2020) 25:626–33. doi: 10.1080/1354750X.2020.1829056

32. He F, Quan Y, Lei M, Liu R, Qin S, Zeng J, et al. Clinical features and risk factors for ICU admission in COVID-19 patients with cardiovascular diseases. *Aging Dis*. (2020) 11:763–9. doi: 10.14336/AD.2020.0622

33. Chen T, Wu D, Chen H, Yan W, Yang D, Chen G, et al. Clinical characteristics of 113 deceased patients with coronavirus disease 2019: retrospective study. *BMJ*. (2020) 368:m1091. doi: 10.1136/bmj.m1091

34. Collman J, Boulatov R, Sunderland C, Fu L. Functional analogues of cytochrome c oxidase, myoglobin, and hemoglobin. *Chem Rev*. (2004) 104:561–88. doi: 10.1021/cr0206059

35. Collinson P, Stubbs P, Kessler A. Multicentre evaluation of the diagnostic value of cardiac troponin T, CK-MB mass, and myoglobin for assessing patients with suspected acute coronary syndromes in routine clinical practice. *Heart*. (2003) 89:280–6. doi: 10.1136/heart.89.3.280

36. Ali A, Kunugi H. Skeletal muscle damage in COVID-19: a call for action. *Med*. (2021) 57:372. doi: 10.3390/medicina57040372

37. de Andrade-Junior M, de Salles I, de Brito C, Pastore-Junior L, Righetti RF, Yamaguti WP. Skeletal muscle wasting and function impairment in intensive care patients with severe COVID-19. *Front Physiol*. (2021) 12:640973. doi: 10.3389/fphys.2021.640973

38. Hendgen-Cotta U, Kelm M, Rassaf T. Myoglobin functions in the heart. *Free Radic Biol Med*. (2014) 73:252–9. doi: 10.1016/j.freeradbiomed.2014.05.005

39. Wang X, Kim H, Szuchman-Sapir A, McMahon A, Dennis JM, Witting PK. Neutrophils recruited to the myocardium after acute experimental myocardial infarct generate hypochlorous acid that oxidizes cardiac myoglobin. *Archiv Biochem Biophys*. (2016) 612:103–14. doi: 10.1016/j.abb.2016.10.013

40. Cao X. COVID-19: immunopathology and its implications for therapy. *Nat Rev Immunol*. (2020) 20:269–70. doi: 10.1038/s41577-020-0308-3

41. Mathew D, Giles J, Baxter A, Oldridge D, Greenplate AR, Wu JE, et al. Deep immune profiling of COVID-19 patients reveals distinct immunotypes with therapeutic implications. *Science*. (2020) 369:eabc8511. doi: 10.1126/science.abc8511

42. Alqahtani J, Oyelade T, Aldhahir A, Alghamdi SM, Almehmadi M, Alqahtani AS, et al. Prevalence, severity and mortality associated with COPD and smoking in patients with COVID-19: a rapid systematic review and meta-analysis. *PLoS ONE*. (2020) 15:e0233147. doi: 10.1371/journal.pone.0233147

43. Bajgain K, Badal S, Bajgain B, Santana M. Prevalence of comorbidities among individuals with COVID-19: a rapid review of current literature. *Am J Infect Control*. (2021) 49:238–46. doi: 10.1016/j.ajic.2020.06.213

44. Oyelade T, Alqahtani J, Canciani G. Prognosis of COVID-19 in patients with liver and kidney diseases: an early systematic review and meta-analysis. *Trop Med Infect Dis*. (2020) 5:80. doi: 10.3390/tropicalmed5020080

45. Pawlotsky J. COVID-19 and the liver-related deaths to come. *Nat Rev Gastroenterol Hepatol*. (2020) 17:523–5. doi: 10.1038/s41575-020-0328-2

46. Chung H, He S, Nasreen S, Sundaram ME, Buchan SA, Wilson SE, et al. Effectiveness of BNT162b2 and mRNA-1273 covid-19 vaccines against symptomatic SARS-CoV-2 infection and severe covid-19 outcomes in Ontario, Canada: test negative design study. *BMJ*. (2021) 374:n1943. doi: 10.1136/bmj.n1943

47. Cornberg M, Buti M, Eberhardt C, Grossi PA, Shouval D. EASL position paper on the use of COVID-19 vaccines in patients with chronic liver diseases, hepatobiliary cancer and liver transplant recipients. *J Hepatol*. (2021) 74:944–951. doi: 10.1016/j.jhep.2021.01.032

48. Chen Y, Klein S, Garibaldi B, Li H, Wu C, Osevala NM, et al. Aging in COVID-19: vulnerability, immunity and intervention. *Ageing Res Rev*. (2021) 65:101205. doi: 10.1016/j.arr.2020.101205

49. Grasselli G, Greco M, Zanella A, Albano G, Antonelli M, Bellani G, et al. Risk factors associated with mortality among patients with COVID-19 in intensive care units in Lombardy, Italy. *JAMA Int Med*. (2020) 180:1345–55. doi: 10.1001/jamainternmed.2020.3539

50. Bellou V, Tzoulaki I, van Smeden M, Moons K, Evangelou E, Belbasis L. Prognostic factors for adverse outcomes in patients with COVID-19: a field-wide systematic review and meta-analysis. *Eur Respir J*. (2021). doi: 10.1101/2020.05.13.20100495. [Epub ahead of print].

14

Clinical Implications of IL-32, IL-34 and IL-37 in Atherosclerosis: Speculative Role in Cardiovascular Manifestations of COVID-19

Ching Chee Law[1], Rajesh Puranik[2], Jingchun Fan[3], Jian Fei[4*], Brett D. Hambly[1] and Shisan Bao[1*]

[1] School of Biomedical Engineering, The University of Sydney, Sydney, NSW, Australia, [2] Department of Cardiology, Royal Prince Alfred Hospital, Sydney, NSW, Australia, [3] School of Public Health, Gansu University of Chinese Medicine, Lanzhou, China, [4] Shanghai Engineering Research Centre for Model Organisms, SMOC, Shanghai, China

*Correspondence:
Shisan Bao
bob.bao@sydney.edu.au
Jian Fei
jfei@tongji.edu.cn

Atherosclerosis, which is a primary cause of cardiovascular disease (CVD) deaths around the world, is a chronic inflammatory disease that is characterised by the accumulation of lipid plaques in the arterial wall, triggering inflammation that is regulated by cytokines/chemokines that mediate innate and adaptive immunity. This review focuses on IL-32, -34 and -37 in the stable vs. unstable plaques from atherosclerotic patients. Dysregulation of the novel cytokines IL-32, -34 and -37 has been discovered in atherosclerotic plaques. IL-32 and -34 are pro-atherogenic and associated with an unstable plaque phenotype; whereas IL-37 is anti-atherogenic and maintains plaque stability. It is speculated that these cytokines may contribute to the explanation for the increased occurrence of atherosclerotic plaque rupture seen in patients with COVID-19 infection. Understanding the roles of these cytokines in atherogenesis may provide future therapeutic perspectives, both in the management of unstable plaque and acute coronary syndrome, and may contribute to our understanding of the COVID-19 cytokine storm.

Keywords: IL-32, IL-34, IL-37, implication, COVID-19

ATHEROSCLEROSIS

Cardiovascular disease (CVD) is the leading cause of death in the world (1). Cerebrovascular disease and coronary artery disease (CAD) are the most prevalent subtypes of cardiovascular disease that result in a high morbidity as well as large economic burden in developing countries (1). Atherogenesis, referring to the development of atherosclerotic plaques, progresses through endothelial dysfunction; leukocytes recruitment; differentiation of monocytes; formation of foam cells; and proliferation of vascular smooth muscle cells (VSMC) (2). The abnormal steps of atherogenesis are regulated by both innate and adaptive immunity *via* cytokines/chemokines modulating the cross-talk between inflammatory and vascular cells (2, 3). Despite the aggressive management of modifiable risks factors for atherosclerosis, for example, lipid-lowering treatments and anti-hypertensives, which promise effective management for atherosclerosis, the mortality and morbidity of CVD are still rather unacceptably high (4). The *Canakinumab Anti-Inflammatory Thrombosis Outcomes Study* is a large-scaled clinical trial which demonstrates a decrease in major adverse cardiovascular events following anti-IL-1β, antibody treatment, supporting the critical role of inflammation during atherogenesis (5).

ATHEROGENESIS

Circulating low-density lipoproteins (LDL) are deposited in the intima at lesion-prone sites and undergo oxidative modification to generate oxidised LDL (OxLDL), which is a potent inflammatory mediator that triggers endothelial dysfunction (6, 7). Endothelial cells respond to OxLDL by expressing adhesion molecules such as ICAM-1 and chemokines including monocyte chemotactic protein-1 (MCP-1/CCL2) for recruitment of leukocytes (7, 8). Macrophages perform a protective role to metabolise lipids *via* scavenger receptors that internalise OxLDL and ATP-binding cassette (ABC) transporters A-1 and G-1 that mediate the efflux of OxLDL (9). However, imbalance of cholesterol influx and efflux results in the accumulation of lipids within macrophages, which contributes to foam cells formation (3, 9). Continuous low grade inflammation within the vessel wall subsequently progressively transforms a fatty streak into a fibro-fatty plaque, which is characterised by a fibrous cap covered by a necrotic core within the grossly thickened arterial intima (3, 10). The fibrous cap is formed by proliferating VSMC that migrate from the media, synthesising and releasing extracellular matrix to stabilise the plaque; whereas the necrotic core is formed by apoptotic macrophages/foam cells that have become exhausted by excessive lipid metabolism (3). Thinning of the fibrous cap is induced by inflammatory mediators triggering apoptosis of VSMC and the production of collagenolytic enzymes that degrade the collagen within the cap (11). Ineffective clearance of apoptotic cells contributes to secondary necrosis, releasing damage-associated molecular patterns (DAMP) to sustain the inflammation, thus enlarging the necrotic core (11). These features characterise the unstable symptomatic plaque that is susceptible to rupture, which results in the release of pro-thrombotic materials to cause intra-vascular thrombosis (10), which in medium sized vessels, such as the major coronary or cerebral vessels, becomes an obstructive atherothrombosis, causing ischaemia and eventual infarction of the tissue perfused by that vessel.

Plaque Phenotypes

Atherosclerotic plaque is classified into stable and unstable phenotypes (3). The stable atherosclerotic plaque is characterised by a thick fibrous cap covering a small necrotic core, which can withstand haemodynamic changes and stresses and is therefore less susceptible to rupture (3, 12). In contrast, the unstable atherosclerotic plaque that is prone to rupture is associated with a thin fibrous cap covering a large necrotic core (10).

IL-32

IL-32, formerly named natural killer cell transcript 4 (NK4), is constitutively produced by peripheral blood mononuclear (PBMC), epithelial and endothelial cells (13, 14). IL-32 consists of eight splice variants, however, only the IL-32α, IL-32β and IL-32γ isoforms have been extensively studied (15). An abundance of IL-32α is found in haematopoietic cells; whereas IL-32β and IL-32γ are the major isoform in endothelial cells and are the most active isoforms, respectively (13, 14, 16) (**Figure 1**).

Overexpression of IL-32 has been reported in rheumatoid arthritis (RA) (17) and Crohn's disease (18), as well as, in human symptomatic atherosclerotic plaques (19), compared to asymptomatic individuals (20). Interestingly, anti-inflammatory activity has been demonstrated in a murine model of asthma with allergic airways inflammation (21). Although the precise explanation for this apparent discrepancy in the activity of IL-32 remains unknown, it may be due to differences in inflammatory regulators between species and/or diseases.

IL-32 and Atherogenesis

IL-32 has been detected in human endothelial cells of atherosclerotic plaques (22) and different isoforms have been demonstrated to exhibit distinct functional roles (23). IL-32α is associated with the suppression of ICAM-1 and VCAM-1 expression on endothelial cells, resulting in attenuation of atherosclerotic lesions, with decreased leukocyte infiltration being observed following overexpression of IL-32α in the IL-32α tg $Apoe^{-/-}$ mouse model of atherosclerosis, suggesting that IL-32α is anti-inflammatory during atherogenesis (24). This is consistent with the finding that IL-32α enhances lipid accumulation and inhibits cholesterol efflux from ox-LDL-exposed THP-1 macrophages *via* the PPARγ-LXRα-ABCA1 pathway (25).

On the other hand, IL-32β promotes vascular inflammation, based on the observation of increased leukocyte adhesion on endothelial cells following overexpression of IL-32β in a transgenic mouse model of atherosclerosis (26), perhaps *via* upregulation of ICAM-1/VCAM-1 expression by IL-32β, as observed on human umbilical vein endothelial cells (HUVECs) following IL-32β stimulation (27). In addition, IL-32 regulates the function of endothelial cells within the aortic, coronary and pulmonary circulations, via IL-1β and other pro-inflammatory cytokines, particularly regulating I-CAM (27).

Thus, taken together, these data support the hypothesis that atherosclerotic development is accelerated by unbalanced expression of IL-32α and IL-32β facilitating vascular inflammation.

Furthermore, IL-32β and IL-32γ have been detected in macrophages of human atherosclerotic plaques, while IL-32γ is associated with greater MCP-1/CCL2 production from monocytic THP-1 cells, suggesting that IL-32γ amplifies local inflammation *via* recruitment of monocytes/macrophages (20). These data are consistent with the finding that IL-32γ enhances monocytes differentiation into macrophage-like cells (28), suggesting that IL-32γ is important for the regulation of the host response against antigens that the immune system detects within atherosclerotic plaques.

It is well known that macrophage heterogeneity is involved in atherogenesis, which consists of pro-inflammatory M1 and anti-inflammatory M2 macrophages (29). Interestingly, M2 macrophages shift towards a pro-atherogenic profile when in a

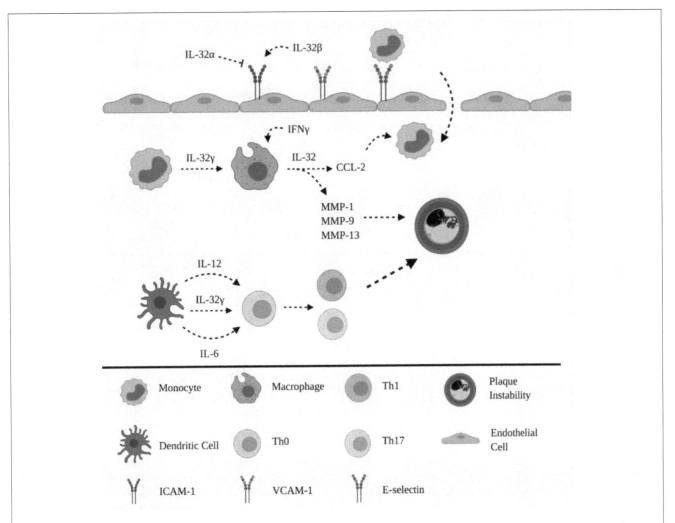

FIGURE 1 | Schematic representation of the roles of IL-32 in atherogenesis. Adhesion molecules are promoted by IL-32β to facilitate monocyte recruitment, whereas recruitment can also be inhibited by IL-32α. The differentiation of monocytes into phagocytic macrophages is induced by IL-32γ, which in turn triggers the release of CCL-2 to recruit circulating monocytes. IL-32γ induces the maturation of DCs, releasing IL-12 and IL-6 to polarise naïve CD4$^+$ T cells into Th1 and Th17 subsets. IL-32γ induces macrophages to produce MMPs leading to atherosclerotic plaque instability. Created with BioRender.com.

pro-inflammatory micro-environment, as reported by the finding that M2 macrophages transform into foam cells *via* upregulation of scavenger receptor CD36 to internalise OxLDL at a higher capacity than M1 macrophages, following their exposure to OxLDL (30). In relation to the IL-32s, M2 rather than M1 macrophages demonstrate a significant upregulation of IL-32 expression in the presence of IFNγ, suggesting that IL-32 is an effector molecule mediating pro-atherogenic responses in the presence of pro-inflammatory stimuli (20). Since IL-32β is a less bioactive form, the upregulation of IL-32β in macrophages may be a form of reverse regulation that is generated by the alternative splicing of the IL-32γ transcript to reduce the overall pro-atherogenic effect (20).

The maturation of murine dendritic cells (DC) is promoted in the presence of rhIL-32γ (31). Specifically, rhIL-32γ increases the production of IL-12 and IL-6 in murine DCs, promoting the polarisation of CD4$^+$ T cells into Th1 and Th17

subsets, accompanied by increased production of IFNγ and IL-17, respectively (31). This is an important mechanism in atherogenesis, in which IFNγ destabilises atherosclerotic plaques *via* the inhibition of VSMC proliferation leading to a thin fibrous cap (10). It is the degradation of the extracellular matrix, i.e., collagen, by matrix metalloproteinases (MMP) that causes thinning of the fibrous cap (3), which can be promoted by IL-32γ *via* increasing the secretion of MMP-1, MMP-9 and MMP-13 from macrophages (20). These data suggest that IL-32 contributes to plaque instability, which supports the finding of a strong correlation between IL-32 and symptomatic plaque phenotype in human atherosclerosis (19).

However, the more controversial role of IL-32, i.e., its anti-inflammatory role, has also been reported. It is well accepted that disruption of the removal of excessive cholesterol in the arterial wall is important in atherogenesis (2), which is regulated by the reverse cholesterol transport (RCT) mechanism *via*

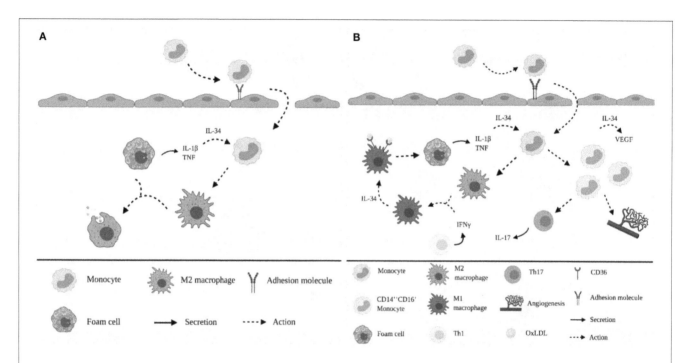

FIGURE 2 | Schematic representation of the roles of IL-34 in atherogenesis. **(A)** In the early stage, TNF and IL-1β produced in the plaque microenvironment stimulate IL-34 production. Infiltrated monocytes are induced by IL-34 to differentiate into M2 macrophages to dampen the inflammatory responses by digesting OxLDL. **(B)** In the advanced stage, IFNγ produced from overwhelming inflammation skews M2 macrophages into an M1 phenotype. These M1 macrophages are induced by IL-34 to upregulate scavenger receptor CD36 to ingest OxLDL, leading to foam cell formation. IL-34 induces the expansion of CD14^bright^CD16^+^ monocytes subpopulations, increasing Th17 polarisation and angiogenesis, together with increased VEGF production. Created with BioRender.com.

high density lipoproteins (HDL) transporting cholesterol to the liver for excretion (32). Increased HDL is associated with ameliorated human coronary atherosclerosis (32). Interestingly, increased HDL has been associated with an IL-32 promoter single nucleotide polymorphism (SNP) in rheumatoid arthritis patients (33), implying an anti-inflammatory role of IL-32 in CVD (33). This is supported by the findings that cholesterol is eliminated *via* ABCA-1, which can be induced by intracellular IL-32γ in hepatocytes (34). In the same study, both IL-32γ and ABCA-1 mRNA have been found in human carotid artery plaques (34). However, this relationship remains to be clarified, since this study did not show that IL-32γ and ABCA-1 can be colocalised *in vivo* in macrophages.

Taken together, the role of IL-32 during the development of atherosclerosis remains to be elucidated. However, we speculate that IL-32 acts differently in different stages of atherogenesis, perhaps depending on the different stimuli occurring within the plaque at various stages of development, based on the data described above. The precise underlying mechanism of IL-32 in atherogenesis, particularly in the presence of M1 vs M2 macrophages warrants further study.

IL-34

IL-34 is a haematopoietic cytokine that shares similar functions with CSF-1/M-CSF, to maintain the viability of the myeloid cells lineage (35). Overexpression of IL-34 is associated with

autoimmune diseases, such as RA (36), inflammatory bowel disease (IBD) (37) and Sjogren's syndrome (38). Upregulated IL-34 is also detected in human atherosclerotic plaques, particularly correlating with unstable plaques (19), suggesting that the pro-inflammatory activities of IL-34 in the advanced stages of plaque development may contribute to acute coronary syndrome and premature death (39). In addition, a substantial circulating IL-34 level has been detected in CAD patients and is associated with the severity of comorbid CAD in heart failure (40, 41) (**Figure 2**).

Roles in Atherogenesis

IL-34 upregulates the scavenger receptor CD36 on murine bone-marrow derived macrophages to promote foam cell formation *via* the internalisation of OxLDL *in vitro* (42). In addition, IL-34 increases the mRNA expression of IL-1β, IL-6 and TNF in murine bone-marrow derived macrophages *in vitro* in the presence of OxLDL (42). These observations are consistent with the finding that IL-34 can elevate the production of chemokines and cytokines, including IL-6, in human PBMC (43). Moreover, IL-34 is upregulated in the presence of TNF and IL-1β (36, 38), suggesting IL-34 may act as a pro-atherogenic factor in both a paracrine and autocrine fashion to enhance foam cell formation in the plaque microenvironment.

Angiogenesis, which is known to promote plaque growth, is promoted in the presence of IL-34 *in vitro* (44, 45). Human PBMCs produce a significant level of VEGF in response to recombinant human (rh) IL-34 (45). Additionally, it is increasingly recognised that monocytes are classified into different subsets based on phenotypic characteristics and have distinct roles during the inflammatory response of atherosclerosis (46), including in relation to angiogenesis. Briefly, these subsets are: classical CD14^{bright}CD16^{-}, intermediate CD14^{bright}CD16^{+} and non-classical CD14^{dim}CD16^{+} monocytes, of which the intermediate CD14^{bright}CD16^{+} monocytes are pro-atherogenic (46). It has also been shown that CD14^{bright}CD16^{+} monocytes express vascular growth factor receptor-2 (VEGFR2) and respond to VEGF, suggesting a pro-angiogenic property (47). Since CD14^{bright}CD16^{+} monocytes are abundantly detected in CAD patients (48), it is reasonable to speculate that IL-34 may promote angiogenesis *via* CD14^{bright}CD16^{+} monocytes stimulation.

In addition, IL-34 induces Th17 polarisation, as evidenced by an increased Th17 cell population following the coculture of IL-34 treated macrophages and naïve CD4^{+} T cells (49). In the presence of IL-34, Th17 polarisation is promoted *via* upregulating IL-6 from human fibroblast-like synoviocytes (50). IL-23 has been shown to be produced by CD14^{bright}CD16^{+} monocytes to induce Th17 polarisation *in vitro* (51). These observations correlate with the high expression of IL-34 in Sjogren's syndrome, in conjunction with an increased expression of IL-17 and IL-23 *in vivo*, suggesting that IL-34 may be linked to the IL-23/Th17 axis (38). Thus, it is reasonable to speculate that IL-34 induces Th17 polarisation during atherogenesis.

In contrast, IL-34 also exhibits an anti-inflammatory capacity. Human monocytes have been shown to differentiate into M2 macrophages in response to IL-34 *in vitro* (44, 52). Interestingly, M2 macrophages that are differentiated in the presence of IL-34, skew towards a pro-inflammatory M1 phenotype in response to IFNγ (52). This finding suggests that IL-34 plays an immunoregulatory role in the early stage of atherogenesis by inducing M2 macrophages to dampen the inflammatory responses and tissue remodelling. This is supported by the report from Boulakirba et al., showing IL-34 promotes M2 polarisation (53).

However, subsequently these M2 macrophages skew towards an M1 phenotype in response to increased IFNγ, which results from overwhelming inflammation in the plaque microenvironment.

Taken together, the role of IL-34 in atherogenesis remains ambiguous due to the complexity of the immune system. However, it is reasonable to suggest that the differential role of IL-34 in different stages of atherogenesis may depend on the specific anti-inflammatory or pro-inflammatory microenvironment in the early or advanced stages of atherogenesis.

IL-37

IL-37 is an anti-inflammatory cytokine member of the IL-1 family (54, 55). IL-37 is constitutively expressed by immune cells including macrophages and DCs, as well as epithelial cells, and is upregulated in response to pro-inflammatory stimuli such as cytokines and TLR ligation (55). IL-37 functions through a heterodimeric receptor, which is composed of IL-18Rα and IL-1R8 (55). Elevated IL-37 expression is detected in autoimmune

diseases such as RA (56) and IBD (57). Elevated IL-37 expression has also been observed in a murine model of atherosclerosis (58) as well as in plasma from acute coronary syndrome patients (59).

IL-37 in Atherogenesis
IL-37 Host Immunity Mediated Atherogenesis
The activity of IL-37 was initially suggested to be pro-atherogenic because high levels of IL-37 are detected in foam cells within atherosclerotic plaques (59). However, interestingly, treatment with recombinant IL-37 has been shown to ameliorate the size of atherosclerotic plaque in diabetic Apoe$^{-/-}$ mice, and is associated with increased anti-inflammatory IL-10, but not pro-inflammatory TNF or IL-18 (60). This striking finding is further supported by another study, showing that plaque size is reduced in IL-37 tg Apoe$^{-/-}$ mice (61) and bone marrow transplanted Ldlr$^{-/-}$ mice with increased endogenous IL-37 expression (62). Moreover, IL-37 reduces atherogenesis *via* decreasing circulating pro-inflammatory and increasing anti-inflammatory cytokines in IL-37 tg Apoe$^{-/-}$ mice (63) and IL-37 treated Apoe$^{-/-}$ mice (58).

Human coronary artery endothelial cells that have been transfected with IL-37 demonstrate downregulation of ICAM-1 in the presence of TLR2 ligand stimuli *in vitro* (64). IL-1β, which is known to upregulate adhesion molecules, is reduced in the presence of IL-37 in OxLDL-treated macrophages *in vitro* (62). These findings, in conjunction with evidence of reduced production of TNF and IL-1β, as well as reduced leukocytes infiltration, in the inflamed colon of IL-37 tg mice with colitis (65), suggest that IL-37 reduces leukocytes recruitment *via* downregulation of TNF and IL-1β during atherogenesis. Furthermore, IL-37-expressing mouse bone marrow-derived macrophages not only reduce uptake of OxLDL, but also decrease macrophage transmigration towards MCP-1 (62). These findings suggest that IL-37 plays an anti-atherogenic role *via* a negative regulatory mechanism to dampen the inflammation in atherosclerosis, perhaps by reducing foam cell formation, pro-inflammatory cytokines, as well as macrophage infiltration. The anti-inflammatory function of IL-37 during atherosclerosis is supported by data from others showing an inverse correlation between IL-37 and M1 macrophage polarisation in human calcified aortic valves (66), as well as in an animal atherosclerotic model (67), perhaps *via* suppressing M1 polarisation. However, while IL-37 reduces systemic inflammation, it does not influence atherosclerosis development in hyperlipidemic LDLr-deficient mice, which might be due to LDLr depletion (68). These mechanisms require future elucidation due to the potential for a major discrepancy between the human and murine context.

IL-37 functions in a dual fashion in DCs to maintain an anti-inflammatory environment by implementing its anti-inflammatory actions intracellularly or by being released as a regulatory cytokine (69). Isolated bone marrow-derived DCs from IL-37 tg mice generate a tolerogenic phenotype in the presence of LPS by downregulating MHC-II and the costimulatory molecule CD40 (70). The findings which show the downregulation of MHC-II and CD86 in DCs from rhIL-37 treated Apoe$^{-/-}$ mice (58) and IL-37 tg Apoe$^{-/-}$ mice (63) suggest that atherogenesis is attenuated *via* reduced antigen presentation (**Figure 3**).

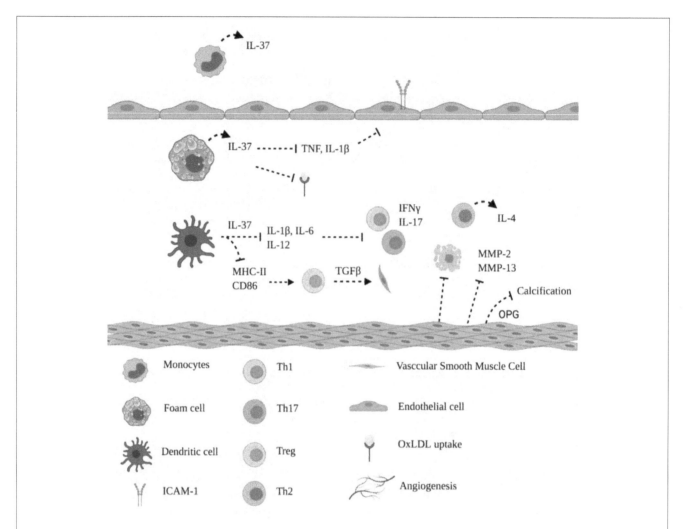

FIGURE 3 | Schematic representation of the roles of IL-37 in atherogenesis. IL-37 is constitutively expressed by monocytes in the unstimulated state. In pathological conditions, IL-37 is upregulated by foam cells to suppress pro-inflammatory cytokines secretion and reduce OxLDL uptake and adhesion molecules expression on endothelial cells. IL-37 downregulates MHC-II and CD86 on dendritic cells to induce Treg activation, promoting collagen deposition via TGFβ production. Additionally, IL-37 reduces IL-1β, IL-6 and IL-12 production, to suppress Th1 and Th17 polarisation accompanied by reduced IFNγ and IL-17 secretion. It remains unclear whether the Th2 population is induced by dendritic cells or IL-37 producing T lymphocytes. IL-37 triggers VSMC to reduce MMP-2 and−13 production, attenuating collagen degradation and inhibiting apoptosis. IL-37 functions closely with VSMC-derived OPG, inhibiting vascular calcification. Created with BioRender.com.

A reduction of Th1 cells is detected in rhIL-37 treated *Apoe*$^{-/-}$ mice (58) and IL-37 tg *Apoe*$^{-/-}$ mice (61), which is consistent with the observed reduction in Th1 cells in IL-37 treated splenic lymphocytes, which is accompanied by decreased IFNγ secretion (58, 61). However, there was no significant reduction of Th17 cells observed in the latter study (61), which suggests that IL-37 promotes Th polarisation during atherogenesis. T regulatory (Treg) cells play an athero-protective role in atherosclerosis *via* IL-10 inhibition of disease progression and TGFβ stimulation of collagen deposition to maintain plaque stability (10). The development of Treg cells is promoted in the presence of isolated bone marrow-derived DCs from IL-37 tg mice *in vitro* (70). This finding is supported by others, showing that Treg cells are increased in rhIL-37 treated *Apoe*$^{-/-}$ mice *in vivo* and increased production of TGFβ and IL-10 is induced

during the coculture of CD4$^+$ T cells with OxLDL plus IL-37-treated bone marrow-derived DCs (58). Interestingly, Th2 cells, but not Treg cells, together with IL-4, are abundant in IL-37 tg *Apoe*$^{-/-}$ mice (61), suggesting that different signalling mechanisms may be exerted by exogenous and/or endogenous IL-37. CD4$^+$ T cells have been shown to be the major source of IL-37 in human atherosclerotic plaques (58, 61). Since Th1 cells shift towards Th2 cells in the presence of IL-37 *in vitro* (61), the hypothesis emerges that Th2 polarisation may be spontaneously induced by CD4$^+$ T cell-derived IL-37 in the plaque microenvironment. These data are in line with others who have shown that IL-37 contributes to the anti-inflammatory response in the development of atherosclerosis, perhaps *via* enhancing Treg cells (71). Interestingly, elevated circulating and local IL-37 in atherosclerotic rabbits is suppressed by atorvastatin (72), suggesting that atorvastatin dampens systemic and local inflammation, resulting in a reduction of IL-37.

IL-37 and Plaque Stability

It is recognised that plaque vulnerability is also promoted by VSMC apoptosis (73). IL-37 inhibits VSMC apoptosis, as evidenced by the reduced apoptotic VSMC area in atherosclerotic plaques of IL-37 tg $Apoe^{-/-}$ mice (61). Such findings are supported by attenuated atherosclerotic plaque in rhIL-37 treated $Apoe^{-/-}$ mice, showing a larger VSMC- and collagen-positive staining area than a mock treated group (58). An increased amount of collagen content, with reduced mRNA expression of MMP-2/-13 within atherosclerotic plaque has been observed in IL-37 tg $Apoe^{-/-}$ mice, compared to $Apoe^{-/-}$ mice only (61), suggesting that IL-37 plays an important role in maintaining plaque stability. VSMC proliferation is reparative and advantageous for atherogenesis in both early and advanced stages, to maintain plaque stability (74). As IL-37 is expressed by VSMC to maintain plaque stability in human atherosclerotic plaques (58, 61), it is reasonable to speculate that IL-37 also induces VSMC proliferation *via* an autocrine mechanism.

Vascular calcification is also one of the key features of atherosclerosis and serves as an independent predictor for acute coronary events (75). Spotty microcalcifications that are dispersed within the necrotic core and fibrous cap drive plaque instability (75). It is well recognised that calcification is driven by VSMC plasticity *via* trans-differentiation into osteoblast, chondrocyte and macrophage-like phenotypes in response to pro-inflammatory cytokines in atherosclerotic plaques, which release pro-calcific factors accompanied by a loss of calcification inhibitors (76). Reduced calcification in the aortic root has been observed in rhIL-37 treated $Apoe^{-/-}$ mice (60), which is consistent with findings in humans, where IL-37 is highly detected in calcified human aortic valve interstitial cells *in vivo*, as well as reduced calcification in calcified human aortic valve interstitial cells in the presence of rIL-37 *in vitro* (77). Osteoprotegrin (OPG), which is a calcification inhibitor, is highly detected in VSMCs of atherosclerotic plaques in rhIL-37 treated $Apoe^{-/-}$ mice (60). However, in the presence of anti-OPG antibody, increased calcified areas are observed, implicating a close relationship between IL-37 and OPG for calcification regulation (60). These finding are indirectly supported by the observation that IL-37 is abundantly detected in human calcified coronary arteries, particularly in VSMCs, compared to normal arteries, suggesting that the purpose of upregulation of IL-37 is to alleviate arterial calcification (78). In addition, a positive correlation between plasma IL-37 and OPG has been detected in patients with severe coronary artery calcification, suggesting that IL-37 is a potential biomarker of arterial calcification (79).

Since an effective treatment to mitigate vascular calcification remains undetermined (75, 76), investigation of the underlying mechanisms of IL-37 in VSMC may provide future therapeutic opportunities.

In addition elevated plasma IL-37 has been detected in acute ischemic stroke patients, and IL-37 is an independent association with poorer prognoses (80), which is consistent with others,

showing elevated circulating IL-37 is associated with a poor outcome in ST-segment elevation acute myocardial infarction in acute coronary syndrome patients (81, 82), although this finding remains controversial (83).

Taken together, IL-37 plays an anti-atherogenic role in atherogenesis. Although the exact mechanism is not well understood, data support speculation that elevation of IL-37 expression is a compensatory mechanism to suppress plaque inflammation, however, inflammatory cells may fail to respond effectively to IL-37 due to exhaustion or the complex nature of the plaque microenvironment, resulting in a continuous release of ineffective IL-37. In relation to COVID-19, IL-37 has been suggested to be a potential treatment based on its anti-inflammatory profile to inhibit IL-1β, IL-6 and TNF, which are the main players of the cytokine storm (84).

CLINICAL IMPLICATIONS OF IL-32, IL-34 AND IL37 IN ATHEROSCLEROSIS

The role of IL-32 during the development of atherosclerosis has been illustrated, showing that IL-32 promotes angiogenesis on endothelial cells, suggesting IL-32 boosts the development of atherosclerosis (85). This is in line with others, showing that the protective role of IL-32 during the development of atherosclerosis is related to a single promoter single-nucleotide polymorphism (SNP) in IL-32, contributing to modified lipid profiles, especially in rheumatoid arthritis patients (33). Furthermore, the benefit of the SNP in IL-32 is related to reduce pro-inflammatory cytokines and increases HDLc concentration (15), further supporting the role of IL-32 during atherogenesis. This may also in line with the findings following influenza viral challenge, showing that increased IL-32 is beneficial against the viral infection (86).

The role of IL-34 during the development of atherosclerosis has been demonstrated, since there is an association between the level of IL-34 and severity of coronary artery disease in patients with heart failure, and IL-34 is an independent risk factor for CAD among heart failure patients, regardless of the systolic function (41). In addition, there is evidence from others, showing that IL-34 is significantly induced in influenza infected patients in an autocrine and paracrine fashion (87), supporting a role for IL-34 in the course of SARS-COV-2 viral infection. Furthermore, the possible mechanisms utilised by IL-34 in atherogenesis have been demonstrated via a linkage among IL-34, obesity, chronic inflammation, and insulin resistance, suggesting that IL-34 enhances atheroma *via* insulin resistance in obese patients (88).

Finally, increased circulating IL-37 levels have been correlated with high coronary calcium score levels, suggesting that IL-37 may contribute to the activation of inflammation. Furthermore, IL-37 has been proposed as a predictor of severe coronary artery disease (79). In addition, the importance of elevated serum and urine IL-37 has been demonstrated in post-ischemic stroke patients (89). However, it is unclear whether the increased IL-37 results from or results in such clinical manifestations. The possible mechanism of the anti-inflammatory role of IL-37 may be by antagonising inflammatory responses while retaining type I interferon, subsequently maintaining the functionalities of vital organs (90). The role of IL-37 in COVID-19 is supported by the findings in influenza viral infection, showing that IL-37 ameliorates influenza pneumonia *in vivo* (91). However, we have reviewed the mechanisms of action of IL-32, -34 and -37 in atherosclerosis, allowing us to speculate on the possible pathogenesis of SARS-CoV-2 involvement in CVD.

SPECULATIVE ROLE OF IL-32, IL-34 AND IL-37 IN ATHEROSCLEROSIS AND COVID-19

COVID-19 is caused by severe acute respiratory syndrome coronavirus 2 (SARS-CoV-2) (92), which is similar to severe acute respiratory syndrome coronavirus (SARS-CoV) (92) and Middle East respiratory syndrome coronavirus (MERS-CoV) (93). SARS-CoV-2 infects host cells by binding to the cell surface receptor angiotensin converting enzyme 2 (ACE2) receptor *via* the viral spike (S) protein (92). The original COVID-19 was first reported in Wuhan (94), then other regions of China (95, 95) and the became a pandemic (96).

Based on the current information available, during the course of COVID-19, particularly in moderate to severe COVID-19 patients, there is likely to be a contribution of COVID-19 in atherosclerosis, perhaps due to the cytokine storm causing vascular dysfunction via the ACE2 pathway, which likely further enhances local inflammation (97) and subsequently results in further activation of endothelial cells in large vessels (98), in addition to the microvascular system. Such insults from the cytokine storm also contribute to hyper-coagulation (99), but this will not be discussed further in the current review.

The role of IL-32 may be induced in local macro-vessels and micro-vessels, which may be due to SARS-COV-2 viral challenge via the ACE2-spike protein pathway. IL-32 may contribute to quench both systemic and local inflammation, which may be effective in moderate COVID-19 patients, but likely fails in severe patients. Subsequently, major organ failure would be induced due to infarction, e.g., heart, lung and kidney (100), particularly in the more susceptible COVID-19 patients. This speculation is supported by others, who have shown that steroids may help to reduce clinical symptoms and shorten the course of COVID-19 (101).

In contrast, IL-34 may contribute to atherosclerosis, but its role in COVID-19 remains unclear. We believe that IL-34 would be secreted by infiltrating inflammatory leucocytes, particularly macrophages and lymphocytes following the cytokine storm in COVID-19 patients (102). More obvious vascular manifestations would then result.

It has been reported that circulating IL-37 is elevated in COVID-19 infected patients. Interestingly, the patients with higher IL-37 had a shorter hospitalisation period than the lower group, suggesting that IL-37 may provide protection during the course of COVID-19 infection (90).

However, there is not yet any solid evidence to clearly state the direct involvement among IL-32, 34 and 37 in the atherogenesis in COVID-19 patients.

In addition there is a strong association between cardiovascular disease (CVD) and the susceptibility to, and the outcomes of, COVID-19 (103), including coronary artery disease (CAD), particularly among those patients with co-existing diabetes mellitus (104). Patients with pre-existing CVD, including hypertension, coronary artery disease (CAD) and diabetes mellitus are more susceptible to SARS-CoV-2 infection and are more likely to develop exaggerated cardiovascular sequelae (105), hence there is a higher prevalence of severe disease in the elderly population (106). A major contributing factor to the higher susceptibility among patients with pre-existing CVD is the higher levels of cell surface expression of ACE2, which makes the patients more vulnerable to SARS-CoV-2 viral infection (106, 107). Additionally, a small proportion of young adults without pre-existing CVD also develop cardiovascular complications following SARS-CoV-2 infection (108), which may be related to their exaggerated host immunity (cytokine storm) (109). One of the key contributing factors for the higher mortality and morbidity in COVID-19 patients is excess local production of pro-inflammatory cytokines, such as IL-1β, IL-6, IL-8 and TNF in key organs (heart, lungs and liver) (110–112), which is termed a cytokine storm (113). Consequently, substantial damage occurs in the heart, lungs, liver and kidneys, which contributes to the disease severity in COVID-19 patients (110). Although the underlying mechanism of SARS-CoV-2 viral attack is not well understood, these findings above suggest that a relationship exists between COVID-19 and CVD outcomes that is both bidirectional and multifactorial (106, 114). Thus, it is reasonable to speculate that many COVID-19-related heart problems are due to a cytokine storm, either in the heart or major arteries (115).

Interestingly, there is some limited data emerging in the literature supporting the view that COVID-19 may increase the rate of acute plaque rupture (116, 117). Respiratory infections such as influenza are known to be capable of triggering acute coronary syndrome (118), so it is likely that COVID-19 will act in a similar manner. A recent case report of an ACS event during COVID-19 infection supports this likelihood (116). Similarly, the likely mechanisms underpinning increased plaque instability during COVID-19 infection have been explored (107, 117).

CONCLUSION

We conclude that IL-32 provides athero-protection *via* differential regulation of polarisation of macrophages in different stages of atherogenesis, perhaps depending on the different stimuli occurring within the plaque at various stages of development. Subsequently IL-32 down-regulates the activities of CCL-2 and MMPs, and finally ABCA1 pathway

IL-34 is pro-atherogenic and its role is stage dependent. In the early stage, recruited monocytes are induced by IL-34 to differentiate into M2 macrophages to dampen the inflammation in the presence of stimuli, e.g., OxLDL, in an autocrine and paracrine fashion. In the advanced stage, particularly in some SNP populations, macrophages are skewed towards the M1 phenotype, especially in the presence of a large amount of IFNγ. IL-34 induced M1 macrophages upregulate scavenger receptor CD36 to ingest OxLDL, leading to foam cell formation. Subsequently, IL-34 induces the expansion of CD14^{bright}CD16^{+} monocytes subpopulations, further boosting the pro-inflammatory responses, including increasing Th17.

IL-37 is also athero-protective. Constitutively expressed IL-37 can be upregulated by foam cells to dampen proinflammatory cytokines secretion, reduce OxLDL uptake and adhesion molecules expression on endothelial cells, as well as downregulate MHC-II and CD86 on dendritic cells to induce Treg activation *via* TGFβ production. In addition, IL-37 reduces IL-1β, IL-6 and IL-12 to suppress Th1/Th17 polarisation, and subsequently down-regulates IFNγ and IL-17 secretion. IL-37 also reduces MMPs on VSMC and attenuates collagen degradation and inhibits apoptosis. Finally, IL-37 inhibits vascular calcification via VSMC-derived OPG.

Finally IL-32 and IL-37 may be protective while IL-34 may contribute to the development of atherosclerosis. In addition, we speculate that the role of IL-32 and 37 may also be beneficial, but IL-34 may be harmful, during the course of COVID-19. Such information highlights gaps in our current understanding for future studies to investigate. Our figures offer a very dynamic summary of these cytokines during the development of atherosclerosis. We believe that our review provides more in-depth information for both basic scientists and clinicians.

AUTHOR CONTRIBUTIONS

CL: conceptualised, drafted, and wrote the manuscript. RP and JFa: conceptualised. JFe: revised the manuscript. BH: revised and edited the manuscript. SB: conceptualised, drafted, and edited the manuscript. All authors contributed to the article and approved the submitted version.

ACKNOWLEDGMENTS

We acknowledge the supporters from SJTU research grant 2019 at the University of Sydney and Science and Technology Commission of Shanghai Municipality (19DZ2280500).

REFERENCES

1. World Health Organisation. *Cardiovascular diseases (CVDs)*. (2017). Available online at: https://www.who.int/news-room/fact-sheets/detail/cardiovascular-diseases-(cvds) (accessed 30 Oct, 2020).
2. Ramji DP, Davies TS. Cytokines in atherosclerosis: Key players in all stages of disease and promising therapeutic targets. *Cytokine & Growth Factor Rev.* (2015) 26:673–85. doi: 10.1016/j.cytogfr.2015.04.003
3. Libby P. Inflammation in atherosclerosis. *Arteriosclerosis, thrombosis, vascular biology.* (2012) 32:2045–51. doi: 10.1161/ATVBAHA.108.179705
4. Martínez GJ, Celermajer DS, Patel S, The NLRP3 inflammasome and the emerging role of colchicine to inhibit atherosclerosis-associated inflammation. *Atherosclerosis.* (2018) 269:262–71. doi: 10.1016/j.atherosclerosis.2017.12.027
5. Ridker PM, Everett BM, Thuren T, MacFadyen JG, Chang WH, Ballantyne C, et al. Antiinflammatory therapy with canakinumab for atherosclerotic disease. *N Engl J Med.* (2017) 377:1119–31. doi: 10.1056/NEJMoa1707914
6. Cinoku II, Mavragani CP, Moutsopoulos HM. Atherosclerosis: Beyond the lipid storage hypothesis. The role of autoimmunity. *Eur J Clin Invest.* (2020) 50:e13195. doi: 10.1111/eci.13195
7. Libby P. Inflammation in atherosclerosis. *Nature.* (2002) 420:868–74. doi: 10.1038/nature01323
8. Tedgui, Mallat Z. Cytokines in Atherosclerosis: Pathogenic and Regulatory Pathways. *Physiological Rev.* (2006) 86:515–81. doi: 10.1152/physrev.00024.2005
9. Schaftenaar F, Frodermann V, Kuiper J, Lutgens E. Atherosclerosis: the interplay between lipids and immune cells. *Curr Opin Lipidol.* (2016) 27:209–15. doi: 10.1097/MOL.0000000000000302
10. Gisterå, Hansson GK. The immunology of atherosclerosis. *Nature Rev Nephrol.* (2017) 13:368–80. doi: 10.1038/nrneph.2017.51
11. Hansson GK, Libby P, Tabas I. Inflammation and plaque vulnerability. *J Internal Med.* (2015) 278:483–93. doi: 10.1111/joim.12406
12. Najib E, Puranik R, Duflou J, Xia Q, Bao S. Age related inflammatory characteristics of coronary artery disease. *Int J Cardiol.* (2012) 154:65–70. doi: 10.1016/j.ijcard.2010.09.013
13. Kim SH, Han SY, Azam T, Yoon DY, Dinarello CA. Interleukin-32: A Cytokine and Inducer of TNFα. *Immunity.* (2005) 22:131–42. doi: 10.1016/S1074-7613(04)00380-2

14. Kobayashi H, Lin PC. Molecular characterization of IL-32 in human endothelial cells. *Cytokine.* (2009) 46:351–58. doi: 10.1016/j.cyto.2009.03.007
15. Damen MSMA, Popa CA, Netea MG, Dinarello CA, Joosten LAB. Interleukin-32 in chronic inflammatory conditions is associated with a higher risk of cardiovascular diseases. *Atherosclerosis.* (2017) 264:83–91. doi: 10.1016/j.atherosclerosis.2017.07.005
16. Choi JD, Bae SY, Hong JW, Azam T, Dinarello CA, Her E, et al. Identification of the most active interleukin-32 isoform. *Immunology.* (2009) 126:535–42. doi: 10.1111/j.1365-2567.2008.02917.x
17. Joosten LAB, Netea MG, Kim SH, Yoon DY, Oppers-Walgreen B, Radstake TRD, et al. IL-32, a proinflammatory cytokine in rheumatoid arthritis. *Proc Natl Acad Sci USA.* (2006) 103:3298–303. doi: 10.1073/pnas.0511233103
18. Netea MG, Azam T, Ferwerda G, Girardin SE, Walsh M, Park JS, et al. IL-32 synergizes with nucleotide oligomerization domain (NOD) 1 and NOD2 ligands for IL-1β and IL-6 production through a caspase 1-dependent mechanism. *Proc Natl Acad Sci USA.* (2005) 102:16309–314. doi: 10.1073/pnas.0508237102
19. Xia Q, Kahramanian A, Arnott C, Bao S, Patel S. Characterisation of novel cytokines in human atherosclerotic plaque. *Int J Cardiol.* (2014) 176:1167–69. doi: 10.1016/j.ijcard.2014.07.252
20. Heinhuis B, Popa CD, van Tits BLJH, Kim S-H, Zeeuwen PL, van den Berg WB, et al. Towards a role of interleukin-32 in atherosclerosis. *Cytokine.* (2013) 64: 433–40. doi: 10.1016/j.cyto.2013.05.002
21. Bang B-R, Kwon H-S, Kim S-H, Yoon S-Y, Choi J-D, Hong GH, et al. Interleukin-32γ suppresses allergic airway inflammation in mouse models of asthma. *Am J Respir Cell Mol Biol.* (2014) 50:1021–30. doi: 10.1165/rcmb.2013-0234OC
22. Yang Z, Shi L, Xue Y, Zeng T, Shi Y, Lin Y, et al. Interleukin-32 increases in coronary arteries and plasma from patients with coronary artery disease. *Clinica Chimica Acta.* (2019) 497:104–09. doi: 10.1016/j.cca.2019.07.019
23. Kang J-W, Park YS, Lee DH, Kim MS, Bak Y, Ham SY, et al. Interaction network mapping among IL-32 isoforms. *Biochimie.* (2014) 101:248–51. doi: 10.1016/j.biochi.2014.01.013
24. Son DJ, Jung YY, Seo YS, Park H, Lee DH, Kim S, et al. Interleukin-32α inhibits endothelial inflammation, vascular smooth muscle cell activation, and atherosclerosis by upregulating timp3 and reck

through suppressing microRNA-205 biogenesis. *Theranostics.* (2017) 7:2186. doi: 10.7150/thno.18407

25. Xu Z, Dong A, Feng Z, Li J. Interleukin-32 promotes lipid accumulation through inhibition of cholesterol efflux. *Exp Ther Med.* (2017) 14:947–52. doi: 10.3892/etm.2017.4596

26. Kobayashi H, Huang J, Ye F, Shyr Y, Blackwell TS, Lin PC. Interleukin-32β propagates vascular inflammation and exacerbates sepsis in a mouse model. *PloS ONE.* (2010) 5:e9458. doi: 10.1371/journal.pone.0009458

27. Nold-Petry CA, Nold MF, Zepp JA, Kim S-H, Voelkel NF, Dinarello CA. IL-32–dependent effects of IL-1β on endothelial cell functions. *Proc Natl Acad Sci USA.* (2009) 106:388–88. doi: 10.1073/pnas.0813334106

28. Netea MG, Lewis EC, Azam T, Joosten LA, Jaekal J, Bae S-Y, et al. Interleukin-32 induces the differentiation of monocytes into macrophage-like cells. *Proc Natl Acad Sci USA.* (2008) 105:3515–20. doi: 10.1073/pnas.0712381105

29. Moore KJ, Tabas I. Macrophages in the pathogenesis of atherosclerosis. *Cell.* (2011) 145:34–355. doi: 10.1016/j.cell.2011.04.005

30. van Tits LJH, Stienstra R, van Lent PL, Netea MG, Joosten LAB, Stalenhoef AFH. Oxidized LDL enhances pro-inflammatory responses of alternatively activated M2 macrophages: A crucial role for Krüppel-like factor 2. *Atherosclerosis.* (2011) 214:345–9. doi: 10.1016/j.atherosclerosis.2010.11.018

31. Jung MY, Son MH, Kim SH, Cho D, Kim TS. IL-32γ induces the maturation of dendritic cells with Th1-and Th17-polarizing ability through enhanced IL-12 and IL-6 production. *J Immunol.* (2011) 186:6848–59. doi: 10.4049/jimmunol.1003996

32. McLaren JE, Michael DR, Ashlin TG, Ramji DP. Cytokines, macrophage lipid metabolism and foam cells: implications for cardiovascular disease therapy. *Prog Lipid Res.* (2011) 50:331–47. doi: 10.1016/j.plipres.2011.04.002

33. Damen SMA, Agca R, Holewijn S, De Graaf J, Dos Santos JC, Van Riel PL, et al. IL-32 promoter SNP rs4786370 predisposes to modified lipoprotein profiles in patients with rheumatoid arthritis. *Sci Rep.* (2017) 7:1–9. doi: 10.1038/srep41629

34. Damen SMA, Dos Santos JC, Hermsen R, van der Vliet JA, Netea MG, Riksen NP, et al. Interleukin-32 upregulates the expression of ABCA1 and ABCG1 resulting in reduced intracellular lipid concentrations in primary human hepatocytes. *Atherosclerosis.* (2018) 271:193–202. doi: 10.1016/j.atherosclerosis.2018.02.027

35. Lin H, Lee E, Hestir K, Leo C, Huang M, Bosch E, et al. Discovery of a Cytokine and Its Receptor by Functional Screening of the Extracellular Proteome. *Science.* (2008) 320:807–11. doi: 10.1126/science.1154370

36. Chemel M, Le Goff B, Brion R, Cozic C, Berreur M, Amiaud J, et al. Interleukin 34 expression is associated with synovitis severity in rheumatoid arthritis patients. *Ann Rheum Dis.* (2012) 71:150. doi: 10.1136/annrheumdis-2011-200096

37. Zwicker S, Gisele Martinez L, Bosma M, Gerling M, Clark R, Majster M, et al. Interleukin 34: a new modulator of human and experimental inflammatory bowel disease. *Clini Sci.* (2015) 129:28–90. doi: 10.1042/CS20150176

38. Ciccia F, Alessandro R, Rodolico V, Guggino G, Raimondo S, Guarnotta C, et al. IL-34 is overexpressed in the inflamed salivary glands of patients with Sjögren's syndrome and is associated with the local expansion of pro-inflammatory CD14brightCD16+ monocytes. *Rheumatology (Oxford).* (2013) 52:1009–17. doi: 10.1093/rheumatology/kes435

39. Fang BA, Dai A, Duflou J, Zhang X, Puranik R, Bao S. Age-related inflammatory mediators in coronary artery disease (II). *Int J Cardiol.* (2013) 168:4839–41. doi: 10.1016/j.ijcard.2013.07.157

40. Li Z, Jin D, Wu Y, Zhang K, Hu P, Cao X, et al. Increased serum interleukin-34 in patients with coronary artery disease. *J Int Med Res.* (2012) 40:1866–70. doi: 10.1177/030006051204000525

41. Fan Q, Yan X, Zhang H, Lu L, Zhang Q, Wang F, et al. IL-34 is associated with the presence and severity of renal dysfunction and coronary artery disease in patients with heart failure. *Sci Rep.* (2016) 6:39324. doi: 10.1038/srep39324

42. Liu Q, Fan J, Bai J, Peng L, Zhang T, Deng L, et al. IL-34 promotes foam cell formation by enhancing CD36 expression through p38 MAPK pathway. *Sci Rep.* (2018) 8:1–10. doi: 10.1038/s41598-018-35485-2

43. Eda H, Zhang J, Keith RH, Michener M, Beidler DR, Monahan JB. Macrophage-colony stimulating factor and interleukin-34 induce chemokines in human whole blood. *Cytokine.* (2010) 52:215–20. doi: 10.1016/j.cyto.2010.08.005

44. Ségaliny AI, Mohamadi A, Dizier B, Lokajczyk A, Brion R, Lanel R, et al. Interleukin-34 promotes tumor progression and metastatic process in osteosarcoma through induction of angiogenesis and macrophage recruitment. *Int J Cancer.* (2015) 137:73–85. doi: 10.1002/ijc.29376

45. Ding LL, Li X, Lei YM, Xia LP, Lu J, Shen H. Effect of Interleukin-34 on secretion of angiogenesis cytokines by peripheral blood mononuclear cells of rheumatoid arthritis. *Immunol Invest.* (2020) 49:81–87. doi: 10.1080/08820139.2019.1649281

46. Idzkowska E, Eljaszewicz A, Miklasz P, Musial WJ, Tycinska AM, Moniuszko M. The role of different monocyte subsets in the pathogenesis of atherosclerosis and acute coronary syndromes. *Scand J Immunol.* (2015) 82:163–73. doi: 10.1111/sji.12314

47. Zawada AM, Rogacev KS, Rotter B, Winter P, Marell R-R, Fliser D, et al. SuperSAGE evidence for CD14++CD16+ monocytes as a third monocyte subset. *Blood.* (2011) 118:e50–e61. doi: 10.1182/blood-2011-01-326827

48. Rogacev KS, Cremers B, Zawada AM, Seiler S, Binder N, Ege P, et al. CD14++CD16+ Monocytes Independently Predict Cardiovascular Events. *J Am Col Cardiol.* (2012) 60:1512–20. doi: 10.1016/j.jacc.2012.07.019

49. Foucher ED, Blanchard S, Preisser L, Descamps P, Ifrah N, Delneste Y, et al. IL-34- and M-CSF-induced macrophages switch memory T cells into Th17 cells via membrane IL-1α. *Eur J Immunol.* (2015) 45:1092–1102. doi: 10.1002/eji.201444606

50. Wang B, Ma Z, Wang M, Sun X, Tang Y, Li M, et al. IL-34 upregulated Th17 production through increased IL-6 expression by rheumatoid fibroblast-Like synoviocytes. *Mediators Inflamm.* (2017) 2017:1567120. doi: 10.1155/2017/1567120

51. Rossol M, Kraus S, Pierer M, Baerwald C, Wagner U. The CD14brightCD16+ monocyte subset is expanded in rheumatoid arthritis and promotes expansion of the Th17 cell population. *Arthritis Rheum.* (2012) 64:671–7. doi: 10.1002/art.33418

52. Foucher ED, Blanchard S, Preisser L, Garo E, Ifrah N, Guardiola P, et al. IL-34 induces the differentiation of human monocytes into immunosuppressive macrophages. antagonistic effects of GM-CSF and IFNγ. *PloS ONE.* (2013) 8. doi: 10.1371/journal.pone.0056045

53. Boulakirba S, Pfeifer A, Mhaidly R, Obba S, Goulard M, Schmitt T, et al. IL-34 and CSF-1 display an equivalent macrophage differentiation ability but a different polarization potential. *Sci Rep.* (2018) 8:256. doi: 10.1038/s41598-017-18433-4

54. McCurdy S, Liu CA, Yap J, Boisvert WA. Potential role of IL-37 in atherosclerosis. *Cytokine.* (2019) 122:154169. doi: 10.1016/j.cyto.2017.09.025

55. Cavalli G, Dinarello CA. Suppression of inflammation and acquired immunity by IL-37. *Immunol Revs.* (2018) 281:179–90. doi: 10.1111/imr.12605

56. Ye L, Jiang B, Deng J, Du J, Xiong W, Guan Y, et al. IL-37 Alleviates Rheumatoid Arthritis by Suppressing IL-17 and IL-17–Triggering Cytokine Production and Limiting Th17 Cell Proliferation. *J Immunol.* (2015) 194:5110–9. doi: 10.4049/jimmunol.1401810

57. Imaeda H, Takahashi K, Fujimoto T, Kasumi E, Ban H, Bamba S, et al. Epithelial expression of interleukin-37b in inflammatory bowel disease. *Clini Exp Immunol.* (2013) 172:410–6. doi: 10.1111/cei.12061

58. Ji Q, Meng K, Yu K, Huang S, Huang Y, Min X, et al. Exogenous interleukin 37 ameliorates atherosclerosis via inducing the Treg response in ApoE-deficient mice. *Sci Rep.* (2017) 7: 3310. doi: 10.1038/s41598-017-02987-4

59. Ji Q, Zeng Q, Huang Y, Shi Y, Lin Y, Lu Z, et al. Elevated Plasma IL-37, IL-18, and IL-18BP concentrations in patients with acute coronary syndrome. *Mediators Inflamm.* (2014) 2014:165742. doi: 10.1155/2014/165742

60. Chai M, Ji Q, Zhang H, Zhou Y, Yang Q, Zhou Y, et al. The protective effect of interleukin-37 on vascular calcification and atherosclerosis in apolipoprotein e-deficient mice with diabetes. *J Interferon Cytokine Res.* (2015) 35:530–9. doi: 10.1089/jir.2014.0212

61. Liu J, Lin J, He S, Wu C, Wang B, Liu J, et al. Transgenic overexpression of IL-37 protects against atherosclerosis and strengthens plaque stability. *Cell Physiol Biochem.* (2018) 45:1034–50. doi: 10.1159/000487344

62. McCurdy S, Baumer Y, Toulmin E, Lee B-H, Boisvert WA. Macrophage-specific expression of IL-37 in hyperlipidemic

mice attenuates atherosclerosis. *J Immunol.* (2017) 199:3604–13. doi: 10.4049/jimmunol.1601907

63. Liu T, Liu J, Lin Y, Que B, Chang C, Zhang J, et al. IL-37 inhibits the maturation of dendritic cells through the IL-1R8-TLR4-NF-κB pathway. *Biochim Biophys Acta.* (2019) 1864:1338–49. doi: 10.1016/j.bbalip.2019.05.009

64. Xie Y, Li Y, Cai X, Wang X, Li J. Interleukin-37 suppresses ICAM-1 expression in parallel with NF-κB down-regulation following TLR2 activation of human coronary artery endothelial cells. *Int Immunopharmacol.* (2016) 38:26–30. doi: 10.1016/j.intimp.2016.05.003

65. McNamee EN, Masterson JC, Jedlicka P, McManus M, Grenz A, Collins CB, et al. Interleukin 37 expression protects mice from colitis. *Proc Natl Acad Sci USA.* (2011) 108:16711–16. doi: 10.1073/pnas.1111982108

66. Zhou P, Li Q, Su S, Dong W, Zong S, Ma Q, et al. Interleukin 37 suppresses M1 macrophage polarization through inhibition of the notch1 and nuclear factor Kappa B pathways. *Front Cell Dev Biol.* (2020) 8:56. doi: 10.3389/fcell.2020.00056

67. Huang J, Hou FL, Zhang AY, Li ZL. Protective effect of the polarity of macrophages regulated by IL-37 on atherosclerosis. *Genet Mol Res.* (2016) 15. doi: 10.4238/gmr.15027616

68. Hoeke G, Khedoe P, van Diepen JA, Pike-Overzet K, van de Ven B, Vazirpanah N, et al. The effects of selective hematopoietic expression of human IL-37 on systemic inflammation and atherosclerosis in LDLr-Deficient mice. *Int J Mol Sci.* (2017) 18:1672. doi: 10.3390/ijms18081672

69. Rudloff, Cho SX, Lao JC, Ngo D, McKenzie M, Nold-Petry CA, et al. Monocytes and dendritic cells are the primary sources of interleukin 37 in human immune cells. *J Leukoc Biol.* (2017) 101:901–911. doi: 10.1189/jlb.3MA0616-287R

70. Luo Y, Cai X, Liu S, Wang S, Nold-Petry CA, Nold MF, et al. Suppression of antigen-specific adaptive immunity by IL-37 via induction of tolerogenic dendritic cells. *Proc Natl Acad Sci USA.* (2014) 111:15178–83. doi: 10.1073/pnas.1416714111

71. Lotfy H, Moaaz M, Moaaz M. The novel role of IL-37 to enhance the anti-inflammatory response of regulatory T cells in patients with peripheral atherosclerosis. *Vascular.* (2020) 28:629–42. doi: 10.1177/1708538120921735

72. Shaoyuan C, Ming D, Yulang H, Hongcheng F. Increased IL-37 in Atherosclerotic Disease could be suppressed by atorvastatin therapy. *Scand J Immunol.* (2015) 82:328–36. doi: 10.1111/sji.12322

73. Clarke MCH, Figg N, Maguire JJ, Davenport AP, Goddard M, Littlewood TD, et al. Apoptosis of vascular smooth muscle cells induces features of plaque vulnerability in atherosclerosis. *Nature Med.* (2006) 12:1075–80. doi: 10.1038/nm1459

74. Bennett MR, Sinha S, Owens GK. Vascular Smooth Muscle Cells in Atherosclerosis. *Circulat Res.* (2016) 118:692–702. doi: 10.1161/CIRCRESAHA.115.306361

75. Nakahara T, Dweck MR, Narula N, Pisapia D, Narula J, Strauss HW. Coronary artery calcification: from mechanism to molecular imaging. *JACC: Cardiovascular Imaging.* (2017) 10:582–93. doi: 10.1016/j.jcmg.2017.03.005

76. Durham AL, Speer MY, Scatena M, Giachelli CM, Shanahan CM. Role of smooth muscle cells in vascular calcification: implications in atherosclerosis and arterial stiffness. *Cardiovasc Res.* (2018) 114:590–600. doi: 10.1093/cvr/cvy010

77. Zeng Q, Song R, Fullerton DA, Ao L, Zhai Y, Li S, et al. Interleukin-37 suppresses the osteogenic responses of human aortic valve interstitial cells in vitro and alleviates valve lesions in mice. *Proc Natl Acad Sci USA.* (2017) 114:1631. doi: 10.1073/pnas.1619667114

78. Yu K, Min X, Lin Y, Huang Y, Huang S, Liu L, et al. Increased IL-37 concentrations in patients with arterial calcification. *Clinica Chimica Acta.* (2016) 461:19–24. doi: 10.1016/j.cca.2016.07.011

79. Chai M, Zhang H-T, Zhou Y-J, Ji Q-W, Yang Q, Liu Y-Y, et al. Elevated IL-37 levels in the plasma of patients with severe coronary artery calcification. *J Geriatr Cardiol.* (2017) 14:285–91. doi: 10.11909/j.issn.1671-5411.2017.05.013

80. Zhang F, Zhu T, Li H, He Y, Zhang Y, Huang N, et al. Plasma interleukin-37 is elevated in acute ischemic stroke patients and probably associated with 3-month functional prognosis. *Clin Interv Aging.* (2020) 15:1285–94. doi: 10.2147/CIA.S230186

81. Liu K, Tang Q, Zhu X, Yang X. IL-37 increased in patients with acute coronary syndrome and associated with a worse clinical outcome after ST-segment elevation acute myocardial infarction. *Clin Chim Acta.* (2017) 468:140–44. doi: 10.1016/j.cca.2017.02.017

82. Yang T, Fang F, Chen Y, Ma J, Xiao Z, Zou S, et al. Elevated plasma interleukin-37 playing an important role in acute coronary syndrome through suppression of ROCK activation. *Oncotarget.* (2017) 8:9686. doi: 10.18632/oncotarget.14195

83. Wang X, Cai X, Chen L, Xu D, Li J. The evaluation of plasma and leukocytic IL-37 expression in early inflammation in patients with acute ST-segment elevation myocardial infarction after PCI. *Mediators Inflamm.* (2015) 2015:626934. doi: 10.1155/2015/626934

84. Conti P, Ronconi G, Caraffa A, Gallenga CE, Ross R, Frydas I, et al. Induction of pro-inflammatory cytokines (IL-1 and IL-6) and lung inflammation by Coronavirus-19 (COVI-19 or SARS-CoV-2): anti-inflammatory strategies. *J Biol Regul Homeost Agents.* (2020) 34:327–31. doi: 10.23812/CONTI-E

85. Nold-Petry CA, Rudloff I, Baumer Y, Ruvo M, Marasco D, Botti P, et al. IL-32 promotes angiogenesis. *J Immunol.* (2014) 192:589–602. doi: 10.4049/jimmunol.1202802

86. Li W, Sun W, Liu L, Yang F, Li Y, Chen Y, et al. IL-32: a host proinflammatory factor against influenza viral replication is upregulated by aberrant epigenetic modifications during influenza A virus infection. *J Immunol.* (2010) 185:5056–65. doi: 10.4049/jimmunol.0902667

87. Yu G, Bing Y, Zhu S, Li W, Xia L, Li Y, et al. Activation of the interleukin-34 inflammatory pathway in response to influenza A virus infection. *Am J Med Sci.* (2015) 349:145–50. doi: 10.1097/MAJ.0000000000000373

88. Chang EJ, Lee SK, Song YS, Jang YJ, Park HS, Hong JP, et al. IL-34 is associated with obesity, chronic inflammation, insulin resistance. *J Clin Endocrinol Metab.* (2014) 99:E1263–71. doi: 10.1210/jc.2013-4409

89. Zafar, Ikram A, Jillella DV, Kempuraj D, Khan MM, Bushnaq S, et al. Measurement of Elevated IL-37 Levels in Acute Ischemic Brain Injury: A Cross-sectional Pilot Study. *Cureus.* (2017) 9:e1767. doi: 10.7759/cureus.1767

90. Li, Ling Y, Song Z, Cheng X, Ding L, Jiang R, et al. Correlation between early plasma interleukin 37 responses with low Inflammatory cytokine levels and benign clinical outcomes in severe acute respiratory syndrome coronavirus 2 infection. *J Infect Dis.* (2021) 223:568–580. doi: 10.1093/infdis/jiaa713

91. Qi F, Liu M, Li F, Lv Q, Wang G, Gong S, et al. Interleukin-37 ameliorates influenza pneumonia by attenuating macrophage cytokine production in a MAPK-Dependent manner. *Front Microbiol.* (2019) 10:2482. doi: 10.3389/fmicb.2019.02482

92. Zhou P, Yang X-L, Wang X-G, Hu B, Zhang L, Zhang W, et al. A pneumonia outbreak associated with a new coronavirus of probable bat origin. *Nature.* (2020) 579:270–3. doi: 10.1038/s41586-020-2012-7

93. Madjid M, Safavi-Naeini, Solomon SD, Vardeny O. Potential effects of coronaviruses on the cardiovascular system: a review. *JAMA Cardiol.* (2020) 5:831–40. doi: 10.1001/jamacardio.2020.1286

94. Leung K, Wu JT, Liu D, Leung GM. First-wave COVID-19 transmissibility and severity in China outside Hubei after control measures, and second-wave scenario planning: a modelling impact assessment. *Lancet.* (2020) 395:1382–93. doi: 10.1016/S0140-6736(20)30746-7

95. Fan J, Liu X, Pan W, Douglas M, Bao S. Epidemiology of Coronavirus Disease in Gansu Province, China, 2020. *Emerg Infect Dis.* (2020) 26:1257. doi: 10.3201/eid2606.200251

96. Fauci AS, Lane HC, Redfield RR. Covid-19 - navigating the uncharted. *N Engl J Med.* (2020) 382:1268–9. doi: 10.1056/NEJMe2002387

97. Chen LYC, Quach TTT. COVID-19 cytokine storm syndrome: a threshold concept. *Lancet Microbe.* (2021) 2:e49–e50. doi: 10.1016/S2666-5247(20)30223-8

98. Riphagen S, Gomez X, Gonzalez-Martinez CN. Wilkinson, and Theocharis, Hyperinflammatory shock in children during COVID-19 pandemic. *Lancet.* (2020) 395:1607–8. doi: 10.1016/S0140-6736(20)31094-1

99. Abou-Ismail MY, Diamond A, Kapoor S, Arafah Y, Nayak L. The hypercoagulable state in COVID-19: Incidence, pathophysiology, and management. *Thromb Res.* (2020) 194:101–15. doi: 10.1016/j.thromres.2020.06.029

100. Lindner D, Fitzek A, Brauninger H, Aleshcheva G, Edler C, Meissner K, et al. Association of cardiac infection with SARS-CoV-2 in confirmed COVID-19 autopsy cases. *JAMA Cardiol.* (2020) 5:1281–5. doi: 10.1001/jamacardio.2020.3551

101. Group RC, Horby, Lim WS, Emberson JR, Mafham M, Bell JL, et al. Dexamethasone in hospitalized Patients with Covid-19. *N Engl J Med.* (2021) 384:693–704. doi: 10.1056/NEJMoa2021436

102. Cron RQ. COVID-19 cytokine storm: targeting the appropriate cytokine. *Lancet Rheumatol.* (2021) 3:E236–E237. doi: 10.1016/S2665-9913(21)00011-4

103. Clerkin Kevin J, Fried Justin A, Raikhelkar J, Sayer G, Griffin Jan M, Masoumi A, et al. COVID-19 and *Cardiovascular Disease. Circulation.* (2020) 141:1648–55. doi: 10.1161/CIRCULATIONAHA.120.046941

104. The Lancet Diabetes. COVID-19 and diabetes: a co-conspiracy? *Lancet Diabetes Endocrinol.* (2020) 8:801. doi: 10.1016/S2213-8587(20)30315-6

105. Gustafson D, Raju S, Wu R, Ching C, Veitch S, Rathnakumar K, et al. Overcoming barriers: the endothelium as a linchpin of coronavirus disease 2019 pathogenesis?. *Arterioscler Thromb Vasc Biol.* (2020) 40:1818–1829. doi: 10.1161/ATVBAHA.120.314558

106. Driggin E, Madhavan MV, Bikdeli B, Chuich T, Laracy J, Biondi-Zoccai G, et al. Cardiovascular considerations for patients, health care workers, and health systems during the covid-19 pandemic. *J Am Col Cardiol.* (2020) 75:2352. doi: 10.1016/j.jacc.2020.03.031

107. Nishiga M, Wang DW, Han Y, Lewis DB, Wu JC. COVID-19 and cardiovascular disease: from basic mechanisms to clinical perspectives. *Nat Rev Cardiol.* (2020) 17:543–58. doi: 10.1038/s41569-020-0413-9

108. Guo T, Fan Y, Chen M, Wu X, Zhang L, He T, et al. Cardiovascular implications of fatal outcomes of patients with coronavirus disease 2019 (COVID-19). *JAMA Cardiology.* (2020) 5:811–8. doi: 10.1001/jamacardio.2020.1017

109. Kowalik MM, Trzonkowski, Łasińska-Kowara M, Mital A, Smiatacz T, Jaguszewski M. COVID-19 - Toward a comprehensive understanding of the disease. *Cardiol J.* (2020) 27:99–114. doi: 10.5603/CJ.a2020.0065

110. Soy M, Keser G, Atagündüz, Tabak F, Atagündüz I, Kayhan S. Cytokine storm in COVID-19: pathogenesis and overview of anti-inflammatory agents used in treatment. *Clini Rheumatol.* (2020) 39:2085–94. doi: 10.1007/s10067-020-05190-5

111. Chen T, Wu D, Chen H, Yan W, Yang D, Chen G, et al. Clinical characteristics of 113 deceased patients with coronavirus disease 2019: retrospective study. *BMJ.* (2020) 368:m1091. doi: 10.1136/bmj.m1091

112. Huang, Wang Y, Li X, Ren L, Zhao J, Hu Y, et al. Clinical features of patients infected with 2019 novel coronavirus in Wuhan, China. *Lancet.* (2020) 395:497–506. doi: 10.1016/S0140-6736(20)30183-5

113. Tisoncik JR, Korth MJ, Simmons CP, Farrar J, Martin TR, Katze MG. Into the eye of the cytokine storm. *Microbiol Mol Biol Rev: MMBR.* (2012) 76:16–32. doi: 10.1128/MMBR.05015-11

114. Corrales-Medina VF, Madjid M, Musher DM. Role of acute infection in triggering acute coronary syndromes. *Lancet Infect Dis.* (2010) 10:83–92. doi: 10.1016/S1473-3099(09)70331-7

115. Akhmerov, Marbán E. COVID-19 and the heart. *Circulat Res.* (2020) 126:1443–55. doi: 10.1161/CIRCRESAHA.120.317055

116. Rey JR, Jimenez Valero S, Poveda Pinedo D, Merino JL, Lopez-Sendon JL, Caro-Codon J. COVID-19 and simultaneous thrombosis of two coronary arteries. *Rev Esp Cardiol (Engl Ed).* (2020) 73:676–7. doi: 10.1016/j.rec.2020.05.021

117. Sheth AR, Grewal US, Patel HP, Thakkar S, Garikipati S, Gaddam J, et al. Possible mechanisms responsible for acute coronary events in COVID-19. *Med Hypotheses.* (2020) 143:110125. doi: 10.1016/j.mehy.2020.110125

118. Kwong JC, Schwartz KL, Campitelli MA. Acute Myocardial Infarction after Laboratory-Confirmed Influenza Infection. *N Engl J Med.* (2018) 378:2540–2541. doi: 10.1056/NEJMc1805679

15

SARS-CoV-2 Infection in Asymptomatic Patients Hospitalized for Cardiac Emergencies: Implications for Patient Management

Thorsten Kessler [1†], Jens Wiebe [1†], Tobias Graf [2], Heribert Schunkert [1], Adnan Kastrati [1†] and Hendrik B. Sager [1*†]

[1] Deutsches Herzzentrum München, Klinik für Herz- und Kreislauferkrankungen, Technische Universität München, Deutsches Zentrum für Herz-Kreislauf-Forschung (DZHK) e.V., Partner Site Munich Heart Alliance, Munich, Germany,
[2] Universitätsklinikum Schleswig-Holstein, Medizinische Klinik II, Deutsches Zentrum für Herz-Kreislauf-Forschung (DZHK) e.V., Partner Site Hamburg/Kiel/Lübeck, Lübeck, Germany

*Correspondence:
Hendrik B. Sager
hendrik.sager@tum.de

†These authors have contributed equally to this work

Background: The coronavirus disease (COVID-19) pandemic imposed diverse challenges on the health care system. Morbidity and mortality of non-COVID-19 emergencies might also have changed because hospitals may not be able to provide optimal care due to restructured resources and uncertainties how to deal with potentially infected patients. It has been recommended to stratify treatment of cardiovascular emergencies according to cardiovascular risk. However, data on the prevalence of asymptomatic SARS-CoV-2 infection in patients presenting with cardiac emergencies remain scarce.

Methods: We retrospectively analyzed patients' data from a tertiary cardiology department between April 15 and May 31, 2020. All patients were screened on admission for COVID-19 symptoms using a questionnaire and body temperature measurements. All hospitalized patients were routinely screened using nasopharyngeal swab testing.

Results: In total, we counted 710 urgent and emergency admissions. Nasopharyngeal swab tests were available in 689 (97%) patients, 409 and 280 of which presented as urgent and emergency admissions, respectively. Among 280 emergency admissions, none tested positive for SARS-CoV-2.

Conclusion: In cardiac emergency patients which were screened negative for COVID-19 symptoms, the prevalence of SARS-CoV-2 infection in regions with a modest overall prevalence is low. This finding might be helpful to better determine timing of emergency procedures and reasonable usage of protective equipment during the COVID-19 crisis and the future.

Keywords: cardiac emergencies, SARS-CoV-2, COVID-19, personal protective equipment (PPE), screening

INTRODUCTION

The coronavirus disease (COVID-19) pandemic imposed diverse challenges on health care providers and hospitals. For instance, hospitals needed to rapidly redistribute and reorganize resources to treat acutely ill COVID-19 patients while keeping up with other emergencies. At the same time outmost attention had to be spent on containing severe acute respiratory syndrome coronavirus 2 (SARS-CoV-2) to protect other patients and staff. Apart from rising numbers of COVID-19 patients, a change in the presentation pattern of non-COVID emergencies was observed. In that light, it was recently shown that hospital admissions for acute coronary syndrome (ACS) declined during the pandemic (1–4). Apart from a decrease in presentations, morbidity and mortality of non-COVID-19 emergencies might have changed because hospitals may not be able to provide optimal care due to restructured resources and uncertainties how to deal with potentially infected patients (5). Position papers consequently recommended to stratify treatment of cardiovascular emergencies according to cardiovascular risk: (1) only high-risk emergencies (e.g., ST elevation myocardial infarction) should be treated immediately with usage of personal protective equipment as in confirmed COVID-19 cases; (2) other emergencies and elective procedures should only be carried out after receiving results of SARS-CoV-2 testing (6–8). A better understanding of the prevalence of asymptomatic SARS-CoV-2 infections may help to guide timely management and reasonable usage of personal protective equipment without affecting the safety of staff and other patients.

We here sought to investigate the prevalence of SARS-CoV-2 infections in asymptomatic patients presenting with cardiac emergencies.

METHODS

Study Cohort

The study protocol was approved by the institutional ethics committee (323/20 S) and conforms to the ethical guidelines of the 1975 Declaration of Helsinki. We retrospectively analyzed patients' data from a tertiary cardiology department which provides 24/7 interventional cardiac care between April 15 and May 31, 2020 (i.e., at the peak of the pandemic's first wave in the region).

Screening of Patients

All patients were screened on admission for COVID-19 symptoms using a questionnaire and had their body temperature measured (ear thermometer). Patients were assigned as COVID-19 asymptomatic when none of the following criteria were met: body temperature $\geq 38.1°C$, coughing, shortness of breath, runny nose, sore throat, or body aches. Additionally, patients were asked whether they had been in contact to a confirmed COVID-19 case or a patient suffering from fever and coughing without proven SARS-CoV-2 infection. Patients reporting shortness of breath were also regarded as COVID-19 asymptomatic if they did not report one of the other criteria. COVID-19 asymptomatic patients were required to wear standard surgical masks (no

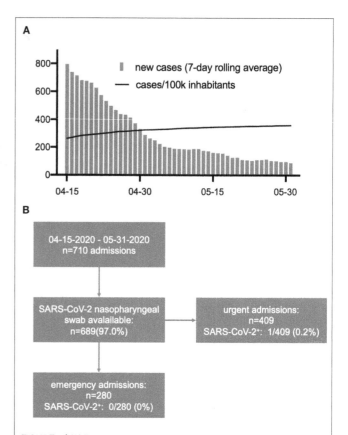

FIGURE 1 | (A) Daily reported cases (Bayerisches Landesamt für Gesundheit und Lebensmittelsicherheit, accessed on 07-15-2020) and prevalence (Daily Situation Report of the Robert Koch Institute, accessed on 07-15-2020) of SARS-CoV-2 infections in the Free State of Bavaria during the study period. (B) Prevalence of asymptomatic SARS-CoV-2 infection.

N95 or FFP2-3) throughout the entire stay. Hospital staff was also required to wear standard surgical masks at all times. These protective measurements were recently shown to reduce in particular the risk of SARS-CoV-2 infection for healthcare workers (9). N95 masks or FFP2-3 masks and further dedicated protective equipment were only used when treating SARS-CoV-2 confirmed or suspected patients.

SARS-CoV-2 Testing

All hospitalized patients were routinely screened for SARS-CoV-2 using nasopharyngeal swab testing (SARS-CoV-2 real-time polymerase chain reaction assay, Mikrogen Diagnostik, Neuried, Germany) since April 15, 2020. Patients without COVID-19 symptoms were only planned to be tested at admission. Repeated testing was performed if patients developed symptoms or if a more recent test result was required for transferal to other treatment facilities.

RESULTS

Until May 31, 2020, a total of 710 patients presented and were included this analysis. **Figure 1A** displays the number of daily infections in the Free State of Bavaria, Germany and the

TABLE 1 | Baseline characteristics and reasons of admission for the patients presenting with cardiac emergencies during the study period.

	Emergency admissions n = 280
Age, years ± SD	68.5 ± 15.0
Female gender, n (%)	103 (36.8)
Comorbidities	
COPD, n (%)	19 (6.8)
Diabetes, n (%)	60 (21.4)
Hypertension, n (%)	189 (67.5)
Coronary artery disease, n (%)	131 (46.8)
Peripheral artery disease, n (%)	26 (9.3)
Cerebrovascular disease, n (%)	34 (12.1)
Cancer, n (%)	30 (10.7)
Chronic renal dysfunction, n (%)	50 (17.9)
Immunodeficiency, n (%)	8 (2.9)
Reasons for admission	
Coronary, n (%)	97 (34.6)
Heart failure, n (%)	23 (8.2)
Structural, n (%)	7 (2.5)
Electrophysiology, n (%)	93 (33.2)
Other, n (%)	60 (21.4)

Coronary includes (suspected) acute coronary syndromes. Electrophysiology includes, e.g., tachycardia and bradycardia. Other includes, e.g., syncope, pulmonary embolism. COPD, chronic obstructive pulmonary disease; SD, standard deviation.

prevalence of SARS-CoV-2 infections per 100,000 inhabitants during the study period. Nasopharyngeal swab tests were available in 689 (97%) patients, 409 and 280 of which presented as urgent [reasons: coronary 116/409 (28.4%), structural 42/409 (10.3%), heart failure 8/409 (2%), electrophysiology 209/409 (51.1%), other 34/409 (8.3%)] and emergency admissions, respectively. As a suspected SARS-CoV-2 infection may have reduced the likelihood of presenting with a non-emergency leading to an underestimation of the actual prevalence, we focused on the 280 patients admitted as cardiac emergencies. Baseline characteristics and reasons for admission are displayed in **Table 1**. None of these COVID-19 asymptomatic patients tested positive for SARS-CoV-2. During the hospital stay, 27 (9.6%) of patients were repeatedly tested with no test revealing a positive result.

In the total cohort, only one patient was diagnosed to be SARS-CoV-2 positive (**Figure 1B**). The patient was sent in home quarantine and treatment was scheduled to be performed after 14 days of quarantine and two subsequent negative nasopharyngeal swabs. This patient remained asymptomatic and no further testing was performed during quarantine.

DISCUSSION

This result needs to be reviewed in the context of the overall SARS-CoV-2 prevalence in the respective region during the observation period. During the study period, ~300 cases per 100,000 citizens were reported in the Free State of Bavaria. Thus, our data indicate that in cardiac emergency patients which were screened negative for COVID-19 symptoms, the prevalence of SARS-CoV-2 infection in regions with a modest overall prevalence is low. Under these circumstances, our findings indicate that a delay/deferral of emergency procedures due to waiting for SARS-CoV-2 test results may not be justified in emergency patients which are screened asymptomatic for COVID-19, but have an unclear SARS-CoV-2 infectious status. While our finding is in line with a recent report from Iceland, where in a random-sample screening of the population, 0.6% tested positive for SARS-CoV-2 (10), a study screening pregnant women admitted for delivery in New York City found that 13.5% of tested women were asymptomatic but tested positive (11).

In summary, the frequency of asymptomatic SARS-CoV-2 carriers among cardiac emergency patients is low when the overall prevalence of COVID-19 is modest. Consequently, emergency but also elective procedures may safely be carried out without delay and waiting for SARS-CoV-2 test results. Importantly, the safety of personnel and patients may be further increased by implementation of rapid or point-of-care tests which despite potential drawbacks [for an overview, see (12)] recently revealed promising results (13).

Our study was performed during a time period in which the prevalence of COVID-19 in Bavaria was rather low and our findings are therefore inherently not applicable in regions with higher prevalence. It was also previously shown that the highest sensitivity of SARS-CoV-2 was reached bronchoalveolar lavage fluid (14) and we may have missed SARS-CoV-2 infection due to only performing nasopharyngeal swab testing. Additional major limitations are the retrospective nature of this analysis and that the data are derived from a single center. The low prevalence of SARS-CoV-2 infection may therefore be due to chance and requires validation in further cohorts to draw definitive conclusions. Our data may nevertheless be helpful to better determine timing of emergency procedures and reasonable usage of protective equipment during the COVID-19 crisis and the future.

AUTHOR CONTRIBUTIONS

AK and HBS designed the study. TK, JW, TG, and HS contributed data. TK, AK, and HBS drafted the manuscript. All authors were involved in critically revising the manuscript.

REFERENCES

1. De Filippo O, D'Ascenzo F, Angelini F, Bocchino PP, Conrotto F, Saglietto A, et al. Reduced rate of hospital admissions for ACS during covid-19 outbreak in Northern Italy. *N Engl J Med.* (2020) 383:88–9. doi: 10.1056/NEJMc2009166

2. Piccolo R, Bruzzese D, Mauro C, Aloia A, Baldi C, Boccalatte M, et al. Population trends in rates of percutaneous coronary revascularization for acute coronary syndromes associated with the COVID-19 outbreak. *Circulation.* (2020) 133:916–8. doi: 10.1161/CIRCULATIONAHA.120.047457

3. De Rosa S, Spaccarotella C, Basso C, Calabrò MP, Curcio A, Filardi PP,

et al. Reduction of hospitalizations for myocardial infarction in Italy in the COVID-19 era. *Eur Heart J.* (2020) 41:2083–8. doi: 10.1093/eurheartj/ehaa409

4. Kessler T, Graf T, Hilgendorf I, Rizas K, Martens E, zur Muhlen von C, et al. Hospital admissions with acute coronary syndromes during the COVID-19 pandemic in German cardiac care units. *Cardiovasc Res.* (2020) 116:1800–1. doi: 10.1093/cvr/cvaa192

5. Rosenbaum L. Facing covid-19 in Italy—ethics, logistics, and therapeutics on the epidemic's front line. *N Engl J Med.* (2020) 382:1873–5. doi: 10.1056/NEJMp2005492

6. Chieffo A, Stefanini GG, Price S, Barbato E, Tarantini G, Karam N, et al. EAPCI position statement on invasive management of acute coronary syndromes during the COVID-19 pandemic. *EuroIntervention.* (2020) 16:233–46. doi: 10.4244/EIJY20M05_01

7. Welt FGP, Shah PB, Aronow HD, Bortnick AE, Henry TD, Sherwood MW, et al. Catheterization laboratory considerations during the coronavirus (COVID-19) pandemic: from the ACC's Interventional Council and SCAI. *J Am Coll Cardiol.* (2020) 75:2372–5. doi: 10.1016/j.jacc.2020.03.021

8. The European Society of Cardiology. *ESC Guidance for the Diagnosis and Management of CV Disease during the COVID-19 Pandemic.* (2020). Avaialble online at: https://www.escardio.org/Education/COVID-19-and-Cardiology/ESC-COVID-19-Guidance (accessed 10 June, 2020).

9. Wang X, Ferro EG, Zhou G, Hashimoto D, Bhatt DL. Association between universal masking in a health care system and SARS-CoV-2 positivity among health care workers. *JAMA.* (2020) 324:703–4. doi: 10.1001/jama.2020.12897

10. Gudbjartsson DF, Helgason A, Jonsson H, Magnusson OT, Melsted P, Norddahl GL, et al. Spread of SARS-CoV-2 in the icelandic population. *N Engl J Med.* (2020) 382:2302–15. doi: 10.1056/NEJMoa2006100

11. Sutton D, Fuchs K, D'Alton M, Goffman D. Universal screening for SARS-CoV-2 in women admitted for delivery. *N Engl J Med.* (2020) 382:2163–4. doi: 10.1056/NEJMc2009316

12. Guglielmi G. Fast coronavirus tests: what they can and can't do. *Nature.* (2020) 585:496–8. doi: 10.1038/d41586-020-02661-2

13. Gibani MM, Toumazou C, Sohbati M, Sahoo R, Karvela M, Hon T-K, et al. Assessing a novel, lab-free, point-of-care test for SARS-CoV-2 (CovidNudge): a diagnostic accuracy study. *Lancet Microbe.* (2020) 1:e300–7. doi: 10.1016/S2666-5247(20)30121-X

14. Wang W, Xu Y, Gao R, Lu R, Han K, Wu G, et al. Detection of SARS-CoV-2 in different types of clinical specimens. *JAMA.* (2020) 323:1843–4. doi: 10.1001/jama.2020.3786

16

Impact of the COVID-19 Pandemic on ST-Elevation Myocardial Infarction Management in Hunan Province, China

Liang Tang[1†], Zhao-jun Wang[1†], Xin-qun Hu[1], Zhen-fei Fang[1], Zhao-fen Zheng[2], Jian-ping Zeng[3], Lu-ping Jiang[4], Fan Ouyang[5], Chang-hui Liu[6], Gao-feng Zeng[7], Yong-hong Guo[8]* and Sheng-hua Zhou[1]*

[1] Department of Cardiology, The Second Xiangya Hospital of Central South University, Changsha, China, [2] Hunan Provincial People's Hospital, The First Affiliated Hospital of Hunan Normal University, Changsha, China, [3] Xiangtan Central Hospital, Xiangtan, China, [4] Changsha Central Hospital, Changsha, China, [5] Zhuzhou Central Hospital, Zhuzhou, China, [6] The First Affiliated Hospital of University of South China, Hengyang, China, [7] The Second Affiliated Hospital of University of South China, Hengyang, China, [8] Department of Geriatric, The Second Xiangya Hospital of Central South University, Changsha, China

*Correspondence:
Yong-hong Guo
guoyonghong@csu.edu.cn
Sheng-hua Zhou
zhoushenghua_guo@163.com

[†] *These authors have contributed equally to this work*

Background: This study aimed to investigate the impact of the COVID-19 pandemic on ST-segment elevation myocardial infarction (STEMI) care in China.

Methods: We conducted a multicenter, retrospective cohort study in Hunan province (adjacent to the epidemic center), China. Consecutive patients presenting with STEMI within 12 h of symptom onset and receiving primary percutaneous coronary intervention, pharmaco-invasive strategy and only thrombolytic treatment, were enrolled from January 23, 2020 to April 8, 2020 (COVID-19 era group). The same data were also collected for the equivalent period of 2019 (pre-COVID-19 era group).

Results: A total of 610 patients with STEMI (COVID-19 era group $n = 286$, pre-COVID-19 era group $n = 324$) were included. There was a decline in the number of STEMI admissions by 10.5% and STEMI-related PCI procedures by 12.7% in 2020 compared with the equivalent period of 2019. The key time intervals including time from symptom onset to first medical contact, symptom onset to door, door-to-balloon, symptom onset to balloon and symptom onset to thrombolysis showed no significant difference between these two groups. There were no significant differences for in-hospital death and major adverse cardiovascular events between these two groups.

Conclusion: During the COVID-19 pandemic outbreak in China, we observed a decline in the number of STEMI admissions and STEMI-related PCI procedures. However, the key quality indicators of STEMI care were not significantly affected. Restructuring health services during the COVID-19 pandemic has not significantly adversely influenced the in-hospital outcomes.

Keywords: COVID-19, ST-segment elevation myocardial infarction, primary percutaneous coronary intervention, thrombolysis, outcomes

INTRODUCTION

In late December 2019, an outbreak of coronavirus disease 2019 (COVID-19) caused by severe acute respiratory syndrome coronavirus 2 (SARS-CoV-2) occurred in Wuhan, China (1, 2). Within 3 months since the outbreak, COVID-19 has emerged as a pandemic and an international public health crisis (3). According to the dynamic real-time information provided by Johns Hopkins University Coronavirus Resource Center, as of January 7, 2022, the pandemic has infected over 303,204,268 people and caused 5,479,893 deaths globally (4). The ongoing pandemic of COVID-19 has imposed a serious threat on public health and the economy worldwide.

ST-segment elevation myocardial infarction (STEMI) remains a leading cause of death worldwide (5). Improvement in clinical outcomes after STEMI depends greatly on the timely effective reperfusion therapy. Primary percutaneous coronary intervention (PPCI) is the preferred reperfusion strategy and is the current standard of care for STEMI (6). However, the COVID-19 pandemic inevitably poses a severe challenge to the emergent care of STEMI patients, as the regional STEMI-network was reorganized to assist COVID-19 patients, and the screening and infectious control of COVID-19 procedures required to prevent nosocomial infection may substantially defer PPCI (7–9). Recently, the American College of Cardiology's Interventional Council and Society of Cardiovascular Angiography and Intervention have issued a statement on the management of STEMI in the context of the COVID-19 pandemic and it continues to recommend PPCI as the standard treatment of STEMI patients with unconfirmed COVID-19 status (10). In contrast, the Chinese Society of Cardiology has issued a consensus on the management of STEMI during the COVID-19 pandemic and recommended a strategy of thrombolytic therapy over PPCI due to concerns of resource allocation, as well as challenges in transfer of patients to facilities that perform PPCI (11).

To date, while there are isolated local and regional level reports that the COVID-19 pandemic is associated with a reduction in both presentations with STEMI and PPCI procedures (7, 8), there have been limited data regarding its impact on real-world reperfusion strategies decision making, key indicators of STEMI care, and clinical outcomes. Therefore, the present investigation was undertaken to investigate the real-world impact of the COVID-19 pandemic on time-sensitive STEMI care delivery in Hunan province, China, a so-called "hot-spot" province (adjacent to the epidemic center Wuhan) where the impact would be expected to be most pronounced and lab results.

MATERIALS AND METHODS

Study Design and Population

We conducted a multicenter, retrospective study involving 13 tertiary care cardiac catheterization centers in Hunan province, China. Consecutive patients, presenting with STEMI within 12 h of symptom onset and receiving reperfusion therapy with PPCI, pharmaco-invasive strategy, and only thrombolytic treatment,

were enrolled from January 23, 2020 to April 8, 2020, when the city of Wuhan was on lockdown to constrain the spread of the virus. A group of STEMI patients from the equivalent period of last year (i.e., January 23, 2019 to April 8, 2019; pre-COVID-19 era group) was used as control.

During the COVID-19 pandemic, all STEMI patients were screened for COVID-19 first. All admitted patients were required to undergo temperature checks and complete an epidemiological survey at prescreening triage station, which was set up at the entrance of the emergency department. For patients with suspected COVID-19 infection, rapid chest scans and routine blood tests were performed. A nasopharyngeal swab was performed if the condition of the patient allows it. Patients were transferred to a COVID-19-designated hospital if COVID-19 is confirmed. In this study, patients with confirmed or suspected COVID-19 were excluded. Besides, Patients were excluded from the analysis if they presented with ischemic time > 12 h or unknown time, combined with neoplastic disease, discharged to other medical facilities within 48 h, received no acute reperfusion, or had records with missing or incomplete data. STEMI patients were classified into two groups: COVID-19 era group and pre-COVID-19 era group according to the time admitted in hospitals. Patients who underwent PCI were further categorized according to whether they received PPCI or pharmaco-invasive strategy to analyze the procedural characteristics and key time indicators. The diagnosis of STEMI was made based on the fourth universal definition (12). The pharmaco-invasive strategy was defined as fibrinolysis combined with routine early PCI strategy (in case of successful fibrinolysis) or rescue PCI (in case of failed fibrinolysis) (6). The study was conducted in accordance with the Declaration of Helsinki and approved by the local hospital Institutional Review Board, and the need for informed consent for using the medical records was waived owing to the retrospective nature of the study.

Data Collection

The clinical data were collected by trained staff reviewing the medical records of all patients. Data were collected retrospectively, in an anonymized fashion without any sensitive data. We collected detailed baseline variables including demographics, cardiovascular risk factors, medical history, physical findings, and Killip classification on admission, early medical treatments (within 24 h after hospital arrival), and laboratory tests. Treatment timelines delay including symptom onset to first medical contact (FMC), symptom onset to door, door to balloon, symptom onset to balloon, and symptom onset to thrombolysis time. In addition, angiographic and procedural characteristics were assessed.

Clinical Outcomes

All adverse clinical events were adjudicated through the use of original source documentation by an independent committee that was unaware of the treatment allocation. The primary outcome of interest was the number of STEMI admissions and STEMI-related PCI (including PPCI, rescue PCI, and routine early PCI) procedures during Wuhan lockdown and the equivalent period in 2019. The secondary outcomes were in-hospital all-cause mortality and major adverse cardiovascular events (MACEs), which were defined as a composite of death, non-fatal reinfarction, target vessel revascularization, new-onset congestive heart failure, and stroke during hospitalization (13, 14).

Statistical Analysis

Continuous data were reported as median with 25th and 75th percentiles (interquartile range, IQR) and compared by the Mann–Whitney U test. Categorical data were expressed as numbers and percentages and compared by the chi-square test or Fisher's exact test. Multivariate logistic regression analysis was used to identify independent predictors of in-hospital mortality and MACEs. All statistical tests were performed using SPSS software, version 24.0 (SPSS Inc., Chicago, IL, United States). A P value of <0.05 was regarded as statistically significant.

RESULTS

Baseline Characteristics

A total of 953 consecutive patients (COVID-19 era group $n = 450$, pre-COVID-19 era group $n = 503$) were admitted for STEMI during the described time frames. Of these, no patient was confirmed or suspected COVID-19 and 610 patients (COVID-19 era group $n = 286$, pre-COVID-19 era group $n = 324$) fit the inclusion criteria for this study (**Figure 1**). Among this study population, 567 (93.0%) patients received PPCI. Forty (6.6%) patients received pharmaco-invasive treatment including routine early PCI ($n = 18$) and rescue PCI ($n = 22$). When comparing the study period of 2020 to the equivalent period of 2019, a reduction of 10.5% in STEMI admissions was observed (**Figure 2**). Also, there was a 12.7% decline in the number of all STEMI-related PCI procedures (including PPCI, rescue PCI and routine early PCI) when compared to the same time interval in 2019 (**Figure 3**). The remaining 3 (0.5%) patients received only thrombolysis treatment.

Demographic, baseline clinical characteristics and laboratory variables of the enrolled patients are listed in **Table 1**. Compared with the pre-COVID-19 era group, the COVID-19 era group was more likely to have a history of previous PCI. Otherwise, there were no significant differences between the two groups in terms of patient demographics, medical history, the prevalence of coronary risk factors, physical findings on admission and concomitant medications. Patients were presented with a slightly higher cardiac troponin I (cTnI) level on admission during the COVID-19 pandemic era compared with the pre-COVID-19 era. Patients in the COVID-19 era group tended to have a lower blood urea nitrogen, low-density lipoprotein cholesterol and C-reactive protein level on admission (**Table 1**).

The baseline angiographic features and procedural data are summarized in **Table 2**. For patients who received PPCI, the time from symptom onset to FMC, symptom onset to door and symptom onset to balloon were not substantially longer during the COVID-19 pandemic era. The door-to-balloon time and the total procedure time were similar between two groups. For

pharmaco-invasive patients, the key time interval, including the time from symptom onset to FMC, symptom onset to door and symptom onset to thrombolysis, showed no significant increase during the COVID-19 pandemic era. Patients who received PPCI were less likely to have a right coronary artery occlusion, multivessel disease, and radial access during the COVID-19 pandemic era compared with the pre-COVID-19 era. Moreover, patients who received PPCI during the COVID-19 pandemic had a greater proportion of direct stenting and thrombus aspiration. Among patients admitted with PPCI, the intra-aortic balloon pump (IABP) use and extracorporeal membrane oxygenation use were no difference during the COVID-19 pandemic and pre-COVID-19 era. A high procedural success rate (97.7 vs. 99.0%) and low complications rate (1.5 vs. 1.3%) were similarly observed between two groups. Among patients who received pharmaco-invasive strategy, no significant difference was observed between the two groups with regard to the location of culprit artery, initial and final TIMI flow grade, and prevalence of multivessel diseases. IABP was less used in these patients during the COVID-19 pandemic era.

Clinical Outcomes

The in-hospital outcomes are shown in **Table 3**. No significant difference was observed in the median hospital length of stay between these two groups. There was no significant difference in in-hospital mortality between these two groups (2.4 vs. 3.4%, $P = 0.490$). One non-fatal myocardial infarction occurred in pre-COVID-19 era group. Two patients in the COVID-19 era group and one in the pre-COVID-19 era group experienced non-fatal stroke in hospital in COVID-19 era group. The rate of in-hospital heart failure decreased from 8.0 to 4.9% during the outbreak period. The rate of target vessel revascularization increased slightly from 0.9 to 2.4% during the outbreak period. Finally, the cumulative MACEs were similar between two groups (9.8 vs. 10.8%, $p = 0.682$). The adjusted odds of in-hospital death and MACEs are shown in **Table 4**. Following adjustment for covariates, no significant differences were found for in-hospital death (odds ratio [OR] 1.180, 95% confidence interval [CI] 0.181–7.679, $P = 0.862$) or MACEs (OR 1.390, 95%CI 0.612–3.161, $P = 0.431$).

DISCUSSION

In response to the COVID-19 pandemic, many countries have implemented strict infection containment measures such as "lockdown" and encouraged a "stay-at-home" lifestyle, to reduce the spread of the pandemic (8, 9, 15). Moreover, the routine hospital services including cardiac catheterization have been restructured in order to increase hospital capacity for COVID-19 patients and prevent cross-infection. These strict restriction measures would inevitably have a profound impact on routine medical care, in particular, acute cardiovascular disease management.

In the present study, we conducted a retrospective analysis in 610 STEMI patients receiving acute reperfusion treatment including PPCI, pharmaco-invasive strategy and systematic

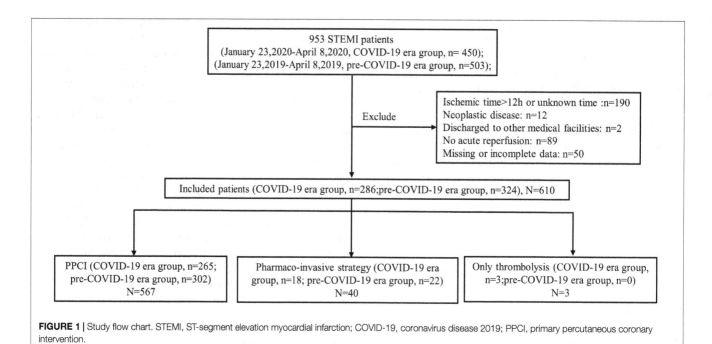

FIGURE 1 | Study flow chart. STEMI, ST-segment elevation myocardial infarction; COVID-19, coronavirus disease 2019; PPCI, primary percutaneous coronary intervention.

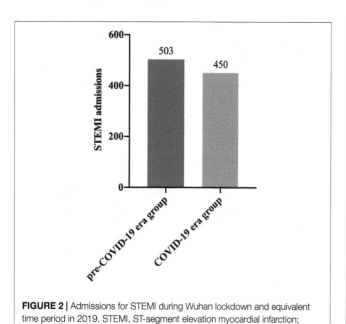

FIGURE 2 | Admissions for STEMI during Wuhan lockdown and equivalent time period in 2019. STEMI, ST-segment elevation myocardial infarction; COVID-19, coronavirus disease 2019.

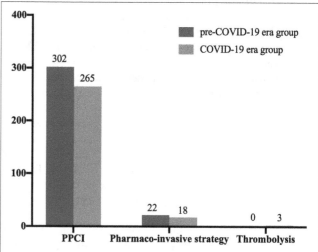

FIGURE 3 | Reperfusion strategy for STEMI patients during Wuhan lockdown and equivalent time period in 2019. STEMI, ST-segment elevation myocardial infarction; COVID-19, coronavirus disease 2019; PPCI, primary percutaneous coronary intervention.

thrombolysis and compared the in-hospital clinical outcomes of patients presenting during the COVID-19 pandemic vs. pre-COVID-19 era. First, we demonstrated a 10.5% drop in STEMI volumes, a 12.7% decline in STEMI-related PCI procedures and a significantly higher cTnI level on admission during the COVID-19 outbreak. Second, in terms of time delay, the pandemic of COVID-19 incurred no additional time delay whether in the PPCI subgroup or pharmaco-invasive strategy subgroup. Finally, there were no differences in clinical outcomes including in-hospital mortality and MACEs before and after lockdown.

Previous studies have reported a common decrease in STEMI admissions while the degree of decline varied considerably among countries affected by the COVID-19 pandemic. During the early phase of the COVID-19 pandemic, Xiang et al. (15) reported a 26.3% reduction in STEMI patients' access to care in non-Hubei provinces in China based on the Chest Pain Center database. A similar reduction of 23% in admissions for STEMI was reported in England (9). Scholz et al. (16) reported a mild decrease in the absolute number of STEM patients treated in systems of STEMI care in Germany (12.6%). Our results supported this finding but presented a relatively milder decrease in STEMI volumes (10.5%). In contrast, reports from other countries (e.g., Singapore, France, and Denmark) report no appreciable decrease and even a modest increase in STEMI volumes (17–19). The largely discrepant reports of

STEMI hospitalization across countries could be partly explained by disparities in healthcare organizations.

Multiple factors might contribute to this decline in admissions of patients with STEMI during the COVID-19 pandemic. One

TABLE 1 | Baseline clinical characteristics.

	COVID-19 group (*n* = 286)	Pre-COVID-19 group (*n* = 324)	Statistic	*P* value
Demographics				
Age (years)	63 (53.5–70)	63 (53–75)	−0.727[‡]	0.467
Male sex, *n* (%)	229 (80.1)	250 (77.2)	0.763[†]	0.383
Cardiovascular risk factors, *n* (%)				
Diabetes mellitus	51 (17.8)	77 (23.8)	3.225[†]	0.073
Hypertension (>140/90 mmHg)	143 (50.0)	148 (45.7)	1.137[†]	0.286
Hyperlipidemia	90 (31.5)	113 (34.9)	0.795[†]	0.373
Current smoker	129 (45.1)	164 (50.6)	1.849[†]	0.174
Number of cardiovascular risk factors			0.658[†]	0.883
≥3	48 (16.8)	60 (18.5)		
2	99 (34.6)	106 (32.7)		
1	90 (31.5)	98 (30.2)		
0	49 (17.1)	60 (18.5)		
Medical history, *n* (%)				
History of PCI	16 (5.6)	6 (1.9)	6.120[†]	0.013
History of CABG	0 (0.0)	0 (0.0)	—	—
Previous MI	8 (2.8)	10 (3.1)	0.440[†]	0.833
Physical findings on admission				
Systolic blood pressure (mm Hg)	126 (110–145.25)	127 (110–141.5)	−0.126[‡]	0.900
Heart rate (beats/min)	77.96 ± 18.083	78.43 ± 17.135	−0.329[*]	0.742
Killip classification on admission, *n* (%)			2.836[†]	0.242
Class I	191 (66.8)	225 (69.4)		
Class II	71 (24.8)	64 (19.8)		
Class III–IV	24 (8.4)	35 (10.8)		
Medication within 24 h of hospital arrival, *n* (%)				
Aspirin	285 (99.7)	322 (99.4)	-	1.000
P2Y12 receptor inhibitor	286 (100.0)	323 (99.7)	-	1.000
GP IIb/IIIa receptor inhibitor	149 (52.1)	151 (46.6)	1.834[†]	0.176
β-blockers	230 (80.4)	279 (86.1)	3.562[†]	0.059
Statins	271 (94.8)	314 (96.9)	1.800[†]	0.180
Angiotensin-converting enzyme inhibitors/Angiotensin receptor blockers	211 (73.8)	240 (74.1)	0.007[†]	0.933
Laboratory tests				
White blood cell × 10⁹/L	9.8 (8.0–12.9)	10.6 (8.0–13.3)	−0.560[‡]	0.575
Neutrophil × 10⁹/L	7.9 (5.7–10.9)	8.4 (5.8–10.7)	−0.402[‡]	0.608
Lymphocyte × 10⁹/L	1.3 (1.0–1.8)	1.3 (0.9–2.0)	−0.553[‡]	0.580
Platelets × 10⁹/L	204.0 (169.0–250.5)	209.5 (177.0–243.3)	−0.097[‡]	0.923
Hs-cTnI (pg/ml)	5.3 (0.8–23.8)	3.0 (0.3–18.2)	−2.707[‡]	0.007
CK (U/L)	877.0 (225.5–2590.7)	939.1 (236.0–2199.0)	−0.243[‡]	0.808
CK-MB (U/L)	92.7 (27.2–232.0)	99.0 (34.6–235.7)	−0.704[‡]	0.482
BNP (pg/ml)	100.0 (31.3–225.1)	105.0 (67.3–419.3)	−1.687[‡]	0.092
NT-proBNP (pg/ml)	560.4 (160.3–1727.5)	392.0 (91.4–1541.0)	−1.534[‡]	0.125
ALT (U/L)	35.2 (24.1–60.0)	39.8 (26.0–61.4)	−1.144[‡]	0.253
AST (U/L)	91.5 (37.9–208.6)	114.5 (38.5–247.9)	−1.378[‡]	0.168
BUN (mmol/L)	5.7 (4.6–7.2)	6.4 (5.0–8.0)	−3.181[‡]	0.001
TC (mmol/L)	4.7 (3.9–5.5)	4.7 (4.0–5.4)	−0.647[‡]	0.517
TG (mmol/L)	1.5 (1.0–2.3)	1.7 (1.1–2.4)	−1.224[‡]	0.221
HDL-C (mmol/L)	1.0 (0.9–1.2)	1.1 (0.9–1.3)	−1.735[‡]	0.083

(Continued)

TABLE 1 | (Continued)

	COVID-19 group (n = 286)	Pre-COVID-19 group (n = 324)	Statistic	P value
LDL-C (mmol/L)	2.8 (2.2–3.5)	3.1 (2.5–3.7)	−2.557[‡]	0.011
Hs-CRP (mg/L)	4.2 (1.7–11.7)	7.6 (2.9–21.4)	−2.737[‡]	0.006
PT (s)	12.5 (11.1–14.6)	12.0 (10.3–15.3)	−2.539[‡]	0.011
APTT (s)	34.1 (27.5–55.5)	32.4 (26.8–41.1)	−2.292[‡]	0.022
D-dimer (mg/L)	0.4 (0.2–1.9)	0.4 (0.2–0.8)	−1.830[‡]	0.067

Data are expressed as mean ± SD, as percentages, or as median (Q1, Q3). *t value; †χ² value; ‡Z value. —: Data not available (Fisher exact test). COVID-19, coronavirus disease 2019; PCI, percutaneous coronary intervention; CABG, coronary artery bypass graft; MI, myocardial infarction; Hs-cTnI, high sensitivity cardiac troponin I; CK, creatine phosphokinase; CK-MB, creatine phosphokinase-MB; BNP, B-type natriuretic peptide; NT-proBNP, N terminal pro-hormone BNP; ALT, alanine transaminase; AST, aspartate transaminase; BUN, blood urea nitrogen; TC, total cholesterol; TG, triglycerides; HDL-C, high-density lipoprotein cholesterol; LDL-C, low-density lipoprotein cholesterol; Hs-CRP, high-sensitivity C-reactive protein; PT, prothrombin time; APTT, activated partial thromboplastin time.

possibility is that the case of misdiagnosis increased because of complex cardiovascular manifestations under the circumstance of COVID-19. It is challenging to differentiate STEMI patients from COVID-19 patients, who might simulate a STEMI manifestation and present with cardiac troponin elevation and/or ST changes (20). Therefore, a proportion of critical STEMI with dyspnea and pulmonary edema could be mistaken with the coronavirus features and managed as a COVID-19 case from the outset. The fear of medical system might be another important factor. The soaring confirmed infections, no effective therapeutic drugs, no vaccines and lack of personal protective equipment may have created an atmosphere of fear. The symptomatic patients might avoid seeking acute medical care for fear of getting in contact with COVID-19 patients (21).

Additionally, our finding showed a decline of 12.7% in STEMI-related PCI procedures, which supports the decline in PCI procedures for STEMI reported in other studies, but we add some additional value to such observations by describing clinical and procedural characteristics and outcomes after the COVID-19 lockdown using last year as a reference. A preliminary analysis from multiple United States centers showed during the early phase of the COVID-19 pandemic, an estimated 38% reduction in cardiac catheterization laboratories activations for STEMI care (22). Another survey of 73 centers in Spain reported a 40% reduction in procedures performed in the STEMI settings (23). Using the British Cardiovascular Intervention Society database, Kwok et al. (24) reported a 43% reduction in all STEMI-related PCI procedures in England in the month after the lockdown. In the present study, we observed a slight decline in STEMI-related PCI procedures. The different degrees of decline in nations and regions indicated the huge differences in terms of local healthcare resources, the pandemic density of the COVID-19 outbreak and changes of the pandemic over time. In China, since Hubei province started lockdown on January 23, 2020, Hunan province had activated Level one major public health emergency response on the same day. With the joint efforts of the government and people, the epidemic was quickly controlled. Subsequently, the government degraded the major public health emergency response to Level two on March 10 due to a sustained decrease in the number of new cases. The regional medical system had the capacity to continue to provide emergency STEMI care according to current clinical practice guidelines.

Undoubtedly, the COVID-19 pandemic is a major burden on the time-dependent emergency healthcare networks and is imposing a change on STEMI care especially in region heavy involvement in the epidemic. An important issue merit consideration is how changes in patients' health-seeking behavior, health service delivery and government strategies to restrict virus spread impact clinical characteristics and outcomes of the patients (24). Our study showed patients admitted during the COVID-19 pandemic were more likely to have a history of previous PCI with a significant increase in the baseline cTnI level compared to a similar time frame last year. Similar observations have also been reported from England and Germany (21, 25). The fear of getting infected within the hospitals and government calls to stay at home and seek medical care only in case of an emergency may lead to patients' delay seeking a doctor, and aggravation of their symptoms (21, 24). As a consequence, a substantial reduction in admissions for STEMI and an increase in the number of out-of-hospital cardiac arrests were observed (26). In the present study, we found relatively fewer patients receiving PCI during the COVID-19 pandemic and no overall increase in in-hospital mortality and MACEs among patients admitted for STEMI. Despite this fact, caution must be exercised in interpreting the results. On the one hand, many patients had STEMI but receive no reperfusion therapy in hospital because of deaths out of hospital. On the other hand, it warrants much investigation to assess whether the long-term clinical outcome was not different before and after the COVID-19 pandemic outbreak.

In present study, there was no difference between two groups in terms of key time interval and short term in-hospital outcomes for STEM patients. This result was in line with studies in other regions of China. A single center report from Beijing by Guan et al. (27) showed door to balloon time, operation time and the incidence of MACEs were similar pre and during COVID-19 pandemic. Similar results were found in Shenzhen, a metropolitan city in southern of China (28). Therefore, above results indicated that safety measures to prevent nosocomial COVID-19 infection did not compromise the in-hospital outcomes as compared with PCI under normal condition. The regional collaborative STEMI treatment network established in China worked well and ensured timely acute cardiac care even in the context of the COVID-19 pandemic.

TABLE 2 | Angiographic characteristics and procedural data.

	PPCI (n = 567)				Pharmaco-invasive (n = 40)			
	COVID-19 era group (n = 265)	Pre-COVID-19 era group (n = 302)	Statistic	P value	COVID-19 era group (n = 18)	Pre-COVID-19 era group (n = 22)	Statistic	P value
Time delays, min								
Symptom onset to FMC	141 (67–282)	147 (70.25–270)	−0.292‡	0.77	88 (30–121.75)	72 (30–193.75)	−0.015‡	0.988
Symptom onset to door	185 (105.75–301)	210 (103–327.5)	−0.668‡	0.504	349 (220–592.5)	382.5 (186.25–579)	−0.184‡	0.854
Door-to-balloon	79 (61–102.5)	77 (55.5–99.5)	−0.855‡	0.393	–	–	–	–
Symptom onset to balloon	274 (177.75–372.75)	278.5 (182.75–425.75)	−0.957‡	0.339	–	–	–	–
Total procedure time	55 (43–72)	53 (42–67)	−1.083‡	0.279	–	–	–	–
symptom onset to thrombolysis	–	–	–	–	139 (70.25–185.5)	120 (70–225.5)	−0.155‡	0.877
Infarct-related artery, n (%)								
LM	18 (6.8)	14 (4.6)	1.233†	0.267	1 (5.6)	0 (0.0)	–	0.45
LAD	150 (56.6)	170 (56.3)	0.006†	0.94	9 (50.0)	14 (63.6)	0.753†	0.385
LCX	69 (26.0)	96 (31.8)	2.262†	0.133	3 (16.7)	5 (22.7)	–	0.632
RCA	124 (46.8)	169 (56.0)	4.751†	0.029	11 (61.1)	11 (50.0)	0.494†	0.482
Multivessel disease Procedural issues, n (%)	77 (29.1)	124 (41.1)	8.887†	0.003	8 (44.4)	12 (54.5)	0.404†	0.525
Procedural issues, n (%)								
Radial access	254 (95.8)	276 (91.4)	4.599†	0.032	17 (94.4)	22 (100.0)	–	0.45
Stent use	236 (89.1)	281 (93.0)	2.794†	0.095	17 (94.4)	22 (100.0)	–	0.45
Direct stenting	100 (37.7)	86 (28.5)	5.489†	0.019	11 (61.1)	16 (72.7)	0.609†	0.435
Thrombus aspiration	34 (12.8)	22 (7.3)	4.876†	0.027	2 (11.1)	0 (0.0)	–	0.196
IABP use	16 (6.0)	22 (7.3)	0.351†	0.554	2 (11.1)	10 (45.5)	5.560†	0.018
ECMO use	2 (0.8)	1 (0.3)	–	0.602	0 (0.0)	0 (0.0)	–	–
Procedural success	259 (97.7)	299 (99.0)	–	0.225	18 (100.0)	22 (100.0)	–	–
Complications	4 (1.5)	4 (1.3)	–	1	1 (5.6)	0 (0.0)	–	0.45
Initial TIMI flow grade (pre-PCI), n (%)								
TIMI flow grade 0–1	223 (84.2)	262 (86.8)	0.774†	0.379	11 (61.1)	16 (72.7)	0.609†	0.435
TIMI flow grade 2–3	42 (15.8)	40 (13.2)			7 (38.9)	6 (27.3)		
Final TIMI flow grade (post-PCI), n (%)								
TIMI flow grade 0–1	2 (0.8)	2 (0.7)	–	1.000	0 (0.0)	0 (0.0)	–	–
TIMI flow grade 2–3	263 (99.2)	300 (99.3)			18 (100.0)	22 (100.0)		

Data are expressed as mean ± SD, as percentages, or as median (Q1, Q3). †χ^2 value; ‡Z value. —: Data not available (Fisher exact test). COVID-19, coronavirus disease 2019; PCI, percutaneous coronary intervention; PPCI, primary PCI; LM, left main; LAD, left anterior descending; LCX, left circumflex; RCA, right coronary artery; IABP, intra-aortic balloon pump; ECMO, extracorporeal membrane oxygenation; TIMI, thrombolysis in myocardial infarction.

TABLE 3 | Clinical outcomes data.

	COVID-19 era group (n = 286)	Pre-COVID-19 era (n = 324)	Statistic	P Value
Length of stay, d	8 (6–10)	8 (6–11)	−0.988‡	0.323
In-hospital death, n (%)	7 (2.4)	11 (3.4)	0.476†	0.490
Non-fatal MI, n (%)	0 (0.0)	1 (0.3)	–	1.000
Non-fatal stroke, n (%)	2 (0.7)	1 (0.3)	–	0.602
Congestive heart failure, n (%)	13 (4.5)	24 (7.4)	2.184†	0.139
Target vessel revascularization, n (%)	7 (2.4)	3 (0.9)	–	0.202
Cumulative MACEs, n (%)	29 (10.1)	40 (12.3)	0.737†	0.391

Data are expressed as mean ± SD, as percentages, or as median (Q₁, Q₃). †χ² value; ‡Z value. —: Data not available (Fisher exact test). COVID-19, coronavirus disease 2019; MI, myocardial infarction; MACEs, major adverse cardiovascular events.

TABLE 4 | Multivariate logistic regression analysis.

	Comparison of COVID-19 era group versus Pre-COVID-19 era group	
	Adjusted OR (95% CI)*	P value
In-hospital death	3.935 (0.511, 30.310)	0.188
MACEs	1.074 (0.416, 2.770)	0.883

COVID-19, coronavirus disease 2019; MACEs, major adverse cardiovascular events. *Adjusted for age, sex, hypertension, hypercholesterolemia, diabetes mellitus, smokers, previous myocardial infarction, previous percutaneous coronary intervention, previous coronary artery bypass graft, aspirin, P2Y12 receptor antagonist, glycoprotein IIb/IIIa inhibitor use, β-blockers, statins, angiotensin converting enzyme inhibitors/Angiotensin II receptor blockers, symptom-to-hospital time, door-to-balloon time, radial access, multivessel disease, vessel of intervention, flow, intra-aortic balloon pump, extracorporeal membrane oxygenation.

Our data demonstrated that a better public communication approach should be adopted to reassure patients in critical conditions to obtain timely medical contact. Public health, political, and physician leaders in China have taken aggressive measures to encourage patients with heart attack symptoms to seek medical care. Social media including WeChat, Weibo, Tik Tok, and so on was applied as a tool for grassroots health promotion initiatives during the COVID-19 pandemic. Based on social media platforms, healthcare professionals reeducated the general population to recognize and act on heart attack signs and symptoms and call an ambulance immediately. Furthermore, it's necessary to stress that the national healthcare system still had the capacity to provide prompt and effective care in a manner that was safe for both patients and healthcare workers. Meanwhile, hospitals had to take appropriate precautions to protect patients and healthcare workers from COVID-19 infection.

STUDY LIMITATIONS

Our study has several limitations. First, although patients affected by COVID-19 were excluded from the final analysis, we cannot definitively exclude the possibility that patients in the COVID-19 era may have COVID-19 infection because it's hard to make an absolutely accurate diagnosis in the early phase of the pandemic. However, we believe this possibility was very small

because all enrolled patients were lack of the epidemiological history and clinical manifestations. Second, we assessed only in-hospital outcomes, as data on post-discharge follow-up are currently not available. Third, the onset of symptoms was a subjective parameter and might not be precisely recorded. Finally, self-report of in-hospital outcomes generally along with early discharge may have resulted in under-reporting of adverse outcomes.

FUTURE DIRECTIONS

Every effort should be made to educate the public to recognize symptoms of life-threatening cardiac conditions and seek appropriate care in a timely fashion. Health authorities should implement strategies to further optimize the STEMI care system in response to emerging infectious diseases like COVID-19.

CONCLUSION

The COVID-19 pandemic outbreak led to a decline in the number of admitted STEMI cases as well as STEMI-related PCI procedures in Hunan province, China. The key quality indicators of reperfusion treatment including median time from symptom onset to FMC, symptom onset to door, door-to-balloon, symptom onset to balloon, and symptom onset to thrombolysis, were not significantly affected during the pandemic outbreak. Restructuring health services during the COVID-19 pandemic has not significantly adversely influenced the in-hospital outcomes.

AUTHOR CONTRIBUTIONS

LT and Z-JW participated in the design of the study, collected clinical data, performed statistical analysis, and drafted the manuscript. X-QH, Z-FF, Z-FZ, J-PZ, L-PJ, FO, C-HL, and G-FZ participated in the treatment for the patients and collected clinical data. Y-HG and S-HZ participated in the design of the study, revised the final version of the manuscript, and supervised the study. All authors participated in the research and reviewed the final version of the manuscript.

REFERENCES

1. Phelan AL, Katz R, Gostin LO. The novel coronavirus originating in Wuhan, China: challenges for global health governance. *JAMA*. (2020) 323:709–10. doi: 10.1001/jama.2020.1097

2. Zhu N, Zhang D, Wang W, Li X, Yang B, Song J, et al. A novel coronavirus from patients with pneumonia in China, 2019. *N Engl J Med*. (2020) 382:727–33. doi: 10.1056/NEJMoa2001017

3. Xiong T-Y, Redwood S, Prendergast B, Chen M. Coronaviruses and the cardiovascular system: acute and long-term implications. *Eur Heart J*. (2020) 41:1798–800. doi: 10.1093/eurheartj/ehaa231

4. Dynamical Change of the Global COVID-19 Cases. *Data in Motion: Friday, January 7, 2022*. (2022). Available online at: https://coronavirus.jhu.edu/ (accessed January 8, 2022).

5. Vogel B, Claessen BE, Arnold SV, Chan D, Cohen DJ, Giannitsis E, et al. ST-segment elevation myocardial infarction. *Nat Rev Dis Primers*. (2019) 5:39. doi: 10.1038/s41572-019-0090-3

6. Ibanez B, James S, Agewall S, Antunes MJ, Bucciarelli-Ducci C, Bueno H, et al. 2017 ESC guidelines for the management of acute myocardial infarction in patients presenting with ST-segment elevation: the task force for the management of acute myocardial infarction in patients presenting with ST-segment elevation of the European society of cardiology (ESC). *Eur Heart J*. (2018) 39:119–77. doi: 10.1093/eurheartj/ehx393

7. De Rosa S, Spaccarotella C, Basso C, Calabrò MP, Curcio A, Filardi PP, et al. Reduction of hospitalizations for myocardial infarction in Italy in the COVID-19 era. *Eur Heart J*. (2020) 41:2083–8. doi: 10.1093/eurheartj/ehaa409

8. Braiteh N, Rehman WU, Alom M, Skovira V, Breiteh N, Rehman I, et al. Decrease in acute coronary syndrome presentations during the COVID-19 pandemic in upstate New York. *Am Heart J*. (2020) 226:147–51. doi: 10.1016/j.ahj.2020.05.009

9. Mafham MM, Spata E, Goldacre R, Gair D, Curnow P, Bray M, et al. COVID-19 pandemic and admission rates for and management of acute coronary syndromes in England. *Lancet*. (2020) 396:381–9. doi: 10.1016/S0140-6736(20)31356-8

10. Mahmud E, Dauerman HL, Welt FGP, Messenger JC, Rao SV, Grines C, et al. Management of acute myocardial infarction during the COVID-19 pandemic: a consensus statement from the society for cardiovascular angiography and interventions (SCAI), the American college of cardiology (ACC), and the American college of emergency physicians (ACEP). *Catheter Cardiovasc Interv*. (2020) 96:336–45. doi: 10.1002/ccd.28946

11. Bu J, Chen M, Cheng X, Dong Y, Fang W, Ge J, et al. [Consensus of Chinese experts on diagnosis and treatment processes of acute myocardial infarction in the context of prevention and control of COVID-19 (first edition)]. *Nan Fang Yi Ke Da Xue Xue Bao*. (2020) 40:147–51. doi: 10.12122/j.issn.1673-4254.2020.02.01

12. Thygesen K, Alpert JS, Jaffe AS, Chaitman BR, Bax JJ, Morrow DA, et al. Fourth universal definition of myocardial infarction (2018). *Circulation*. (2018) 138:e618–51. doi: 10.1161/CIR.0000000000000617

13. Cutlip DE, Windecker S, Mehran R, Boam A, Cohen DJ, van Es G-A, et al. Clinical end points in coronary stent trials: a case for standardized definitions. *Circulation*. (2007) 115:2344–51. doi: 10.1161/CIRCULATIONAHA.106.685313

14. Tang L, Chen P-F, Hu X-Q, Shen X-Q, Zhao Y-S, Fang Z-F, et al. Effect of Chinese national holidays and weekends versus weekday admission on clinical outcomes in patients with STEMI undergoing primary PCI. *J Geriatr Cardiol*. (2017) 14:604–13. doi: 10.11909/j.issn.1671-5411.2017.10.003

15. Xiang D, Xiang X, Zhang W, Yi S, Zhang J, Gu X, et al. Management and outcomes of patients with STEMI during the COVID-19 pandemic in China. *J Am Coll Cardiol*. (2020) 76:1318–24. doi: 10.1016/j.jacc.2020.06.039

16. Scholz KH, Lengenfelder B, Thilo C, Jeron A, Stefanow S, Janssens U, et al. Impact of COVID-19 outbreak on regional STEMI care in Germany. *Clin Res Cardiol*. (2020) 109:1511–21. doi: 10.1007/s00392-020-01703-z

17. Chew NW, Sia CH, Wee HL, Benedict LJ, Rastogi S, Kojodjojo P, et al. Impact of the COVID-19 pandemic on door-to-balloon time for primary percutaneous coronary intervention- results from the Singapore western STEMI network. *Circ J*. (2021) 85:139–49. doi: 10.1253/circj.CJ-20-0800

18. Montagnon R, Rouffilange L, Agard G, Benner P, Cazes N, Renard A. Impact of the COVID-19 pandemic on emergency department use: focus on patients requiring urgent revascularization. *J Emerg Med*. (2021) 60:229–36. doi: 10.1016/j.jemermed.2020.09.042

19. Ostergaard L, Butt JH, Kragholm K, Schou M, Phelps M, Sorensen R, et al. Incidence of acute coronary syndrome during national lock-down: insights from nationwide data during the coronavirus disease 2019 (COVID-19) pandemic. *Am Heart J*. (2021) 232:146–53. doi: 10.1016/j.ahj.2020.11.004

20. Chieffo A, Stefanini GG, Price S, Barbato E, Tarantini G, Karam N, et al. EAPCI position statement on invasive management of acute coronary syndromes during the COVID-19 pandemic. *EuroIntervention*. (2020) 16:233–46. doi: 10.4244/EIJY20M05_01

21. Rattka M, Baumhardt M, Dreyhaupt J, Rothenbacher D, Thiessen K, Markovic S, et al. 31 days of COVID-19-cardiac events during restriction of public life-a comparative study. *Clin Res Cardiol*. (2020) 109:1476–82. doi: 10.1007/s00392-020-01681-2

22. Garcia S, Albaghdadi MS, Meraj PM, Schmidt C, Garberich R, Jaffer FA, et al. Reduction in ST-segment elevation cardiac catheterization laboratory activations in the United States during COVID-19 pandemic. *J Am Coll Cardiol*. (2020) 75:2871–2. doi: 10.1016/j.jacc.2020.04.011

23. Rodríguez-Leor O, Cid-Álvarez B, Pérez de Prado A, Rossello X, Ojeda S, Serrador A, et al. Impact of COVID-19 on ST-segment elevation myocardial infarction care. The Spanish experience. *Revista Espanola Cardiologia (English Ed)*. (2020) 73:994–1002. doi: 10.1016/j.rec.2020.08.002

24. Kwok CS, Gale CP, Kinnaird T, Curzen N, Ludman P, Kontopantelis E, et al. Impact of COVID-19 on percutaneous coronary intervention for ST-elevation myocardial infarction. *Heart*. (2020) 106:1805–11. doi: 10.1136/heartjnl-2020-317650

25. Abdelaziz HK, Abdelrahman A, Nabi A, Debski M, Mentias A, Choudhury T, et al. Impact of COVID-19 pandemic on patients with ST-segment elevation myocardial infarction: insights from a British cardiac center. *Am Heart J*. (2020) 226:45–8. doi: 10.1016/j.ahj.2020.04.022

26. Baldi E, Sechi GM, Mare C, Canevari F, Brancaglione A, Primi R, et al. Out-of-hospital cardiac arrest during the Covid-19 outbreak in Italy. *N Engl J Med*. (2020) 383:496–8. doi: 10.1056/NEJMc2010418

27. Guan X, Zhang J, Li Y, Ma N. Safety measures for COVID-19 do not compromise the outcomes of patients undergoing primary percutaneous coronary intervention: a single center retrospective study. *Sci Rep*. (2021) 11:9959. doi: 10.1038/s41598-021-89419-6

28. Zhu S, Jiang G, Fan Z, Yi L, Wu C, Zhou Q, et al. [Effects of COVID-19 epidemic on patients with acute myocardial infarction with ST-segment elevation in a grade-A tertiary hospital in Shenzhen]. *Chin J Hygiene Rescue (Electron Ed)*. (2020) 6:257–61.

17

Thromboinflammation and COVID-19: The Role of Exercise in the Prevention and Treatment

Helena Angelica Pereira Batatinha[1], Karsten Krüger[2] and José Cesar Rosa Neto[1]*

[1] Immunometabolism Research Group, Biomedical Science Institute, University of São Paulo, São Paulo, Brazil, [2] Department of Exercise Physiology and Sports Therapy, University of Giessen, Giessen, Germany

*Correspondence:
José Cesar Rosa Neto
josecesar23@hotmail.com

Keywords: COVID-19, exercise, pandemic, thromboinflammation, cytokine storm

INTRODUCTION

The coronavirus disease 2019 (COVID-19) pandemic is currently the biggest public health concern across the globe. On a global scale, from December 2019 to September 2020, more than 34,114,000 people were infected with the disease, with 1,016,000 deaths recorded (1). Although the etiology of the disease has long been investigated, it is still a harsh challenge for the medical and scientific community.

COVID-19 infection is complex, and the risk factors are different from the known viral respiratory infections. People with chronic inflammatory diseases (such as obesity, hypertension, diabetes, and cardiovascular disorder) are at a huge risk of developing moderate to severe symptoms and being hospitalized in the intensive care unit (ICU) (2, 3). The most common phenomena among these conditions are chronic low-grade inflammation and increased cardiovascular complications. Several evidences have been put forward to support the association between COVID-19 and thromboinflammation (3, 4). Specifically, venous thrombosis has been found to be causally related to pulmonary embolism in many cases (5).

Exercise is well-known for having a prophylactic and therapeutic effect on chronic inflammatory diseases, with a high impact on the vascular system. Furthermore, it has been reported that exercise may decrease the severity of infectious diseases and number of days of disease symptoms (6). Consistent with this, it is speculated that regular exercise represents a protective factor against the severity of COVID-19 relating to thromboinflammation and its complications.

EXERCISE AS A TOOL FOR DECREASING CHRONIC INFLAMMATION AND IMPROVING ANGIOGENESIS AND IMMUNE RESPONSE

The vascular system is largely affected by COVID-19 infection. Although pulmonary failure is not directly related to the loss of pulmonary alveoli, lack of blood flow in this area can induce a collapse of the alveoli, as recently demonstrated by Ackermann et al. (7). Furthermore, kidneys are highly vascularized organs that also may be affected by this infection (2).

Venous thrombosis is usually found in coagulopathies and also observed in arterial thrombosis and stroke (7). Clinical markers of the coagulation cascade, such as D-dimer and fibrinogen, are elevated in those with moderate and severe forms of COVID-19 (8). Low innate antiviral defense and high inflammatory cytokine release contribute to the severity of COVID-19 (9), suggesting that it can be an important trigger for thrombotic complications. High amounts of pro-inflammatory cytokines contribute to the activation of thrombotic pathways. For instance, it was demonstrated that interleukin (IL)-6 induces thrombin generation and that IL-1 and tumor necrosis factor (TNF)-α inhibit anticoagulant pathways (8).

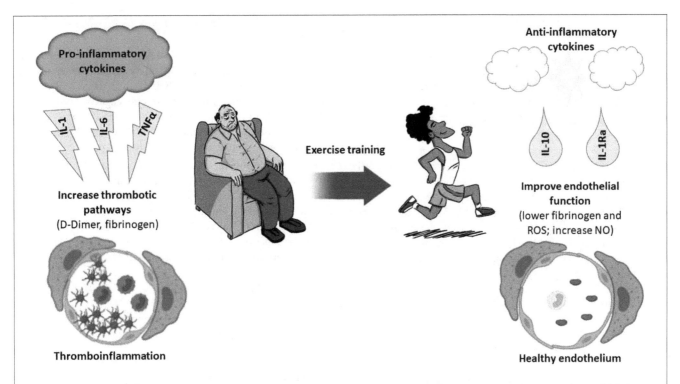

FIGURE 1 | Thromboinflammation and the effect of exercise. A sedentary lifestyle leads to an increase in the release of pro-inflammatory cytokines, which induce a low-grade chronic inflammation. These inflammatory mediators enhance the thrombotic pathways that facilitate thromboinflammation, which has been associated with poor prognosis in coronavirus disease 2019 (COVID-19) patients. Exercise decreases inflammation by many pathways, including the release of anti-inflammatory cytokines. Regular exercise is associated with lower levels of fibrinogen and reactive oxygen species and increased amounts of nitric oxide (NO) production, thus inducing a healthy endothelium environment.

Exercise, especially in the form of regular aerobic activities, have the potential of dampening chronic inflammation by stimulating anti-inflammatory pathways and associated improvement of cardiovascular functions. Accordingly, by decreasing the basal concentration of inflammatory cytokines and reducing the percentage of pro-inflammatory T effector memory CD45+ re-expressing T cells (T-EMRA cells), exercise indirectly prevents the activation of thrombotic pathways (10).

Exercise has been shown to directly affect coagulation. While acute and strenuous activities can culminate in pro-coagulative stimuli, regular activity has been shown to diminish platelet activation under resting conditions (11). Exercise reduces fibrinogen level and enhances the plasma volume without increasing the erythrocyte volume (11). Also, exercise was used as a treatment for deep venous post-thrombotic syndrome (12). Heart failure patients with reduced fraction of ejection, when treated with moderate endurance exercise, showed a reduction in vascular endothelial damage as well as suppression of inflammation and oxidative stress (13).

The intensity and duration of aerobic exercise are correlated with the increase in nitric oxide production and reduction of reactive oxygen species, which lead to an improvement in endothelial function. Moreover, aerobic exercise reduces hypertension on coronary arteries and vascular stiffness (14).

In parallel, regular exercise can enhance the innate and adaptive immune defense system, thus improving the response against viral infections. While it can only be speculated that exercise has a protective effect against severe acute respiratory syndrome coronavirus 2 (SARS-CoV-2) infection, regular activity has been shown to decrease the severity of infectious episodes and number of days of the symptom in other infectious diseases (6). Concerning influenza infection, exercise is associated with a lower excess risk of mortality (15). Similarly, in murine models, it was proven that moderate exercise reduces mortality in the initial days after an influenza virus infection (16). Moreover, moderate aerobic training has been shown to enhance T cell count, which is found to be decreased in the blood of SARS-CoV-2-infected patients (21), increase anti-inflammatory cytokines, improve endothelial function, and repair (**Figure 1**), enhance VO2peak, and have beneficial effects on clinical outcomes (22). A minimum of 150 min per week (30 min−5 days/week) of moderate aerobic exercise (5–7 on a scale of 0–10, where 0 is super easy and 10 is exhaustive) was recommended by the American College of Sports Medicine to achieve the health benefits of exercise. Moderate aerobic exercise is applied to improve immunity and metabolic complications that can reduce the poor prognosis of COVID-19 (23).

Therefore, we hypothesized that moderate intensity of aerobic training could be a protective factor against severe courses of

COVID-19 (17) (**Figure 1**). Therefore, we can draw the attention of physicians toward assessment of the fitness level of COVID-19 patients.

THE POTENTIAL ROLE OF EXERCISE IN THE RECOVERY OF THOSE INFECTED WITH CORONAVIRUS DISEASE 2019

In 2016, the WHO proposed "functioning" as a third clinical outcome indicator, such that diseases that are not fully cured are accompanied by some dysfunctions. Improving functional life while recovering from a disease is a key sign of medical effectiveness and overall health. Many patients who are recovering from COVID-19, especially those presenting severe symptoms during the infection phase, are not able to return to the normal life of caring for themselves after being discharged (18).

As discussed above, poor vascularization could cause alveoli collapse, thus leading to pulmonary failure. Several individuals infected by SARS-CoV-2 have presented respiratory problems with impairment of pulmonary ventilation function and air exchange in the alveoli, which lead to chest tightness, dyspnea, and pulmonary fibrosis (18). Pulmonary fibrosis is directly associated with high mortality rates. Furthermore, dyspnea, which is often associated with loss of skeletal muscle mass, is responsible

for a decreased exercise capacity due to a reduction of daily leaving activities (19).

Several studies have investigated the role of exercise in the treatment of chronic lung disease and pulmonary fibrosis patients. A meta-analysis recently published stated that aerobic training significantly improves exercise capacity and health-related quality of life of patients with chronic respiratory disease and/or pulmonary fibrosis and that aerobic training improved the dyspnea scores when combined with breathing exercises (20).

It is important to remember that most of the benefits promoted by physical exercise in the rehabilitation of respiratory and cardiovascular diseases can be gradually lost if the patient does not continue to exercise in the long run (18). However, the practice of exercise for the improvement of medical conditions should be supervised. In conclusion, regular exercise could be an adjuvant for the prevention and treatment of COVID-19.

AUTHOR CONTRIBUTIONS

All authors listed have made a substantial, direct and intellectual contribution to the work, and approved it for publication.

ACKNOWLEDGMENTS

The authors thank Luciano Proença for helping with the design of the figure and FAPESP and CNPQ.

REFERENCES

1. Johns Hopkins Coronavirus Resource Center. *Johns Hopkins Coronavirus Resource Center.* Available online at: https://coronavirus.jhu.edu/ (accessed June 19, 2020).
2. Gémes K, Talbäck M, Modig K, Ahlbom A, Berglund A, Feychting M, et al. Burden and prevalence of prognostic factors for severe COVID-19 in Sweden. *Eur J Epidemiol.* (2020) 35:401–9. doi: 10.1007/s10654-020-00646-z
3. Harenberg J, Favaloro E. COVID-19: progression of disease and intravascular coagulation—present status and future perspectives. *Clin Chem Lab Med.* (2020) 58:1029–36. doi: 10.1515/cclm-2020-0502
4. Lillicrap D. Disseminated intravascular coagulation in patients with 2019-nCoV pneumonia. *J Thromb Haemost.* (2020) 18:786–7. doi: 10.1111/jth.14781
5. Barton LM, Duval EJ, Stroberg E, Ghosh S, Mukhopadhyay S. COVID-19 autopsies, Oklahoma, USA. *Am J Clin Pathol.* (2020) 153:725–33. doi: 10.1093/ajcp/aqaa062
6. Grande AJ, Keogh J, Silva V, Scott AM. Exercise versus no exercise for the occurrence, severity, and duration of acute respiratory infections. *Cochrane Database Syst Rev.* (2020) 4:CD010596. doi: 10.1002/14651858.CD010596.pub3
7. Ackermann M, Verleden SE, Kuehnel M, Haverich A, Welte T, Laenger F, et al. Pulmonary vascular endothelialitis, thrombosis, and angiogenesis in covid-19. *N Engl J Med.* (2020) 383:120–8. doi: 10.1056/NEJMoa2015432
8. Levi M, Thachil J, Iba T, Levy JH. Coagulation abnormalities and thrombosis in patients with COVID-19. *Lancet Haematol.* (2020) 7:e438–40. doi: 10.1016/S2352-3026(20)30145-9
9. Blanco-Melo D, Nilsson-Payant BE, Liu W-C, Uhl S, Hoagland D, Møller R, et al. Imbalanced host response to SARS-CoV-2 drives development of COVID-19. *Cell.* (2020) 181:1036–45.e9. doi: 10.1016/j.cell.2020.04.026

10. Philippe M, Gatterer H, Burtscher M, Weinberger B, Keller M, Grubeck-Loebenstein B, et al. Concentric and eccentric endurance exercise reverse hallmarks of T-cell senescence in pre-diabetic subjects. *Front Physiol.* (2019) 10:684. doi: 10.3389/fphys.2019.00684
11. Heber S, Volf I. Effects of physical (in)activity on platelet function. *BioMed Res Int.* (2015) 2015:165078. doi: 10.1155/2015/165078
12. Kahn SR, Shrier I, Shapiro S, Houweling AH, Hirsch AM, Reid RD, et al. Six-month exercise training program to treat post-thrombotic syndrome: a randomized controlled two-centre trial. *CMAJ.* (2011) 183:37–44. doi: 10.1503/cmaj.100248
13. Hsu C-C, Fu T-C, Huang S-C, Wang J-S. High-intensity interval training recuperates capacity of endogenous thrombin generation in heart failure patients with reduced ejection fraction. *Thromb Res.* (2020) 187:159–65. doi: 10.1016/j.thromres.2020.01.013
14. Roque FR, Briones AM, García-Redondo AB, Galán M, Martínez-Revelles S, Avendaño MS, et al. Aerobic exercise reduces oxidative stress and improves vascular changes of small mesenteric and coronary arteries in hypertension. *Br J Pharmacol.* (2013) 168:686–703. doi: 10.1111/j.1476-5381.2012.02224.x
15. Wong C-M, Lai H-K, Ou C-Q, Ho S-Y, Chan K-P, Thach T-Q, et al. Is exercise protective against influenza-associated mortality? *PLoS ONE.* (2008) 3:e2108. doi: 10.1371/journal.pone.0002108
16. Lowder T, Padgett DA, Woods JA. Moderate exercise protects mice from death due to influenza virus. *Brain Behav Immun.* (2005) 19:377–80. doi: 10.1016/j.bbi.2005.04.002
17. Channappanavar R, Zhao J, Perlman S. T cell-mediated immune response to respiratory coronaviruses. *Immunol Res.* (2014) 59:118–28. doi: 10.1007/s12026-014-8534-z
18. Giallauria F, Piccioli L, Vitale G, Sarullo FM. Exercise training in patients with chronic heart failure: a new challenge for Cardiac Rehabilitation

Community. *Monaldi Arch Chest Dis Arch Monaldi Mal Torace*. (2018) 88:987. doi: 10.4081/monaldi.2018.987

19. Dixit S. Can moderate intensity aerobic exercise be an effective and valuable therapy in preventing and controlling the pandemic of COVID-19? *Med Hypotheses*. (2020) 143:109854. doi: 10.1016/j.mehy.2020.109854

20. Zbinden-Foncea H, Francaux M, Deldicque L, Hawley JA. Does high cardiorespiratory fitness confer some protection against pro-inflammatory responses after infection by SARS-CoV-2? *Obes Silver Spring Md*. (2020) 28:1378–81. doi: 10.1002/oby.22849

21. Li J. Rehabilitation management of patients with COVID-19. Lessons learned from the first experiences in China. *Eur J Phys Rehabil Med*. (2020) 24:9. doi: 10.23736/S1973-9087.20.06292-9

22. Dyspnea. Mechanisms, assessment, and management: a consensus statement. American Thoracic Society. *Am J Respir Crit Care Med*. (1999) 159:321–40. doi: 10.1164/ajrccm.159.1.ats898

23. Hanada M, Kasawara KT, Mathur S, Rozenberg D, Kozu R, Hassan SA, et al. Aerobic and breathing exercises improve dyspnea, exercise capacity and quality of life in idiopathic pulmonary fibrosis patients: systematic review and meta-analysis. *J Thorac Dis*. (2020) 12:1041–55. doi: 10.21037/jtd.2019.12.27

18

Quantifying the Excess Risk of Adverse COVID-19 Outcomes in Unvaccinated Individuals with Diabetes Mellitus, Hypertension, Ischaemic Heart Disease or Myocardial Injury

Sher May Ng [1†], Jiliu Pan [2†], Kyriacos Mouyis [3], Sreenivasa Rao Kondapally Seshasai [4], Vikas Kapil [5], Kenneth M. Rice [6] and Ajay K. Gupta [5*]

[1] St. Bartholomew's Hospital, London, United Kingdom, [2] Royal Brompton and Harefield Hospitals, London, United Kingdom, [3] Royal Free London NHS Foundation Trust, London, United Kingdom, [4] Cardiovascular Clinical Academic Group, Molecular and Clinical Sciences Research Institute, St. George's University of London, St. George's University Hospitals NHS Foundation Trust, London, United Kingdom, [5] William Harvey Research Institute, Queen Mary University London, London, United Kingdom, [6] Department of Biostatistics, University of Washington, Seattle, WA, United States

*Correspondence:
Ajay K. Gupta
ajay.gupta@qmul.ac.uk

[†] These authors have contributed equally to this work

Background: More than 80% of individuals in low and middle-income countries (LMICs) are unvaccinated against coronavirus disease 2019 (COVID-19). In contrast, the greatest burden of cardiovascular disease is seen in LMIC populations. Hypertension (HTN), diabetes mellitus (DM), ischaemic heart disease (IHD) and myocardial injury have been variably associated with adverse COVID-19 outcomes. A systematic comparison of their impact on specific COVID-19 outcomes is lacking. We quantified the impact of DM, HTN, IHD and myocardial injury on six adverse COVID-19 outcomes: death, acute respiratory distress syndrome (ARDS), invasive mechanical ventilation (IMV), admission to intensive care (ITUadm), acute kidney injury (AKI) and severe COVID-19 disease (SCov), in an unvaccinated population.

Methodology: We included studies published between 1st December 2019 and 16th July 2020 with extractable data on patients ≥18 years of age with suspected or confirmed SARS-CoV-2 infection. Odds ratios (OR) for the association between DM, HTN, IHD and myocardial injury with each of six COVID-19 outcomes were measured.

Results: We included 110 studies comprising 48,809 COVID-19 patients. Myocardial injury had the strongest association for all six adverse COVID-19 outcomes [death: OR 8.85 95% CI (8.08–9.68), ARDS: 5.70 (4.48–7.24), IMV: 3.42 (2.92–4.01), ITUadm: 4.85 (3.94–6.05), AKI: 10.49 (6.55–16.78), SCov: 5.10 (4.26–6.05)]. HTN and DM were also significantly associated with death, ARDS, ITUadm, AKI and SCov. There was substantial heterogeneity in the results, partly explained by differences in age, gender, geographical region and recruitment period.

Conclusion: COVID-19 patients with myocardial injury are at substantially greater risk of death, severe disease and other adverse outcomes. Weaker, yet significant associations are present in patients with HTN, DM and IHD. Quantifying these associations is important for risk stratification, resource allocation and urgency in vaccinating these populations.

Systematic Review Registration: https://www.crd.york.ac.uk/prospero/, registration no: CRD42020201435 and CRD42020201443.

Keywords: **COVID-19, cardiovascular risk factors, myocardial injury, ischaemic heart disease, diabetes, hypertension, adverse outcomes**

INTRODUCTION

The global coronavirus disease 2019 (COVID-19) pandemic has impacted healthcare systems and economies worldwide. It has laid bare health inequalities and magnified unequal effects of public health measures implemented across the world, with associated ramifications on global health. This is well-exemplified by the global COVID-19 vaccine inequality, where only 14.4% of individuals in low-income countries have received one dose of COVID-19 vaccine, as of March 2022 (1).

Low and middle-income countries (LMICs) are plagued by the difficult decision between strict non-pharmaceutical interventions such as national lockdowns and their socioeconomic impact, particularly on the urban poor. Moreover, these countries suffer from increased COVID-19 associated mortality owing to insufficient healthcare resources and poorly funded emergency response programmes (2, 3).

While high-income countries (HICs) have made significant progress in vaccination rollout programmes, LMICs continue to lag behind. Importantly, studies from HIC populations have suggested the COVID-19 incidence and hospitalization rates among unvaccinated individuals are approximately 2 and 5-times that of vaccinated (but without a booster) individuals respectively (4).

Multiple observational studies have shown associations between cardiovascular (CV) risk factors such as hypertension (HTN), diabetes mellitus (DM), previous ischaemic heart disease (IHD), myocardial injury and outcomes such as mortality or severe disease due to COVID-19 (SCov). Other studies have challenged these findings, showing heterogeneous associations between these risk factors and COVID-19 related death (5, 6). In addition, there remains a lack of consensus on the impact of myocardial injury and CV risk factors on other important COVID-19 adverse outcomes such as acute respiratory distress syndrome (ARDS), invasive mechanical ventilation (IMV) and intensive care admission (ITUadm).

Therefore, quantifying the risk of COVID-19-related adverse outcomes attributable to CV risk factors, IHD and myocardial injury in unvaccinated persons is essential, not only for patient-specific care but also for risk stratification and planning of healthcare delivery in already stretched LMICs. This is especially relevant where the greatest burden of cardiovascular disease is amongst LMICs. In this meta-analysis, we quantify the association between CV risk factors, IHD and myocardial injury, and specific adverse clinical outcomes in unvaccinated adults with COVID-19 infection.

METHODS

The protocol for this meta-analysis with pre-specified aims and objectives was prospectively registered on PROSPERO (CRD42020201435 and CRD42020201443). The aim of the meta-analysis was to study the impact of pre-specified cardiovascular risk factors (HTN, DM, previous IHD, and presence of myocardial injury) on adverse COVID-19 outcomes [all-cause mortality, ARDS, IMV, admission to intensive care (ITUadm), AKI, and study-defined severe COVID-19 disease (SCoV)]. We included studies published (in print or pre-print version) during the early phase of the COVID-19 pandemic, prior to widespread use of COVID-19 vaccinations.

Population Selection

We included studies that reported prevalence of pre-existing cardiovascular risk factors in adult patients ($\geq$18 years of age) with suspected or confirmed COVID-19 disease and any one of the COVID-19 related adverse outcomes.

Search Strategy

We searched databases of published (MEDLINE, CINAHL, Embase, EMCARE, British Nursing Index) and pre-print (medRxiv) articles without language restrictions, between 1st December 2019 and 16th July 2020. We also searched data from the COVID-19 specific World Health Organization (WHO) global research database. Duplicate studies were identified and removed initially through a Mendeley folder (AT) followed by manual de-duplication by two authors working independently (JP and SMN). The final study list was agreed by consensus. Three authors (JP, KM, SMN) screened references of full-text studies, review articles and existing meta-analyses for additional studies. **Appendix A** gives the full search strategy.

Selection Criteria

Studies were included if they had extractable data on (i) patients $\geq$ 18 years of age with suspected or confirmed SARS-CoV-2 infection (COVID-19); (ii) pre-existing CV risk factors, specifically HTN and DM, IHD, or evidence of myocardial injury (defined as serum troponin level above the 99th percentile upper reference limit); and (iii) COVID-19 related outcomes, in particular all-cause mortality, ARDS, IMV, admission to intensive care (ITUadm), AKI, and study-defined severe COVID-19 disease (SCoV). Data from Chinese studies were translated and extracted by JP. Studies reporting only on special populations (e.g., dialysis patients, pregnant women, elderly patients or

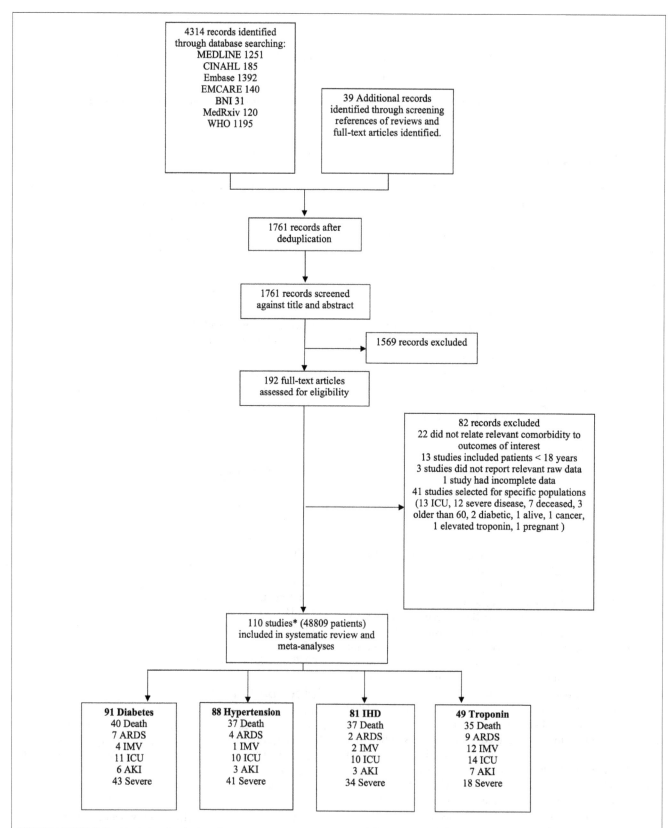

FIGURE 1 | PRISMA flow chart of study selection. *Three studies reported different outcomes on the same cohort. Therefore, 208 patients have been excluded from the total number of patients as they were considered to be a duplicate cohort.

children) were excluded (**Appendix C**). Case reports, case series, review articles and meta-analyses were also excluded. **Figure 1** shows the PRISMA flow chart for study selection.

Three authors (KM, JP, SMN) independently screened all titles and abstracts, reviewed full text articles, extracted data onto pre-specified forms and performed risk of bias assessments. Disagreements were resolved by consensus. Risk of bias assessment for individual studies was performed using the Newcastle-Ottawa Scale (NOS) (**Appendix D**). The quality of body of evidence for each outcome was assessed using Grading of Recommendations, Assessment, Development and Evaluation (GRADE) working group approach (**Appendix E**).

Statistical Analysis

Associations between disease status and COVID-19 outcomes were quantified using odds ratios (OR) which were combined using fixed-effects meta-analysis (7). Random-effects analysis was also performed as an alternative assessment of the impact of heterogeneity on the analyses. Results presented were derived from the fixed-effects model if no notable difference from the random-effects analysis was identified. Heterogeneity around the fixed-effects (inverse-variance weighted) average effect was assessed using the I^2 statistic (8) and where larger numbers of studies were present, fixed-effects meta-regression. Meta-regression was used to assess the effect-modification of disease status on COVID-19 outcomes by age, geographic region, date of last recruitment and proportion of male participants. In sensitivity analyses to address miscalibration of inference due to small sample sizes, we compared meta-analysis results to those with higher-order accuracy (9).

RESULTS

We identified 110 studies comprising 49,017 patients with COVID-19. The full list of included and excluded studies are detailed in **Appendices B, C**. As three studies reported on the same cohort of patients, we excluded 208 individuals from the meta-analysis, leaving 48,809 patients (**Figure 1**). The mean age was 56.7 years and 57% were male. A median of three risk factors and outcomes were reported per study. In total 20% had DM, 37% had HTN, 10% had IHD and 12% had evidence of myocardial injury. Death and severe COVID-19 disease were the commonest reported outcomes; overall, there were 7,150 deaths, 2,180 cases of ARDS, 3,162 individuals needing IMV, 2,950 admissions to intensive care, 3119 patients with AKI and 4,804 severe COVID-19 cases. **Table 1** summarizes the characteristics of included studies, categorized by risk factors.

Presence of Diabetes, Hypertension and Ischaemic Heart Disease and COVID-19 Outcomes

Table 2 summarizes the associations between the four studied risk factors and six outcomes of interest.

Presence of DM (40 studies, 18,979 patients, 3,791 with DM), HTN (37 studies, 17,995 patients, 6,695 with HTN) or IHD (37 studies, 19,968 patients, 2,619 with IHD) was strongly associated with death from COVID-19 [DM: OR 2.16 (95% confidence interval, CI: 1.97–2.36), HTN: 2.72 (2.51–2.97) and IHD: 3.29 (3.00–3.63), respectively]. These cardiovascular risk factors were also associated with severe COVID-19 disease (**Figure 2**).

Fewer studies explored the association between DM, HTN and IHD with ARDS, IMV, ITUadm and AKI. Nevertheless, we observed significant associations between these CV risk factors, IHD and ITUadm as well as AKI. While DM and HTN were significant risk factors for developing ARDS, a similar association was not observed in patients with pre-existing IHD [OR 1.42 (0.49–4.10), $p = 0.30$], though only 2 studies involving 310 patients (15 with IHD) were included in this meta-analysis. Only one study (393 patients) explored the association between HTN and IMV, finding no significant association [OR 1.25 (0.82–1.90)].

There was some discrepancy between the fixed-effects and random-effect analysis of the association between IHD and ITUadm. However, the odds ratio and confidence intervals from the fixed-effects model are entirely within the confidence intervals from the random-effect analysis. This would be expected when a random-effect analysis is simply a less efficient estimate of the same parameter or a numerically similar one estimated by the fixed-effects analysis.

Presence of Myocardial Injury and COVID-19 Outcomes

Forty-nine studies reported on the risks of death and other adverse outcomes associated with the presence of myocardial injury at baseline in patients with COVID-19. Presence of myocardial injury was associated with all six adverse COVID-19 outcomes (**Figure 2**). There was a near 9-fold increase in the risk of death [OR 8.85; (8.08–9.68)] amongst those with myocardial injury (vs. those without) in 35 studies including 21,707 patients, where 5,225 had myocardial injury and 2,197 patients died. In a meta-analysis of 7 studies comprising 1,777 patients, those with myocardial injury had more than 10-fold increased risk of AKI [OR 10.5; (6.55–16.8)]. Similarly, myocardial injury was also associated with ARDS [OR 5.70; (4.48–7.24)], IMV [3.42; (2.91–4.01)], ITUadm [4.85; (3.93–6.05)] and SCov [OR 5.10 (4.26–6.05)]. Apart from the association between myocardial injury and acute kidney injury, there was substantial heterogeneity in association between studies for all other outcomes (10).

The mean NOS score for all studies combined was 6.95, indicating that they were of satisfactory quality (**Appendix D**). Moderate to substantial heterogeneity was observed in the majority of meta-analyses. Only four meta-analyses had insignificant heterogeneity ($I^2 < 10\%$), all with small numbers of included studies.

We performed a meta-regression to assess the effect modification by age, gender, publication date and geographic region, on the association of cardiovascular risk factors and myocardial injury on death and severe COVID-19 disease. Overall, advanced age, studies conducted in Asia and male gender showed stronger association between cardiovascular risk factors, ischaemic heart disease and myocardial injury with

TABLE 1 | Characteristics of included studies reporting COVID-19 related outcomes, categorized by risk factors.

Outcome by risk factor	Number of studies	Total number of patients	N patients with risk factor* No. (%)	N patients with outcome** No. (%)	Mean age	Male no. (%)	Region of study	N patients with risk factor and outcome No. (%)	% of patients exposed to risk factor reaching outcome
Death									
Diabetes mellitus	40	18,979	3,791 (20)	3,194 (17)	60	61	24 Asia, 11 Europe, 5 USA	984 (5)	26
Hypertension	37	17,995	6,695 (37)	3,063 (17)	59.1	60	22 Asia, 10 Europe, 5 USA	1,698 (9)	25
Ischaemic heart disease	37	19,968	2,619 (13)	3,521 (18)	60.3	60	21 Asia, 11 Europe, 5 USA	928 (5)	35
Myocardial injury	35	21,707	5,225 (24)	3,259 (15)	58.2	54	26 Asia, 5 Europe, 4 USA	2,197 (10)	42
ARDS									
Diabetes mellitus	7	1,428	257 (18)	404 (28)	57	750 (53)	6 Asia, 1 Europe	112 (8)	44
Hypertension	4	476	154 (32)	172 (36)	56.5	287 (60)	3 Asia, 1 Europe	65 (14)	42
Ischaemic heart disease	2	310	15 (5)	137 (44)	53	187 (60)	2 Asia	8 (3)	53
Myocardial injury	9	2,189	584 (27)	615 (28)	57.8	1,128 (52)	6 Asia, 2 Europe, 1 USA	348 (16)	60
IMV									
Diabetes mellitus	4	1,345	275 (20)	214 (16)	58.7	1,376 (52)	3 Asia, 1 USA	65 (5)	24
Hypertension	1	393	197 (50)	130 (33)	61.5	238 (61)	1 USA	70 (18)	36
Ischaemic heart disease	2	8,831	777 (9)	689 (8)	59.6	4,782 (54)	2 USA	109 (1)	14
Myocardial injury	12	10,424	2,796 (26)	836 (8)	57.3	5,625 (54)	9 Asia, 1 Europe, 2 USA	553 (5)	20
ITU									
Diabetes mellitus	11	2,487	482 (19)	432 (17)	56.9	1,376 (55)	7 Asia, 3 Europe, 1 USA	133 (5)	28
Hypertension	10	1,891	761 (40)	394 (21)	57.2	1,089 (58)	6 Asia, 3 Europe, 1 USA	211 (11)	28
Ischaemic heart disease	10	1,891	259 (14)	394 (21)	57.2	1,089 (58)	6 Asia, 3 Europe, 1 USA	63 (3)	24
Myocardial injury	14	2,753	698 (25)	644 (23)	56	1,487 (54)	9 Asia, 4 Europe, 1 USA	309 (11)	44
AKI									
Diabetes mellitus	6	7,018	2,124 (30)	2,205 (31)	59.6	4,081 (58)	4 Asia, 2 USA	914 (13)	43
Hypertension	3	6,066	3,332 (55)	2,140 (35)	61.5	3,618 (60)	1 Asia, 2 USA	1,419 (23)	43

(Continued)

TABLE 1 | Continued

Outcome by risk factor	Number of studies	Total number of patients	N patients with risk factor* No. (%)	N patients with outcome** No. (%)	Mean age	Male No. (%)	Region of Study	N patients with risk factor and outcome No. (%)	% of patients exposed to risk factor reaching outcome
Ischaemic heart disease	3	6,066	673 (11)	2,140 (35)	61.5	3,618 (60)	1 Asia, 2 USA	318 (5)	47
Myocardial injury	7	1,777	410 (23)	153 (9)	57.4	914 (51)	5 Asia, 1 Europe, 1 USA	113 (6)	28
Severe disease									
Diabetes mellitus	43	11,495	2,171 (19)	3,444 (30)	52.3	6,215 (54)	41 Asia, 2 USA	959 (8)	44
Hypertension	41	10,653	3,774 (35)	3,206 (30)	50.8	5,800 (54)	39 Asia, 2 USA	1,602 (15)	42
Ischaemic heart disease	34	10,149	1,325 (13)	3,001 (30)	53.3	5,531 (54)	32 Asia, 2 USA	644 (6)	48
Myocardial injury	18	4,731	925 (20)	1,461 (31)	53.2	2,456 (52)	16 USA, 1 Europe, 1 USA	549 (12)	59

*Risk factors are defined as presence of diabetes, hypertension, ischaemic heart disease or myocardial injury. ARDS, acute respiratory distress syndrome; IMV, invasive mechanical ventilation; ITU, admission to intensive care; AKI, acute kidney injury. **Total number of patients with specific outcomes presented in this table include only studies which reported outcomes according to risk factors of interest. Reported outcomes that were not explicitly associated with risk factors are not included in this table. Therefore, these numbers may not reflect the total number of adverse COVID-19 outcomes in all included studies.

TABLE 2 | Odds Ratio [Confidence Intervals] for COVID-19 adverse outcomes according to risk exposure.

Risk exposure	COVID-19 adverse outcome Odds ratio [95% confidence interval]																		
	Death	p-value	I^2	ARDS	p-value	I^2	IMV	p-value	I^2	ITU	p-value	I^2	AKI	p-value	I^2	Severe Disease	p-value	I^2
Diabetes mellitus	2.15 [1.97, 2.36]	<0.001	68.6	2.48 [1.82, 3.32]	<0.001	43.9	1.77 [1.25, 2.51]	0.0014	66.3	1.65 [1.26, 2.16]	<0.001	60.1	1.84 [1.65, 2.05]	<0.001	0.0	1.80 [1.63, 1.99]	<0.001	48.0
Hypertension	2.72 [2.51, 2.97]	<0.001	67.8	1.68 [1.07, 2.63]	0.025	0.0	1.24 [0.82, 1.90]	0.30	N/A	1.55 [1.20, 1.99]	<0.001	66.3	1.90 [1.70, 2.12]	<0.001	88.5	2.14 [1.93, 2.34]	<0.001	73.4
Ischaemic heart disease	3.29 [3.00, 3.63]	<0.001	51.2	1.42 [0.49, 4.10]	0.49	7.1	1.99 [1.58, 2.48]	<0.001	0.0	1.51 [1.05, 2.16]	0.024	69.3	1.75 [1.49, 2.05]	<0.001	37.6	2.20 [1.93, 2.51]	<0.001	40.2
Myocardial injury	8.85 [8.08, 9.68]	<0.001	77.1	5.70 [4.48, 7.24]	<0.001	82.7	3.42 [2.92, 4.01]	<0.001	70.1	4.85 [3.94, 6.05]	<0.001	75.7	10.49 [6.55, 16.78]	<0.001	10.8	5.10 [4.26, 6.05]	<0.001	73.5

ARDS, acute respiratory distress syndrome; IMV, invasive mechanical ventilation; ITU, admission to intensive care; AKI, acute kidney injury.

the COVID-19 outcomes of interest. Gender did not appear to affect the association between myocardial injury and death whereas age did not modify the association between myocardial injury and COVID-19 disease severity. All four modifiers also partly accounted for the observed heterogeneity between studies. Importantly, the GRADE assessment shows low to moderate levels of certainty for associations studied (**Appendix E**). We did not identify apparent publication bias in our meta-analyses (**Appendix F**).

DISCUSSION

The co-existence of HTN, DM, IHD and/or myocardial injury among patients with COVID-19 has been considered to be a harbinger of adverse clinical outcomes. By undertaking this meta-analysis, we confirmed a significant association between four risk factors (HTN, DM, IHD and myocardial injury) and six important adverse COVID-19 outcomes: death, ARDS, IMV, ITUadm, AKI and SCoV. Furthermore, we demonstrated the differential impact of these risk factors on individual COVID-19 outcomes, with myocardial injury emerging as the most adverse indicator of all. These findings may be considered when risk-stratifying unvaccinated patients and unexposed individuals for potential of severe unfavorable outcomes of COVID-19, as well as prioritization of vaccination rollout programmes.

It is worth reviewing the pathogenesis of COVID-19 disease to better understand the detrimental effects of cardiovascular risk factors and myocardial injury on COVID-19 related outcomes. Entry of SARS-CoV-2 into host cells relies on the surface glycoprotein, spike (S) protein, which has a receptor-binding domain (RBD) mediating direct contact with angiotensin-converting enzyme 2 (ACE2). In addition, the betacoronavirus also contains an S1/S2 polybasic cleavage site that is cleaved by cellular transmembrane protease serine 2 (TMPRSS2) and cathepsin L, which further facilitate viral entry. Whilst the predominant tissue tropism of SARS-CoV-2 is that of the alveolar epithelial cells, ACE2 is widely expressed in other organs such as the gastrointestinal tract, myocardium, kidneys and vascular endothelial cells (11). The latter likely contributes to the extrapulmonary manifestations commonly seen in severe COVID-19 disease. Viral replication within alveolar pneumocytes results in the activation of immune cells and release of inflammatory cytokines resulting in a cytokine storm. This is further exacerbated by the downregulation of ACE2 on cell surface membranes, which have a lung-protective and anti-inflammatory effect via the PIP3/Akt signaling pathway. Overall, the propagation of pro-inflammatory cytokine release accelerates clinical deterioration resulting in severe respiratory complications such as ARDS and multiorgan dysfunction (12).

Cardiovascular Risk Factors, IHD and COVID-19 Outcomes

Pre-existing DM, HTN and IHD were associated with a higher risk of death and severe COVID-19 disease in our meta-analysis, each comprising data from more than 30 studies. These findings concur with pre-existing studies showing worse COVID-19 outcomes in patients with DM and HTN. We further quantified

risks of developing specific COVID-19 adverse outcomes, namely death, ARDS, IMV, ITUadm, SCov and AKI in patients with these co-morbidities.

Whilst patients with DM were at an increased risk of developing all six adverse outcomes, the strongest association was seen between DM and the development of ARDS. The pathogenic mechanism underlying severe respiratory complications in patients with DM and COVID-19 is speculated to be due to alveolar-capillary microangiopathy and interstitial fibrosis, resulting from overactive pro-inflammatory pathways and vascular inflammation. A proposed key player to the ongoing inflammation and endothelial damage in DM is interleukin-6 (IL-6), a pro-inflammatory cytokine suggested as a severity predictor of lung disease in DM (13, 14). These pathophysiological changes have previously been associated with obstructive and restrictive lung pathology in patients with DM.

The development of a cytokine storm in patients with severe COVID-19 is well-described (15). Previous studies have found elevated levels of IL-6 in COVID-19 patients, which were independent predictors of COVID-19 disease severity (16). Thus, it is plausible that increased oxidative stress resulting from higher IL-6 levels can lead to rapid progression of microvascular and macrovascular complications in DM patients with pre-existing low-grade vascular inflammation, resulting in increased risk of ARDS and COVID-19 mortality in this cohort (17). This, in part, may account for the observed beneficial effects of IL-6 inhibitor, tocilizumab in hospitalized patients with COVID-19. One could extrapolate the increased odds of IMV and ITUadm in patients with DM and COVID-19 to be due to the requirement for respiratory support in context of ARDS. In addition, multi-organ dysfunction as a consequence of a cytokine storm in DM may contribute further to the need for organ support in intensive care units, especially considering the increased risk for myocardial injury and AKI in patients with DM and SARS-CoV-2 infection. The pre-existing low-grade inflammation coupled with dysregulated immunomodulation in DM patients raises the question of whether a lower threshold or earlier use of IL-6 inhibitors should be considered in this at-risk cohort.

Similarly, patients with pre-existing HTN are at increased odds of COVID-19 related death, SCov and AKI. This may reflect the interlink between SARS-CoV-2 cell entry via angiotensin converting enzyme 2 (ACE2) binding, the renin-angiotensin-aldosterone system (RAAS) and the ubiquity of ACE2 in multiple organs including the lungs, myocardium, kidneys and gastrointestinal tract. Chronic mechanical stress on the vascular wall as a result of increased intraluminal pressure in hypertension leads to endothelial dysfunction, release of reactive oxygen species and a pro-coagulant state. In conjunction with RAAS dysfunction following SARS-CoV-2 infection, this facilitates a pro-inflammatory state, cytokine release syndrome and progression to multi-organ involvement in COVID-19 resulting in more severe disease and adverse outcomes (18).

Whilst also at increased odds of respiratory complications such as ARDS and requirement for IMV, patients with HTN and COVID-19 appear to be at a lower risk of these complications when compared to DM patients. Here, it may be worth raising whether there is a protective role of regular antihypertensives such as ACE-inhibitors and angiotensin

Quantifying the Excess Risk of Adverse COVID-19 Outcomes in Unvaccinated Individuals with Diabetes...

127

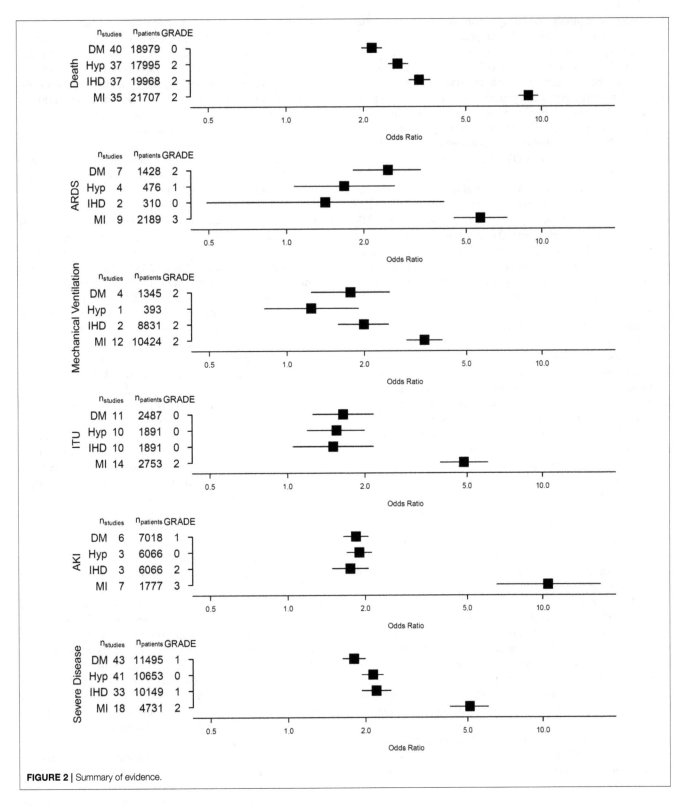

FIGURE 2 | Summary of evidence.

receptor blockers (ARB). The reduction in angiotensin-2 levels and suppression of angiotensin-2 binding to angiotensin-I receptors (AT1R) by ACE-inhibitors and ARBs, respectively, may in fact prevent the downstream pro-inflammatory and vasoconstrictive effects of angiotensin-2, lowering the risk of respiratory complications such as ARDS. Indeed, large cohort-based population studies have suggested a protective effect of ACE-inhibitors and ARBs (as compared to calcium channel blockers) against SCoV, death and IMV in patients with hypertension (19).

Another commonly raised question is whether optimal glycaemic control in DM or blood pressure management in HTN have a protective role against adverse COVID-19 outcomes. Certainly, infection with SARS-CoV-2 leads to dysregulated glucose metabolism that can result in elevated IL-6 levels as compared to normoglycaemic patients. Optimal glucose control significantly lowers levels of pro-inflammatory cytokines with improved outcomes in COVID-19 patients with or without diabetes (20). Further studies have also demonstrated adverse effects of hyperglycaemia on COVID-19 outcomes and reduction in the effectiveness of tocilizumab in patients with COVID-19 and hyperglycaemia (21). What remains unclear is whether prior glycaemic control in patients with known diabetes affect outcomes in COVID-19. Population-based studies in the UK have shown an increased risk of COVID-19 mortality with higher glycated hemoglobin (HbA1c) levels (22). This is in contrast to hospital-based cohort studies that have not demonstrated an association between prior glycaemic control with COVID-19-related mortality or invasive mechanical ventilation (23). In our opinion, the increased risk of COVID-19 adverse outcomes in patients with DM are likely reflective of the associated chronic end-organ microvascular and macrovascular complications exacerbated by acute infective sequelae such as increased insulin resistance and an exaggerated inflammatory response. The potential role of antidiabetic medications such as dipeptidylpeptidase-4 (DPP4) inhibitors and glucagon-like peptide 1 (GLP-1) analogs for optimal glycaemic control and their anti-inflammatory properties should be explored in both the acute and chronic stages of COVID-19 infection.

Whilst one may assume patients with poorly controlled blood pressure to be at increased risk of adverse COVID-19 outcomes, this was interestingly not the case in a large observational study of more than 45,000 symptomatic COVID-19 patients with hypertension. Sheppard et al. (24) observed that patients with recent uncontrolled blood pressure had lower odds of COVID-19 related mortality as compared to patients with well-controlled blood pressure. This may suggest a greater role of chronic hypertensive end-organ damage as risk factors for worse COVID-19 outcome.

Importantly, it is worth remembering that many patients have more than one of these studied risk factors. The combined effect of DM and HTN, as well as other components of the "metabolic syndrome" such as dyslipidaemia and obesity is likely greater than its individual components with regards to increased odds of adverse COVID-19 outcome, as demonstrated in specific meta-analyses studying the risk of metabolic syndrome on SCov and death (25). Other comorbidities beyond CV risk factors may play a significant role in adverse COVID-19 outcomes also, as suggested through a prior meta-analysis finding association between cerebrovascular disease and chronic liver disease with IMV in COVID-19 (26).

Myocardial Injury and COVID-19 Outcomes

Of the four studied risk predictors, myocardial injury had the strongest association with all six adverse COVID-19 outcomes. One could argue this may be a marker of multi-organ involvement and disease severity, rather than a direct pathogenic

mechanism. Also, pre-existing cardiovascular diseases such as HTN and IHD increase odds of developing myocardial injury in context of COVID-19 disease (27). Autopsy studies have also suggested an upregulation of ACE2 expression in cardiomyocytes of patients with DM, increasing susceptibility to SARS-CoV-2 entry and myocardial injury in this patient cohort (28). As such, it is not be unreasonable to assume that myocardial injury, as indicated by raised serum troponin levels may simply be a surrogate to the increased odds of adverse COVID-19 outcomes in patients with DM, HTN and IHD. However, Shi et al. (29) and Chen et al. (30) have previously demonstrated that myocardial injury is an independent predictor of mortality in COVID-19. Subsequent multivariable analyses by Wang et al. (31) however showed that this association was only significant on univariate analysis. To date, it remains unclear whether myocardial injury represents a cause or consequence of severe COVID-19 disease.

In our study, we found that 67% (2,197/3,259) of the deceased patients had evidence of myocardial injury, which was associated with a near 9-fold increased odds of COVID-19 related death. Further, our study explores the association between myocardial injury and AKI, demonstrating patients with COVID-19 and myocardial injury are at 10-fold increased odds of developing AKI. 28% of patients with myocardial injury developed AKI as compared to 2.4% of patients without myocardial injury.

The exact mechanism linking myocardial injury with ARDS and AKI in COVID-19 infection is poorly understood. Several hypotheses include a bystander process with cytokine storm and hyperinflammation in severe COVID-19 disease as the driver of multi-organ involvement, endothelial damage and thrombo-inflammation secondary to ACE2-mediated entry of SARS-CoV-2 into endothelial cells of multiple vascular beds and right ventricular dysfunction secondary to increased afterload from raised pulmonary artery pressures in ARDS, thereby causing dysregulated renal blood flow (32, 33).

Strengths and Limitations

Our meta-analysis pools data from studies across the world and focuses on COVID-19 outcomes in the early phase of the pandemic, before effective evidence-based treatments and vaccines were commonplace. The geographical diversity of included studies overcomes concerns regarding generalisability of earlier meta-analyses, while avoiding biases introduced by novel therapies and vaccines in later stages of the pandemic. Our meta-analysis comprehensively explores the multiple associations between CV risk factors, IHD and myocardial injury with specific COVID-19 outcomes and complications such as AKI and ARDS alongside more commonly reported outcomes such as mortality and IMV.

The generalisability of findings from our meta-analysis was enhanced by not setting language restrictions in our search strategy and by including studies from conventional as well as novel databases (e.g., medRxiv and the WHO COVID-19 database). Moreover, risk of bias was minimized by excluding studies involving specific population cohorts or pre-selected COVID-19 outcomes. By undertaking meta-regression analyses, we were able to explore sources of heterogeneity including age, gender, study recruitment date and geographic region.

Our study has several limitations. Firstly, it is limited in its scope, focusing on outcomes of COVID-19 in a relatively unexposed population in the immediate months following its initial outbreak. Its applicability to populations with high vaccination or herd immunity rates may be limited. Indeed, the emergence of variants with significant mutations affecting virulence features such as transmissibility and pathogenesis may alter aspects of the natural history of COVID-19. At the same time, variants could affect effectiveness of current vaccines (34). In order to delineate the associations between cardiometabolic risk factors and myocardial injury with significant outcomes of COVID-19, we focused on the pre-vaccine phase of the pandemic when rates of adverse outcomes were high and bias arising from access to treatments and vaccines was comparably less pronounced. A necessary trade-off limiting broader applicability to vaccinated populations and potential future variants was accepted.

In addition, the majority of included studies explored adverse outcomes in hospitalized COVID-19 patients. This introduces an inherent selection bias as patients presenting with mild symptoms were likely excluded. Unvaccinated, non-hospitalized individuals with mild COVID-19 symptoms remain an important cohort to study, particularly with the changing trends of disease severity with different SARS-CoV-2 variants.

As our meta-analysis focused specifically on the pre-vaccination phase of the pandemic, we are unable to comment on the association between DM, HTN, IHD and myocardial injury with biomarkers of disease severity including coagulation indicators such as fibrinogen degradation products, prothrombin time, D-dimer and platelets, as these were infrequently reported in earlier studies included. Indeed, the pro-coagulation state in COVID-19 disease is now well-recognized and biomarkers such as D-dimer are used to guide routine use of anticoagulants in COVID-19 patients (35). Whilst findings from the REMAP-CAP trial have not shown a protective effect of antiplatelets in patients with critically-ill patients with COVID-19, it would be interesting to further stratify whether empirical antiplatelet and anticoagulant therapy in patients with different risk profiles (e.g., DM vs. non-DM) will improve overall outcomes (36).

The inclusion of studies conducted at different centers across geographical regions also results in considerable between-study heterogeneity. This could be due to multiple reasons including different sociodemographic factors, varying definitions of outcomes (e.g., ARDS, severe COVID-19 disease) and variations in clinical practice between the countries (we therefore assessed for the effect of geographical variation through meta-regression). For outcomes with fewer studies (ARDS, IMV and AKI), the level of certainty of evidence is low owing to the small study size and wide confidence intervals, limiting the veracity of these findings.

Notwithstanding the above limitations, our meta-analysis quantifies the excess risk of adverse COVID-19 outcomes in unvaccinated patients with pre-existing CV risk factors, IHD and myocardial injury. In addition, we demonstrate the differential impact of these factors on six important adverse COVID-19 outcomes. Our findings will help inform clinicians, policymakers and patients in terms of risk prediction, stratification and resource allocation. Our meta-analysis contributes to the expanding body of evidence reporting on risk factors for poor COVID-19 outcomes, which could inform public health advice regarding social isolation guidelines and vaccine prioritization strategies, especially relevant for LMICs.

Future studies evaluating the altered impact of cardiovascular risk factors such as HTN, DM and IHD on COVID-19 outcomes in a post-vaccination population are required. In addition, the immunogenicity of different COVID-19 vaccines in these patient groups remain poorly elucidated and should be better characterized to guide design of vaccination programmes and choice of vaccine.

CONCLUSION

In summary, our meta-analysis demonstrates a significant association between myocardial injury and adverse clinical outcomes in COVID-19 patients. To a lesser extent, we also found that DM, HTN and IHD predict poorer outcomes, especially for death and severe disease. These findings provide comprehensive quantitative data that can be used in risk prediction and risk stratification by clinicians as well as policymakers. It also provides the underpinning evidence for the vaccination policies targeting vulnerable patients.

AUTHOR CONTRIBUTIONS

SN, SK, VK, and AG designed the study. SN, JP, and KM identified studies and extracted data. KR performed the statistical analysis. SN, JP, KM, SK, VK, KR, and AG wrote the manuscript. All authors contributed to the article and approved the submitted version.

ACKNOWLEDGMENTS

The authors would like to acknowledge Mr. Adam Tocock for assisting with the search of databases for this meta-analysis.

REFERENCES

1. Ritchie H, Mathieu E, Rodés-Guirao L, Appel C, Giattino C, Ortiz-Ospina E, et al. *Coronavirus Pandemic (COVID-19)*. Our World in Data (2020) Mar 5. Available online at: https://ourworldindata.org/ (accessed March 27, 2022).
2. Gyawali N, Al-Amin HM. Living and dying with COVID-19 in South Asian low- and middle-income countries. *Front Public Health.* (2021) 9:600878. doi: 10.3389/fpubh.2021.600878
3. Biccard BM, Gopalan PD, Miller M, Michell WL, Thomson D, Ademuyiwa A, et al. Patient care and clinical outcomes for patients with COVID-19 infection admitted to African high-care or intensive care units (ACCCOS): a multicentre, prospective, observational cohort study. *Lancet.* (2021) 397:1885–94. doi: 10.1016/S0140-6736(21)00441-4
4. Danza P. SARS-CoV-2 Infection and Hospitalization Among Adults Aged ≥18 Years, by Vaccination Status, Before and During SARS-CoV-2 B.1.1.529 (Omicron) Variant Predominance — Los Angeles County, California,

November 7, 2021–January 8, 2022. *MMWR Morb Mortal Wkly Rep.* (2022) 71:177–81. doi: 10.15585/mmwr.mm7105e1

5. Hu H, Yao N, Qiu Y. Comparing rapid scoring systems in mortality prediction of critically ill patients with novel coronavirus disease. *Acad Emerg Med.* (2020) 27:461–8. doi: 10.1111/acem.13992

6. Du R-H, Liu L-M, Yin W, Wang W, Guan L-L, Yuan M-L, et al. Hospitalization and critical care of 109 decedents with COVID-19 Pneumonia in Wuhan, China. *Ann Am Thorac Soc.* (2020) 17:839–46. doi: 10.1513/AnnalsATS.202003-225OC

7. Lin DY, Zeng D. On the relative efficiency of using summary statistics versus individual-level data in meta-analysis. *Biometrika.* (2010) 97:321–32. doi: 10.1093/biomet/asq006

8. Higgins JPT, Thompson SG, Deeks JJ, Altman DG. Measuring inconsistency in meta-analyses. *BMJ.* (2003) 327:557–60. doi: 10.1136/bmj.327.7414.557

9. Qijun Li K, Rice K. Improved inference for fixed-effects meta-analysis of 2 × 2 tables. *Res Synth Methods.* (2020) 11:387–96. doi: 10.1002/jrsm.1401

10. *Cochrane Handbook for Systematic Reviews of Interventions. Version 5.1.0.* Available online at: https://handbook-5-1.cochrane.org/chapter_9/9_5_2_identifying_and_measuring_heterogeneity.htm - Google Search (accessed March 27, 2022).

11. Harrison AG, Lin T, Wang P. Mechanisms of SARS-CoV-2 transmission and pathogenesis. *Trend Immunol.* (2020) 41:1100–15. doi: 10.1016/j.it.2020.10.004

12. Chen R, Lan Z, Ye J, Pang L, Liu Y, Wu W, et al. cytokine storm: the primary determinant for the pathophysiological evolution of COVID-19 deterioration. *Front Immunol.* (2021) 12:589095. doi: 10.3389/fimmu.2021.589095

13. Sardu C, Gargiulo G, Esposito G, Paolisso G, Marfella R. Impact of diabetes mellitus on clinical outcomes in patients affected by COVID-19. *Cardiovasc Diabetol.* (2020) 19:76. doi: 10.1186/s12933-020-01047-y

14. Khateeb J, Fuchs E, Khamaisi M. Diabetes and lung disease: a neglected relationship. *Rev Diabet Stud.* (2019) 15:1–15. doi: 10.1900/RDS.2019.15.1

15. Ragab D, Salah Eldin H, Taeimah M, Khattab R, Salem R. The COVID-19 cytokine storm; what we know so far. *Front Immunol.* (2020) 11:1446. doi: 10.3389/fimmu.2020.01446

16. Zeng Z, Yu H, Chen H, Qi W, Chen L, Chen G, et al. Longitudinal changes of inflammatory parameters and their correlation with disease severity and outcomes in patients with COVID-19 from Wuhan, China. *Crit Care.* (2020) 24:525. doi: 10.1186/s13054-020-03255-0

17. Lim S, Bae JH, Kwon H-S, Nauck MA. COVID-19 and diabetes mellitus: from pathophysiology to clinical management. *Nat Rev Endocrinol.* (2021) 17:11–30. doi: 10.1038/s41574-020-00435-4

18. Muhamad S-A, Ugusman A, Kumar J, Skiba D, Hamid AA, Aminuddin A. COVID-19 and hypertension: the what, the why, and the how. *Front Physiol.* (2021) 12:665064. doi: 10.3389/fphys.2021.665064

19. Semenzato L, Botton J, Drouin J, Baricault B, Vabre C, Cuenot F, et al. Antihypertensive drugs and COVID-19 risk. *Hypertension.* (2021) 77:833–42. doi: 10.1161/HYPERTENSIONAHA.120.16314

20. Sardu C, D'Onofrio N, Balestrieri ML, Barbieri M, Rizzo MR, Messina V, et al. Outcomes in patients with hyperglycemia affected by COVID-19: can we do more on glycemic control? *Diabetes Care.* (2020) 43:1408–15. doi: 10.2337/dc20-0723

21. Marfella R, Paolisso P, Sardu C, Bergamaschi L, D'Angelo EC, Barbieri M, et al. Negative impact of hyperglycaemia on tocilizumab therapy in COVID-19 patients. *Diabetes Metab.* (2020) 46:403–5. doi: 10.1016/j.diabet.2020.05.005

22. Holman N, Knighton P, Kar P, O'Keefe J, Curley M, Weaver A, et al. Risk factors for COVID-19-related mortality in people with type 1 and type 2 diabetes in England: a population-based cohort study. *Lancet Diabetes Endocrinol.* (2020) 8:823–33. doi: 10.1016/S2213-8587(20)30271-0

23. Bloomgarden Z. Does glycemic control affect outcome of COVID-19? *J Diabetes.* (2020) 12:868–9. doi: 10.1111/1753-0407.13116

24. Sheppard JP, Nicholson BD, Lee J, McGagh D, Sherlock J, Koshiaris C, et al. Association between blood pressure control and coronavirus disease 2019 outcomes in 45 418 symptomatic patients with hypertension. *Hypertension.* (2021) 77:846–55. doi: 10.1161/HYPERTENSIONAHA.120.16472

25. Rico-Martín S, Calderón-García JF, Basilio-Fernández B, Clavijo-Chamorro MZ, Sánchez Muñoz-Torrero JF. Metabolic syndrome and its components in patients with COVID-19: severe acute respiratory syndrome (SARS) and mortality. a systematic review and meta-analysis. *J Cardiovasc Dev Dis.* (2021) 8:162. doi: 10.3390/jcdd8120162

26. Patel U, Malik P, Usman MS, Mehta D, Sharma A, Malik FA, et al. Age-adjusted risk factors associated with mortality and mechanical ventilation utilization amongst COVID-19 hospitalizations-a systematic review and meta-analysis. *SN Compr Clin Med.* (2020) 2:1740–9. doi: 10.1007/s42399-020-00476-w

27. Fan Q, Zhu H, Zhao J, Zhuang L, Zhang H, Xie H, et al. Risk factors for myocardial injury in patients with coronavirus disease 2019 in China. *ESC Heart Failure.* (2020) 7:4108–17. doi: 10.1002/ehf2.13022

28. D'Onofrio N, Scisciola L, Sardu C, Trotta MC, De Feo M, Maiello C, et al. Glycated ACE2 receptor in diabetes: open door for SARS-CoV-2 entry in cardiomyocyte. *Cardiovasc Diabetol.* (2021) 20:99. doi: 10.1186/s12933-021-01286-7

29. Shi S, Qin M, Shen B, Cai Y, Liu T, Yang F, et al. Association of cardiac injury with mortality in hospitalized patients with COVID-19 in Wuhan, China. *JAMA Cardiol.* (2020) 5:802–10. doi: 10.1001/jamacardio.2020.0950

30. Chen C, Yan JT, Zhou N, Zhao JP, Wang DW. [Analysis of myocardial injury in patients with COVID-19 and association between concomitant cardiovascular diseases and severity of COVID-19]. *Zhonghua Xin Xue Guan Bing Za Zhi.* (2020) 48:567–71. doi: 10.3760/cma.j.cn112148-20200225-00123

31. Wang L, He W, Yu X, Hu D, Bao M, Liu H, et al. Coronavirus disease 2019 in elderly patients: characteristics and prognostic factors based on 4-week follow-up. *J Infect.* (2020) 80:639–45. doi: 10.1016/j.jinf.2020.03.019

32. Gupta A, Madhavan MV, Sehgal K, Nair N, Mahajan S, Sehrawat TS, et al. Extrapulmonary manifestations of COVID-19. *Nat Med.* (2020) 26:1017–32. doi: 10.1038/s41591-020-0968-3

33. Varga Z, Flammer AJ, Steiger P, Haberecker M, Andermatt R, Zinkernagel AS, et al. Endothelial cell infection and endotheliitis in COVID-19. *Lancet.* (2020) 395:1417–8. doi: 10.1016/S0140-6736(20)30937-5

34. Saxena SK, Kumar S, Ansari S, Paweska JT, Maurya VK, Tripathi AK, et al. Transmission dynamics and mutational prevalence of the novel severe acute respiratory syndrome coronavirus-2 Omicron variant of concern. *J Med Virol.* (2022) 94:2160–6. doi: 10.1002/jmv.27611

35. Sardu C, Gambardella J, Morelli MB, Wang X, Marfella R, Santulli G. Hypertension, thrombosis, kidney failure, and diabetes: is COVID-19 an endothelial disease? a comprehensive evaluation of clinical and basic evidence. *J Clin Med.* (2020) 9:1417. doi: 10.3390/jcm9051417

36. REMAP-CAP Writing Committee for the REMAP-CAP Investigators, Bradbury CA, Lawler PR, Stanworth SJ, McVerry BJ, McQuilten Z, et al. Effect of antiplatelet therapy on survival and organ support-free days in critically Ill patients with COVID-19: a randomized clinical trial. *JAMA.* (2022) 327:1247–59. doi: 10.1001/jama.2022.2910

19

Comparison of the Characteristics, Management and Outcomes of STEMI Patients Presenting With vs. Those of Patients Presenting without COVID-19 Infection

Yanjiao Wang [1,2†], Linlin Kang [1,2†], Ching-Wen Chien [2], Jiawen Xu [2], Peng You [2], Sizhong Xing [1*] and Tao-Hsin Tung [3*]

[1] Shenzhen Bao'an District Traditional Chinese Medicine Hospital, Shenzhen, China, [2] Institute for Hospital Management, Tsing Hua University, Shenzhen, China, [3] Evidence-Based Medicine Center, Taizhou Hospital of Zhejiang Province Affiliated to Wenzhou Medical University, Linhai, China

*Correspondence:
Tao-Hsin Tung
ch2876@gmail.com
Sizhong Xing
xsz7220@163.com

†These authors have contributed equally to this work and share first authorship

Objectives: This study aimed to investigate the differences in the characteristics, management, and clinical outcomes of patients with and that of those without coronavirus disease 2019 (COVID-19) infection who had ST-segment elevation myocardial infarction (STEMI).

Methods: Databases including Web of Science, PubMed, Cochrane Library, and Embase were searched up to July 2021. Observational studies that reported on the characteristics, management, or clinical outcomes and those published as full-text articles were included. The Newcastle-Ottawa Scale (NOS) was used to assess the quality of all included studies.

Results: A total of 27,742 patients from 13 studies were included in this meta-analysis. Significant delay in symptom onset to first medical contact (SO-to-FMC) time (mean difference = 23.42 min; 95% CI: 5.85–40.99 min; $p = 0.009$) and door-to-balloon (D2B) time (mean difference = 12.27 min; 95% CI: 5.77–18.78 min; $p = 0.0002$) was observed in COVID-19 patients. Compared to COVID-19 negative patients, those who are positive patients had significantly higher levels of C-reactive protein, D-dimer, and thrombus grade ($p < 0.05$) and showed more frequent use of thrombus aspiration and glycoprotein IIbIIIa (Gp2b3a) inhibitor ($p < 0.05$). COVID-19 positive patients also had higher rates of in-hospital mortality (OR = 5.98, 95% CI: 4.78–7.48, $p < 0.0001$), cardiogenic shock (OR = 2.75, 95% CI: 2.02–3.76, $p < 0.0001$), and stent thrombosis (OR = 5.65, 95% CI: 2.41–13.23, $p < 0.0001$). They were also more likely to be admitted to the intensive care unit (ICU) (OR = 4.26, 95% CI: 2.51–7.22, $p < 0.0001$) and had a longer length of stay (mean difference = 4.63 days; 95% CI: 2.56–6.69 days; $p < 0.0001$).

Conclusions: This study revealed that COVID-19 infection had an impact on the time of initial medical intervention for patients with STEMI after symptom onset and showed that COVID-19 patients with STEMI were more likely to have thrombosis and had poorer outcomes.

Keywords: COVID-19, SARS-CoV-2, mortality, ST-segment elevation myocardial infarction, STEMI

INTRODUCTION

An eventual pandemic brought by the coronavirus disease 2019 (COVID-19) caused by severe acute respiratory syndrome coronavirus 2 (SARS-CoV-2) resulted in plenty of deaths and has had a strong impact on the world's healthcare system (1–3). Although the disease is predominantly characterized by respiratory symptoms, including pneumonia, dyspnea, and cough (4), various extrapulmonary features, such as myocardial damage, arrhythmia, thrombotic events, and renal injury have also been observed (5, 6).

A type of heart attack called ST-segment elevation myocardial infarction (STEMI) is usually caused by thrombotic occlusion at the site of a ruptured plaque in the coronary artery (7). Although the survival rates of STEMI patients have improved, it is still associated with high morbidity and mortality worldwide with a 1-year mortality rate of up to 10% (8–10). The COVID-19 pandemic may lead to a decrease in the number of STEMI admissions and could have a significant impact on the reperfusion strategy for patients with STEMI (11, 12). The tendency of patients with COVID-19 to be predisposed to cardiac arrest and coronary thrombosis due to increased inflammation, platelet activation, endothelial dysfunction, and SARS-CoV-2 invasion of cardiomyocytes has been reported (13–15). Moreover, data regarding the characteristics, management strategies, and clinical outcomes including in-hospital mortality and cardiogenic shock in patients presenting with STEMI concurrent with COVID-19 infection are limited (16). Accordingly, we aimed to conduct a systematic review and meta-analysis to compare the characteristics, management, and clinical outcomes between the COVID-19 and non-COVID-19 patients concomitant STEMI.

METHODS

Literature Search

We performed a literature search using databases including Web of Science (Beijing), PubMed (Bethesda), Cochrane Library (UK), and Embase (Amsterdam) for relevant papers without language limitation on July 31, 2021. The search strategy included a mix of MeSH and free-text terms relevant to the critical concept of "STEMI" and "COVID-19" (**Table 1**). The protocol for this meta-analysis was registered at PROSPERO under the number CRD42021283880.

Study Selection

Studies were included if they met the following inclusion criteria: (i) studies involving STEMI patients; (ii) the exposure group included patients diagnosed with COVID-19 using PCR test or had a high index of clinical suspicion, and the control group included patients without COVID-19; (iii) studies that reported at least one of the following information: characteristics, management strategy, or clinical outcomes; (iv) relevant cohort studies, cross-sectional studies, case series, and case-control studies. Two independent authors screened the titles and abstracts of all relevant studies and identified whether they met the inclusion criteria by reviewing the full text of each potential study. Any discrepancy was resolved through consensus with a third author.

Data Extraction and Quality Assessment

Relevant data from all included studies were extracted by two authors independently, and any disagreement was resolved by discussion with a third author. The following data were extracted: authors, publication year, country, study design, study subject, sample size, mean age of patients/subjects, sex, comparison period, participant characteristics, management strategies, and clinical outcomes. The Newcastle–Ottawa Scale (NOS), which includes participant selection, comparability, and outcome, was used to assess the quality of the included studies. Likewise, all included studies were rated by two authors independently, and any discrepancy was adjudicated by consensus.

Statistical Analysis

We used Review Manager 5.4 (The Nordic Cochrane Center, Cochrane Collaboration, 2020, Denmark) to perform the statistical analysis. If studies only reported median values and interquartile ranges (IQR), means and SDs were calculated according to the Box-Cox method (17). Categorical variables were presented as odds ratios (ORs), including 95% CIs, and continuous variables were presented as the mean difference (MD) or standardized mean difference (SMD), including 95% CI. Heterogeneity was assessed using the I^2 statistic and the p-value of the chi-square test. The I^2 statistic $> 50\%$ indicates significant heterogeneity. The choice between the fixed and random effects models depended on the comparability among the studies. A two-tailed p-value of < 0.05 was interpreted to be statistically significant. The risk of publication bias was evaluated using the funnel plots.

RESULTS

Characteristics of Included Studies

A total of 2,702 articles were retrieved through electronic database searches, of which 1,371 were duplicates. After screening the titles and abstracts, 24 potential articles were assessed for eligibility after a full-text review, and 13 articles (18–30) with a total of 27,742 patients were finally included

TABLE 1 | Search strategy.

Database	Searching key words	
PubMed	(1) "ST Segment Elevation Myocardial Infarction": 9451	(10) SARS-CoV-2: 106826
	(2) "ST Elevated Myocardial Infarction": 317	(11) "Coronavirus disease 19": 1603
	(3) STEMI: 28060	(12) "Severe Acute Respiratory Syndrome Coronavirus 2": 16865
	(4) "Acute myocardial infarction": 61630	(13) "novel coronavirus": 9766
	(5) AMI: 25165	(14) "2019 novel coronavirus": 1550
	(6) "Acute coronary syndromes": 13188	(15) #1 or #2 or #3 or #4 or #5 or #6 or #7: 208085
	(7) ACS: 116546	(16) #8 or #9 or #10 or #11 or #12 or #13 or #14: 169136
	(8) "SARSCoV-2 pandemic": 120	(17) #15 and #16: 1340
	(9) COVID-19: 168784	
Web of science	(1) "ST Segment Elevation Myocardial Infarction": 17531	(10) SARS-CoV-2: 127748
	(2) "ST Elevated Myocardial Infarction": 1899	(11) "Coronavirus disease 19": 3460
	(3) STEMI: 23388	(12) "Severe Acute Respiratory Syndrome Coronavirus 2": 58794
	(4) "Acute myocardial infarction": 145384	(13) "novel coronavirus": 14678
	(5) AMI: 44201	(14) "2019 novel coronavirus": 2224
	(6) "Acute coronary syndromes": 27560	(15) #1 or #2 or #3 or #4 or #5 or #6 or #7: 248982
	(7) ACS: 58425	(16) #8 or #9 or #10 or #11 or #12 or #13 or #14: 262441
	(8) "SARSCoV-2 pandemic": 25	(17) #15 and #16: 1098
	(9) COVID-19: 248069	
Cochrane library	(1) "ST Segment Elevation Myocardial Infarction": 4031	(10) SARS-CoV-2: 322
	(2) "ST Elevated Myocardial Infarction": 156	(11) "Coronavirus disease 19": 43
	(3) STEMI: 3616	(12) "Severe Acute Respiratory Syndrome Coronavirus 2": 631
	(4) "Acute myocardial infarction": 9325	(13) "novel coronavirus": 497
	(5) AMI: 3603	(14) "2019 novel coronavirus": 55
	(6) "Acute coronary syndromes": 2562	(15) #1 or #2 or #3 or #4 or #5 or #6 or #7: 19050
	(7) ACS: 4853	(16) #8 or #9 or #10 or #11 or #12 or #13 or #14: 6784
	(8) "SARSCoV-2 pandemic": 52	(17) #15 and #16: 31
	(9) COVID-19: 6666	
Embase	('acute myocardial infarction':ti,ab,kw OR ami:ti,ab,kw OR 'acute coronary syndromes':ti,ab,kw OR acs:ti,ab,kw OR 'st segment elevation myocardial infarction':ti,ab,kw OR 'st elevated myocardial infarction':ti,ab,kw OR stemi:ti,ab,kw) AND ('sarscov-2 pandemicor COVID-19':ti,ab,kw OR 'sars cov 2':ti,ab,kw OR 'coronavirus disease 19':ti,ab,kw OR 'novel coronavirus':ti,ab, kw OR 'severe acute respiratory syndrome coronavirus 2':ti,ab,kw) AND [1-1-1900]/sd NOT [1-8-2021]/sd; result = 233	

(**Figure 1**). A summary of the main characteristics of these 13 studies and the baseline characteristics of all study subjects is presented in **Tables 2A,B**. One study originated from Poland (19), two each from the United Kingdom (24, 28), France (18, 21), Turkey (20, 30), Italy (25, 26), and Spain (27, 29), and the remaining two studies (22, 23) were international studies. The NOS score for all included studies varied from 5 to 8 points.

Delays

The symptom onset to first medical contact (SO-to-FMC) time among STEMI, which was reported in four studies (19, 20, 27, 30), was significantly different between the COVID-19 group and the non-COVID-19 group (MD = 23.42 min, 95% CI: 5.85 to 40.99 min, $p = 0.009$; **Figure 2A**). Furthermore, seven studies (18, 22–25, 28, 30) reported the time from door to balloon (D2B) and found that D2B was significantly longer in the COVID-19 group (MD = 12.27 min, 95% CI: 5.77 to 18.78 min, $p = 0.0002$; **Figure 2B**) than in the non-COVID-19 group. *3.3 Laboratory values.*

The meta-analysis showed that compared to the non-COVID-19 group, the COVID-19 group had significantly higher levels of C-reactive protein (CRP), white blood cell count (WBC), and D-dimer (SMD = 0.76, 95% CI: 0.38 to 1.13, $p < 0.0001$; SMD = 0.39, 95% CI: 0.1 to 0.69, $p = 0.009$; SMD = 0.79, 95% CI: 0.36 to 1.22, $p = 0.0003$, respectively, **Figures 3A–C**), and had significantly lower level of lymphocyte count (SMD = −0.52, 95% CI: −0.69, −0.36, $p < 0.0001$, **Figure 3D**).

Management and Procedural Characteristic

There was no significant difference in the rate of primary angioplasty between the two groups (OR = 0.28, 95% CI: 0.08 to 1.01, $p = 0.05$; **Figure 4A**). Myocardial infarction with no obstructive coronary atherosclerosis (MINOCA) was more frequently observed, and the rate of stent implantation was lower in patients with COVID-19 infection (OR = 9.57, 95% CI: 2.14 to 42.83, $p = 0.003$; OR = 0.28, 95% CI: 0.11 to 0.71, $p = 0.008$, respectively, **Figures 4B,C**). Baseline thrombus grade > 3 and modified thrombus grade > 3 were significantly higher in the COVID-19 group than in the non-COVID-19 group (OR = 3.09, 95% CI: 1.83 to 5.23, $p < 0.0001$; OR = 5.84, 95% CI: 1.36 to 25.06, $p = 0.02$, respectively; **Figures 4D,E**). Intracoronary thrombus was angiographically identified and scored in 0–5 grades as previously described (31). In patients initially presenting with grade 5, thrombus grade will be reclassified into one of the other categories after flow achievement (32). After reclassification and based on clinical outcomes, the thrombus burden can be divided into 2 categories: low thrombus grade for thrombus < grade 4, and high thrombus grade for thrombus grade 4 (32). Consistent with this, the COVID-19 group showed a higher use of thrombus aspiration and glycoprotein IIbIIIa (Gp2b3a) inhibitor (OR = 1.68, 95% CI: 1.25 to 2.26, $p = 0.0007$; OR = 2.86, 95% CI: 1.78 to 4.62, $p < 0.0001$, respectively; **Figures 4F,G**). Moreover, thrombolysis in myocardial infarction (TIMI)-3 flow post-procedure was less common in the COVID-19 group than in the non-COVID-19 group (OR = 0.6, 95% CI: 0.42 to 0.84, $p = 0.003$, **Figure 4H**).

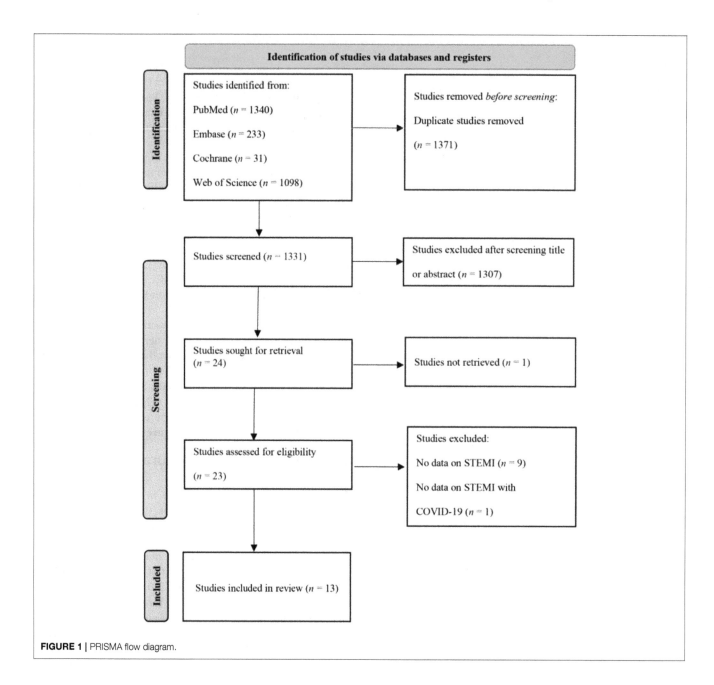

FIGURE 1 | PRISMA flow diagram.

In-Hospital Outcomes
In-hospital mortality among patients with COVID-19 was significantly higher than that in patients without COVID-19 (OR = 5.98, 95% CI: 4.78 to 7.48, $p < 0.0001$, **Figure 5A**). The rates of cardiogenic shock as well as stent thrombosis were also higher in the COVID-19 group than in the non-COVID-19 group (OR = 2.75, 95% CI: 2.02 to 3.76, $p < 0.0001$; OR = 5.65, 95% CI: 2.41 to 13.23, $p < 0.0001$, respectively; **Figures 5B,C**). Although bleeding was more common in STEMI patients with COVID-19, there was no significant difference between the two groups (OR = 2.82, 95% CI: 0.88 to 9.05, $p = 0.08$, **Figure 5D**). In addition, patients with COVID-19 were more likely to be admitted to the intensive care unit (ICU) and had a longer length of hospital stay (OR = 4.26, 95% CI: 2.51 to 7.22, $p < 0.0001$; MD =

4.63 days, 95% CI: 2.56 to 6.69 days, $p < 0.0001$, respectively, **Figures 5E,F**).

Grade Summary of Findings
The GRADE summary of findings tool was used to evaluate the quality of evidence, and the assessment for each outcome is presented in **Table 3**. In addition to in-hospital mortality, which moderates the quality of evidence, other outcomes had low or very low quality of evidence because all included studies were observational.

Sensitivity Analysis and Publication Bias
The leave-one-out approach was applied for sensitivity analysis to evaluate the impact of a single study on

TABLE 2A | Characteristics of included studies.

References	Country	Study design	Study group	Participants characteristics	Comparison period	COVID-19 diagnosis approach/time to diagnosis	Major findings
Popovic et al. (18)	France	Monocentric cohort study	COVID-19 STEMI	n = 11, age 63.6 ± 17.4 years, 63.9% males	26/2/2020–10/5/2020	RT-PCR or typical clinical features plus CT results/NA	D2B time, Laboratory values, Primary angioplasty, MINOCA, Stent implantation, Gp2b3a inhibitor use, TIMI status, In-hospital mortality
			Non-COVID-19 STEMI	n = 72, age 62.5 ± 12.6 years, 73.6% males	26/2/2020–10/5/2020		
Siudak et al. (19)	Poland	Multicentric cohort study	COVID-19 STEMI	n = 145, age 63.19 ± 12.55 years, 71.33% males	13/3/2020–13/5/2020	Swabs for molecular RT-PCR testing/NA	SO-to-FMC time
			Non-COVID-19 STEMI	n = 2276, age 65.43 ± 12.23 years, 67.65% males	13/3/2020–13/5/2020		
Kiris et al. (20)	Turkey	Multicentric cross-sectional study	COVID-19 STEMI	n = 65, age 66.8 ± 12.0 years, 68% males	11/3/2020–15/5/2020	Nasal/pharyngeal swabs or symptoms plus radiological imaging/NA	SO-to-FMC time, Laboratory values, Primary angioplasty, Thrombus aspiration, Gp2b3a inhibitor use, Baseline thrombus grade, Modified thrombus grade, TIMI status, In-hospital mortality, Bleeding, Stent thrombosis, Cardiogenic shock
			Non-COVID-19 STEMI	n = 668, age 60.0 ± 12.3 years, 78% males	11/3/2020–15/5/2020		
Koutsoukis et al. (21)	France	Multicentric cross-sectional study	COVID-19 STEMI	n = 17, age 63.4 ± 13.2 years, 70% males	1/4/2020–22/4/2020	RT-PCR on nasopharyngeal samples/NA	Laboratory values, Primary angioplasty, Thrombus aspiration, MINOCA, Stent implantation, Gp2b3a inhibitor use, In-hospital mortality
			Non-COVID-19 STEMI	n = 99, age 63.8 ± 13.9 years, 67% males	1/4/2020–22/4/2020		
Garcia et al. (22)	USA & Canada	Multicentric cohort study	COVID-19 STEMI	n = 230, 71% males	1/1/2020–6/12/2020	Confirmed COVID+ by any commercially available test/NA	D2B time, Primary angioplasty, MINOCA, In-hospital mortality, LOS
			Non-COVID-19 STEMI	n = 460, 68% males	1/2015–12/2019		
Kite et al. (23)	Data from 55 international centers	Multicentric cohort study	COVID-19 STEMI	n = 144, age 63.1 ± 12.6 years, 77.8% males	1/3/2020–31/7/2020	RT-PCR or clinical status plus CXR or CT findings/NA	D2B time, Laboratory values, Thrombus aspiration, In-hospital mortality, Bleeding, Cardiogenic shock, LOS
			Non-COVID-19 STEMI	n = 24961, age 65.6 ± 13.4 years, 72.2% males	2018–2019		
Little et al. (24)	UK	Multicentric cohort study	COVID-19 STEMI	n = 46, age 61.80 ± 7.95 years, 80.4% males	1/3/2020–30/4/2020	RT-PCR on oro/nasopharyngeal throat swabs or typical symptoms plus radiographic appearances and characteristic blood test/NA	D2B time, Laboratory values, Thrombus aspiration, Gp2b3a inhibitor use, TIMI status, In-hospital mortality, Cardiogenic shock, ICU admission, LOS

(Continued)

TABLE 2A | Continued

References	Country	Study design	Study group	Participants characteristics	Comparison period	COVID-19 diagnosis approach/time to diagnosis	Major findings
Marfella et al. (25)	Italy	Multicentric cohort study	Non-COVID-19 STEMI	n = 302, age 64.18 ± 13.41 years, 79.8% males	1/3/2020–30/4/2020		
			COVID-19 STEMI	n = 46, age 56.13 ± 6.21 years, 67.4% males	2/2020–11/2020	RT-PCR on nasal/pharyngeal swabs/NA	D2B time, Laboratory values, Gp2b3a inhibitor use, Modified thrombus grade, TIMI status, In-hospital mortality, LOS, ICU admission, Cardiogenic shock
			Non-COVID-19 STEMI	n = 130, age 68.43 ± 6.46 years, 66.2% males	2/2020–11/2020		
Pellegrini et al. (26)	Italy	Monocentric cohort study	COVID-19 STEMI	n = 24, age 69.63 ± 11.00 years, 83.3% males	8/3/2020–20/4/2020	RT-PCR on nasal swab or endotracheal aspirate/3–6 h	Thrombus aspiration, MINOCA, Stent implantation, Gp2b3a inhibitor use, In-hospital mortality, Cardiogenic shock, Bleeding
			Non-COVID-19 STEMI	n = 26, age 64.65 ± 13.04 years, 84.6% males	8/3/2020–20/4/2020		
Rodriguez-Leor et al. (27)	Spain	Multicentric cohort study	COVID-19 STEMI	n = 91, age 64.8 ± 11.8 years, 84.4% males	14/3/2020–30/4/2020	PCR assay/NA	SO-to-FMC time, Primary angioplasty, Thrombus aspiration, MINOCA, Stent implantation, Gp2b3a inhibitor use, TIMI status, In-hospital mortality, Cardiogenic shock, Stent thrombosis, bleeding
			Non-COVID-19 STEMI	n = 919, age 62.5 ± 13.1 years, 78.4% males	14/3/2020–30/4/2020		
Choudry et al. (28)	UK	Monocentric cohort study	COVID-19 STEMI	n = 39, age 61.7 ± 11.0 years, 84.6% males	1/3/2020–20/5/2020	PT-PCR on nasal/pharyngeal swabs/NA	D2B time, Laboratory values, Primary angioplasty, Thrombus aspiration, Gp2b3a inhibitor use, Baseline thrombus grade, Modified thrombus grade, TIMI status, In-hospital mortality, Stent thrombosis
			Non-COVID-19 STEMI	n = 76, age 61.7 ± 12.6 years, 75% males	1/3/2020–20/5/2020		
Biasco et al. (29)	Spain	Monocentric cross-sectional study	COVID-19 STEMI	n = 5, age 62 ± 14 years, 80% males	23/3/2020–11/4/2020	RT-PCR on nasopharyngeal and throat swab samples/NA	Laboratory values
			Non-COVID-19 STEMI	n = 50, age 58 ± 12 years, 88% males	7/2015–12/2015		
Güler et al. (30)	Turkey	Monocentric cross-sectional study	COVID-19 STEMI	n = 62, age 60.2 ± 9.5 years, 66.1% males	11/3/2020–10/1/2021	RT-PCR on nasopharyngeal swabs/NA	SO-to-FMC time, D2B time, Laboratory values, Thrombus aspiration, Gp2b3a inhibitor use, Baseline thrombus grade, TIMI status, In-hospital mortality, ICU admission, LOS
			Non-COVID-19 STEMI	n = 64, age 63 ± 8 years, 70.3% males	11/3/2020–10/1/2021		

UK, United Kingdom; NOS, Newcastle-Ottawa Scale; D2B, door to balloon; MINOCA, myocardial infarction with non-obstructive coronary arteries; TIMI, thrombolysis in myocardial infarction; SO-to-FMC, symptom onset to first medical contact; LOS, length of stay; ICU, intensive care unit; RT-PCR, reverse transcriptase-polymerase chain reaction; CT, computed tomography; CXR, chest x-ray.

Comparison of the Characteristics, Management and Outcomes of STEMI Patients Presenting...

137

TABLE 2B | Baseline characteristics of study subjects.

References	Study group	Total subjects (n)	Age (years) (mean ± SD)	Male (%)	Body mass index (kg/m²)	Diabetes mellitus (%)	Hypertension (%)	Dyslipidemia (%)	Smoking (%)	Multivessel desease (%)	Previous myocardial infarction (%)
Popovic et al. (18)	COVID-19 STEMI	11	63.6 ± 17.4	63.9	25.1 ± 8.1	18.2	45.5	27.3	36.4	0	NA
	Non-COVID-19 STEMI	72	62.5 ± 12.6	73.6	27.02 ± 4.8	19.4	43.1	38.9	55.6	12.5	NA
Siudak et al. (19)	COVID-19 STEMI	145	63.19 ± 12.55	71.33	NA	14.48	46.21	NA	37.24	NA	12.41
	Non-COVID-19 STEMI	2,276	65.43 ± 12.23	67.65	NA	16.86	57.55	NA	31.08	NA	15.94
Kiris et al. (20)	COVID-19 STEMI	65	66.8 ± 12.0	68	NA	26	48	NA	34	44	NA
	Non-COVID-19 STEMI	668	60.0 ± 12.3	78	NA	29	42	NA	33	40	NA
Koutsoukis et al. (21)	COVID-19 STEMI	17	63.4 ± 13.2	70	NA	NA	NA	NA	NA	30.7	NA
	Non-COVID-19 STEMI	99	63.8 ± 13.9	67	NA	NA	NA	NA	NA	61.2	NA
Garcia et al. (22)	COVID-19 STEMI	230	18–55 yrs: 23%; 55–65 yrs: 32%; 66–75 yrs: 28%; >75 yrs: 17%	71	29.3 ± 7.6	46	73	46	44	0	13
	Non-COVID-19 STEMI	460	18–55 yrs: 26%; 55–65 yrs: 30%; 66–75 yrs: 27%; >75 yrs: 17%	68	29.5 ± 6.4	28	69	60	59	16	24
Kite et al. (23)	COVID-19 STEMI	144	63.1 ± 12.6	77.8	27.3 ± 4.5	34	64.8	46	31.7	NA	16.4
	Non-COVID-19 STEMI	24,961	65.6 ± 13.4	72.2	27.8 ± 5.5	20.9	44.8	28.9	33.7	NA	13
Little et al. (24)	COVID-19 STEMI	46	61.80 ± 7.95	80.4	NA	32.6	54	52.2	41.3	NA	10.9
	Non-COVID-19 STEMI	302	64.18 ± 13.41	79.8	NA	23.5	50.7	33.1	41.7	NA	12.6
Marfella et al. (25)	COVID-19 STEMI	46	56.13 ± 6.21	67.4	27.09 ± 1.81	17.4	39.1	15.2	6.5	NA	NA
	Non-COVID-19 STEMI	130	68.43 ± 6.46	66.2	29.55 ± 1.97	29.2	55.4	23.7	29.2	NA	NA
Pellegrini et al. (26)	COVID-19 STEMI	24	69.63 ± 11.00	83.3	26.60 ± 3.36	41.7	70.8	62.5	29.2	45.8	29.2
	Non-COVID-19 STEMI	26	64.65 ± 13.04	84.6	26.11 ± 3.43	15.4	53.9	65.4	38.5	28.6	19.2
Rodriguez-Leor et al. (27)	COVID-19 STEMI	91	64.8 ± 11.8	84.4	NA	23.1	51.7	48.4	18.7	37.4	NA
	Non-COVID-19 STEMI	919	62.5 ± 13.1	78.4	NA	20.9	53.3	46.9	45.5	37.1	NA
Choudry et al. (28)	COVID-19 STEMI	39	61.7 ± 11.0	84.6	26.7 (24.8–30.7)	46.2	71.8	61.6	61.6	NA	15.4
	Non-COVID-19 STEMI	76	61.7 ± 12.6	75	26.7 (24.8–30.7)	46.2	42.1	36.8	46.1	NA	3.9
Blasco et al. (29)	COVID-19 STEMI	5	62 ± 14	80	28.0 (27.3–30.1)	0	80	0	40	NA	NA
	Non-COVID-19 STEMI	50	58 ± 12	88	27.6 (24.9–30.3)	8	42	52	78	NA	NA
Güler et al. (30)	COVID-19 STEMI	62	60.2 ± 9.5	66.1	NA	48.4	59.7	43.5	51.6	NA	9.7
	Non-COVID-19 STEMI	64	63 ± 8	70.3	NA	54.7	57.8	34.3	56.3	NA	28.1

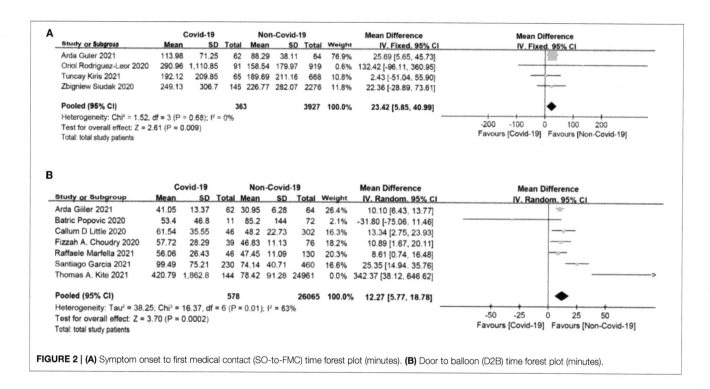

FIGURE 2 | (A) Symptom onset to first medical contact (SO-to-FMC) time forest plot (minutes). **(B)** Door to balloon (D2B) time forest plot (minutes).

outcomes with a high degree of heterogeneity. As shown in **Table 4**, the overall results were relatively robust and not influenced by a single study, except for primary angioplasty, stent implantation, and modified thrombus grade. An asymmetrical plot was observed in some funnel plots, suggesting that publication bias may exist (**Figures 6A–9F**).

DISCUSSION

Clinical Implications

This is the first meta-analysis to compare the characteristics, management, and clinical outcomes of patients with STEMI presenting with COVID-19 infection and that of those patients without COVID-19 infection. Compared to the non-COVID-19 group, the COVID-19 group had significant delays in SO-to-FMC and D2B times. Among the two groups, laboratory values, such as CRP, WBC, and D-dimer, were elevated in the COVID-19 group, while lymphocyte count was found to be lower compared to the non-COVID-19 group. In addition, STEMI concomitant with COVID-19 infection was characterized by a higher rate of MINOCA, lower rate of stent implantation, and higher thrombus grade, and associated higher use of thrombus aspiration and Gp2b3a inhibitors. Furthermore, we found that the COVID-19 group had an increased rate of in-hospital mortality, cardiogenic shock, stent thrombosis, ICU admission, longer length of hospital stays, and decreased TIMI flow post-procedure.

The COVID-19 pandemic started in late 2019 and has caused severe delays in the treatment of patients with STEMI compared to the pre-COVID-19 era, and this is mostly explained by the limited access to emergency medical services

(EMS) and the lack of effective organization of healthcare systems (33, 34). Several studies reported that the time from SO-to-FMC and D2B was longer in STEMI patients with COVID-19 than in those without COVID-19, which may be related to the following factors: a higher rate of respiratory symptoms without chest pain as a clinical manifestation in COVID-19 patients may result in an unclear diagnosis of heart attack and lead to a delay in seeking medical service (35), Furthermore, interventional procedures may be more complex in COVID-19 patients than in non-COVID-19 patients (24).

The reperfusion strategy for patients with STEMI during the COVID-19 pandemic remains controversial. The Chinese Cardiac Society and the Canadian Association of Interventional Cardiology recommend thrombolysis as the preferred reperfusion strategy for patients with STEMI (36, 37). In contrast, the American College of Cardiology (ACC) and the Society for Cardiovascular Angiography and Interventions (SCAI) still suggested the use of primary percutaneous coronary intervention (PPCI) as the main treatment for all patients with STEMI during the COVID-19 crisis (1, 2). Rashid et al. reported that STEMI patients with COVID-19 were less likely to receive PPCI than STEMI patients without COVID-19 (38). However, in this study, we did not find a significant difference in the rate of primary angioplasty between both groups. Moreover, we found that the COVID-19 group had a lower rate of stent implantation, which may be associated with a higher rate of MINOCA.

Previous studies have shown that COVID-19 may lead to a prothrombotic state and that a high thrombus burden is more common in STEMI patients with COVID-19 (39–42). SARS-CoV-2 causes a systemic inflammatory response, resulting

Comparison of the Characteristics, Management and Outcomes of STEMI Patients Presenting...

139

TABLE 3 | GRADE summary of findings.

Effects of COVID-19 in STEMI patients

Patient or population: STEMI Patients
Setting: Europe, Asian, North America
Intervention: COVID-19
Comparison: Non-COVID-19

Outcomes	Anticipated absolute effects* (95% CI)		Relative effect (95% CI)	No of participants (studies)	Certainty of the evidence (GRADE)	Comments
	Risk with Non-COVID-19	Risk with COVID-19				
Symptom-to-FMC time	The mean symptom-to-FMC time was 0	MD 23.42 higher (5.85 higher to 40.99 higher)	–	4,290 (4 observational studies)	⊕◯◯◯ Very low	NA
D2B time	The mean D2B time was 0	MD 12.27 higher (5.77 higher to 18.78 higher)	–	26,643 (7 observational studies)	⊕◯◯◯ Very low	NA
CRP	–	SMD 0.76 higher (0.38 higher to 1.13 higher)	–	1,576 (7 observational studies)	⊕◯◯◯ Very low	NA
WBC	–	SMD 0.39 higher (0.1 higher to 0.69 higher)	–	1,205 (5 observational studies)	⊕◯◯◯ Very low	NA
D-Dimer	–	SMD 0.79 higher (0.36 higher to 1.22 higher)	–	324 (3 observational studies)	⊕◯◯◯ Very low	NA
Lymphocyte count	–	SMD 0.52 lower (0.69 lower to 0.36 lower)	–	848 (5 observational studies)	⊕⊕◯◯ Low	NA
Primary angioplasty	942 per 1,000	820 per 1,000 (566 to 943)	OR 0.28 (0.08 to 1.01)	2,796 (7 observational studies)	⊕◯◯◯ Very low	NA
MINOCA	55 per 1,000	356 per 1,000 (110 to 712)	OR 9.57 (2.14 to 42.83)	1,949 (5 observational studies)	⊕◯◯◯ Very low	NA
Stent implantation	895 per 1,000	704 per 1,000 (483 to 858)	OR 0.28 (0.11 to 0.71)	1,264 (4 observational studies)	⊕◯◯◯ Very low	NA
Baseline thrombus grade > 3	677 per 1,000	866 per 1,000 (793 to 916)	OR 3.09 (1.83 to 5.23)	974 (3 observational studies)	⊕◯◯◯ Very low	NA
Modified thrombus grade > 3	350 per 1,000	759 per 1,000 (423 to 931)	OR 5.84 (1.36 to 25.06)	1,024 (3 observational studies)	⊕◯◯◯ Very low	NA
Thrombus aspiration	204 per 1,000	301 per 1,000 (243 to 367)	OR 1.68 (1.25 to 2.26)	2,498 (7 observational studies)	⊕⊕◯◯ Low	NA
Gp2b3a inhibitor	176 per 1,000	379 per 1,000 (275 to 496)	OR 2.86 (1.78 to 4.62)	2,757 (9 observational studies)	⊕◯◯◯ Very low	NA
TIMI-3 Flow	892 per 1,000	832 per 1,000 (776 to 874)	OR 0.60 (0.42 to 0.84)	2,572 (7 observational studies)	⊕⊕◯◯ Low	NA
In-hospital mortality	57 per 1,000	265 per 1,000 (224 to 311)	OR 5.98 (4.78 to 7.48)	25,266 (11 observational studies)	⊕⊕⊕◯ Moderate	NA
Cardiogenic shock	84 per 1,000	201 per 1,000 (156 to 256)	OR 2.75 (2.02 to 3.76)	24,085 (5 observational studies)	⊕⊕◯◯ Low	NA
Stent thrombosis	10 per 1,000	52 per 1,000 (23 to 114)	OR 5.65 (2.41 to 13.23)	1,858 (3 observational studies)	⊕⊕◯◯ Low	NA
Bleeding	5 per 1,000	13 per 1,000 (4 to 39)	OR 2.82 (0.88 to 9.05)	15,850 (4 observational studies)	⊕◯◯◯ Very low	NA
ICU admission	83 per 1,000	277 per 1,000 (184 to 394)	OR 4.26 (2.51 to 7.22)	650 (3 observational studies)	⊕◯◯◯ Very low	NA
Length of stay	The mean length of stay was 0	MD 4.63 higher (2.56 higher to 6.69 higher)	–	26,445 (5 observational studies)	⊕◯◯◯ Very low	NA

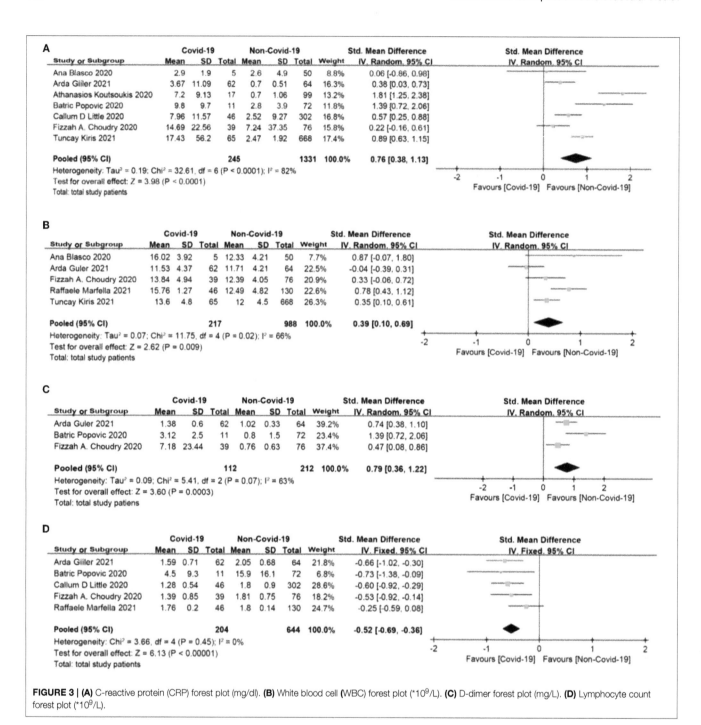

FIGURE 3 | (A) C-reactive protein (CRP) forest plot (mg/dl). **(B)** White blood cell (WBC) forest plot (*10^9/L). **(C)** D-dimer forest plot (mg/L). **(D)** Lymphocyte count forest plot (*10^9/L).

in endothelial and hemostatic activation, which involves the activation of platelets and the coagulation cascade (43). In addition, our study found that the time from SO-to-FMC and D2B was longer in STEMI patients with COVID-19 than in those without COVID-19. The studies of Duman et al. (44) and Ge et al. (45) reported that the delay in SO-to-FMC and D2B would prolong the time for opening infarct-related vessels which may account for a higher thrombus burden. Therefore, in the COVID era, it is of great significance that novel technologies should be developed so as to achieve more

efficient thrombus aspiration in patients with very high intra-coronary thrombus burden such as patients with STEMI and coexistent COVID-19 infection (46). Furthermore, strategies to reduce reperfusion delay times such as educating the public about the recognition and diversity of coronary symptoms and optimizing interventional procedures are essential. In keeping with the high thrombus burden, the COVID-19 group had elevated CRP, WBC, and D-dimer levels and a lower lymphocyte count compared to the non-COVID-19 group. High thrombus grade, reduced TIMI flow, high rate of MINOCA, and stent

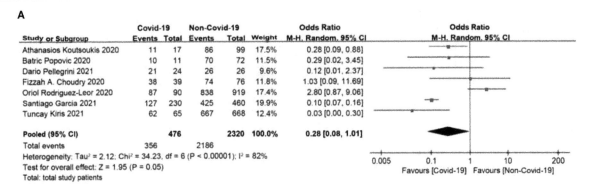

FIGURE 4 | Continued

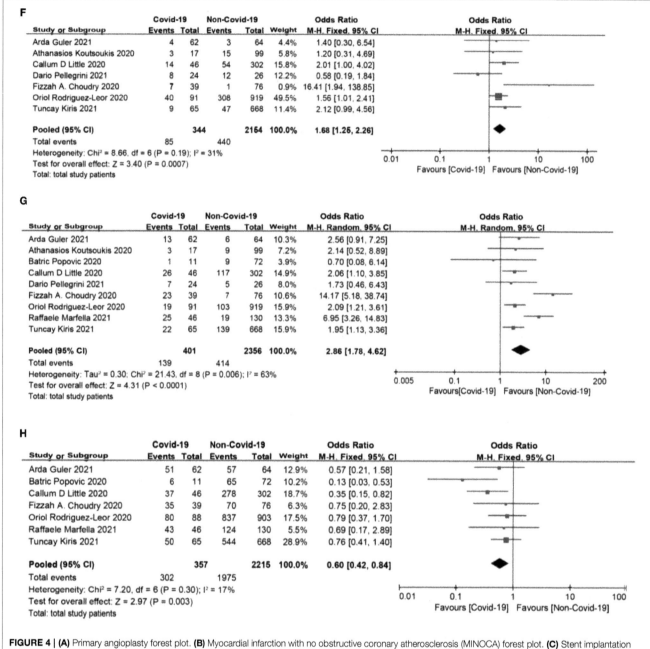

FIGURE 4 | (A) Primary angioplasty forest plot. **(B)** Myocardial infarction with no obstructive coronary atherosclerosis (MINOCA) forest plot. **(C)** Stent implantation forest plot. **(D)** Baseline thrombus grade forest plot. **(E)** Modified thrombus grade forest plot. **(F)** Thrombus aspiration forest plot. **(G)** Glycoprotein IIbIIIa (Gp2b3a) inhibitor use forest plot. **(H)** Thrombolysis in myocardial infarction (TIMI)-3 flow forest plot.

thrombosis may be the result of the intense inflammatory and heightened thrombus burden observed in COVID-19 patients (18, 27, 28, 34). Consistently, the data presented here demonstrated a more aggressive use of thrombus aspiration and a Gp2b3a inhibitor in STEMI patients with concomitant SARS-CoV-2 infection. The use of a Gp2b3a inhibitor may also increase the risk of bleeding (47), but this study showed no significant difference between the two groups in terms of bleeding.

Hospital-mortality was dramatically higher in STEMI patients who presented with COVID-19 than in those without COVID-19. Longer ischemia time, higher thrombus burden, and increased rate of adverse cardiovascular events, including cardiogenic shock, may also be contributory (48, 49). Current studies (50, 51) have reported that STEMI patients with concomitant COVID-19 have higher ICU admission rates and longer lengths of stay, and the results of this meta-analysis support this finding. An

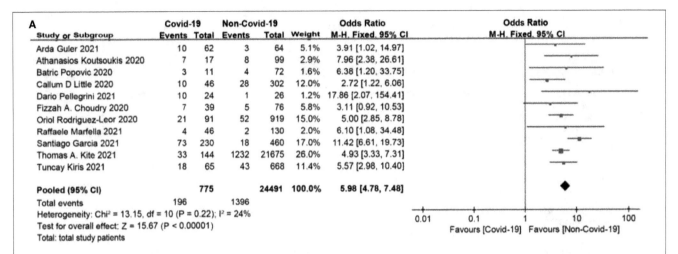

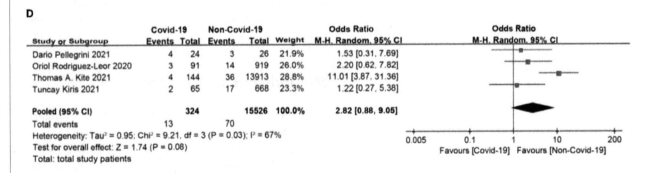

FIGURE 5 | Continued

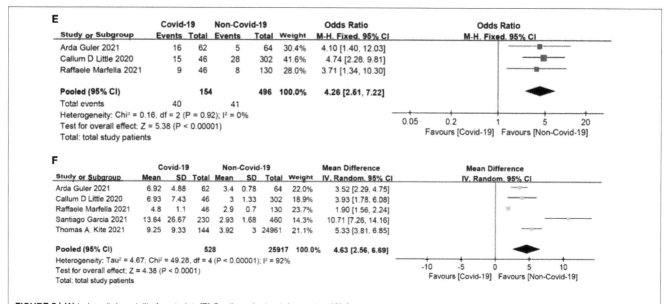

FIGURE 5 | (A) In-hospital mortality forest plot. (B) Cardiogenic shock forest plot. (C) Stent thrombosis forest plot. (D) Bleeding forest plot. (E) Intensive care unit (ICU) admission rate forest plot. (F) Length of stay forest plot (days).

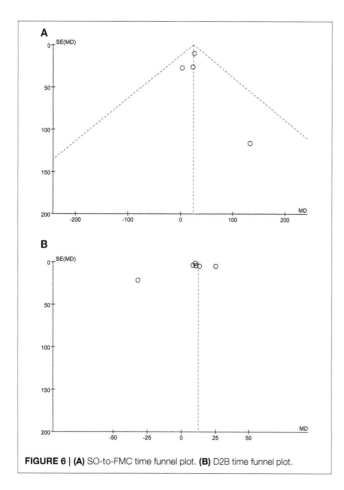

FIGURE 6 | (A) SO-to-FMC time funnel plot. (B) D2B time funnel plot.

increased ICU admission rate and length of stay may have a significant impact on hospital resources. Taken

together, COVID-19 status may have great implications on the characteristics, management, and outcomes of patients with STEMI.

Heterogeneity of Meta-Analysis

In a meta-analysis, heterogeneity may exist while the sample estimates for the population risk were of different magnitudes (52). The I^2 statistic means the percentage of total variation across effect size estimates that is due to heterogeneity rather than chance. In our study, there are significant and high degrees of heterogeneity for some outcomes. The existing heterogeneity can partly result from different sample sizes, study designs, study times, study scope (nation and region), diagnostic methods, the severity of the disease. We aggregate studies that are different methodologies, but the heterogeneity in the results is still inevitable.

Methodological Considerations

To our knowledge, this is the first meta-analysis that summarizes the comparison of clinical information on STEMI patients presenting with vs. those presenting without COVID-19 infection. We included multiple studies that were conducted in Asia, Europe, and North America, so that our findings can provide a broad overview of COVID-19 infection in patients with STEMI. However, our study has several limitations. First, the delay time, laboratory values, and length of stay were reported in terms of median values and IQR in many studies, which have been adjusted to means and SDs using the Box-Cox method.

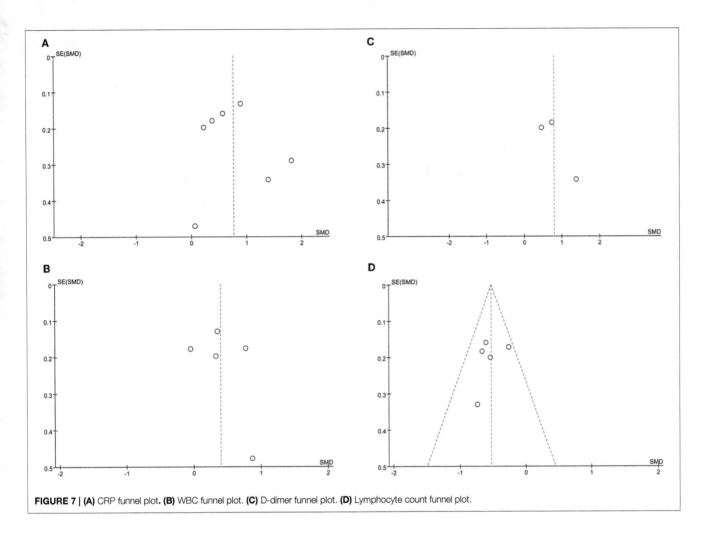

FIGURE 7 | (A) CRP funnel plot. **(B)** WBC funnel plot. **(C)** D-dimer funnel plot. **(D)** Lymphocyte count funnel plot.

Nevertheless, using this method to calculate SDs may entail inaccuracy and make the SDs greater than the mean in some cases, which is an inherent feature of the method (17). Second, the disparity in study size may affect the weighting of the studies and the pooled effect size, which is innate to meta-analyses (53, 54). Third, a high degree of heterogeneity was observed in some outcomes. Due to inadequate information for the included studies, it is difficult to conduct a subgroup analysis to explain the heterogeneity. We performed a sensitivity analysis to assess the reliability of our findings and used the random-effects model when I^2 statistics were more than 50%. Fourth, we were unable to compare the rate of thrombosis and elective PCI and the revascularization rate of patients undergoing primary angioplasty between the two groups due to a lack of sufficient data. Future studies are needed to further investigate these outcomes. Finally, our data were limited to in-hospital outcomes. Long-term follow-up is required to explore the association between SARS-CoV-2 infection and poor outcomes in patients with STEMI.

CONCLUSION

In patients with STEMI, COVID-19 has had a deep impact on their therapeutic management and clinical outcomes. A longer time from SO-to-FMC and D2B was observed in STEMI patients with COVID-19 in our study. Moreover, patients with STEMI who also had COVID-19 had more severe thrombotic events adverse outcomes. Further studies are required to explore the mechanism of coronary thrombus burden and the optimal treatment for patients with STEMI and COVID-19.

AUTHOR CONTRIBUTIONS

YW, LK, C-WC, SX, and T-HT: conception. YW, LK, C-WC, JX, PY, SX, and T-HT: methodology. YW, LK, JX, PY, and T-HT: analysis. YW, LK, JX, and PY: interpretation and writing. C-WC, SX, and T-HT: supervision. All authors have read and agreed to the published version of the manuscript.

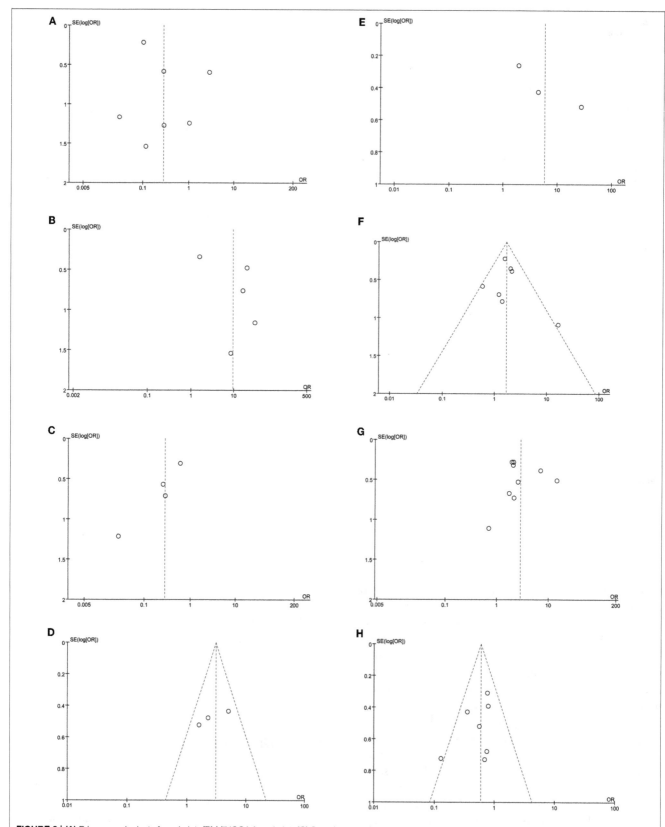

FIGURE 8 | (A) Primary angioplasty funnel plot. **(B)** MINOCA funnel plot. **(C)** Stent implantation funnel plot. **(D)** Baseline thrombus grade funnel plot. **(E)** Modified thrombus grade funnel plot. **(F)** Thrombus aspiration funnel plot. **(G)** Gp2b3a inhibitor use funnel plot. **(H)** TIMI-3 flow funnel plot.

Comparison of the Characteristics, Management and Outcomes of STEMI Patients Presenting...

147

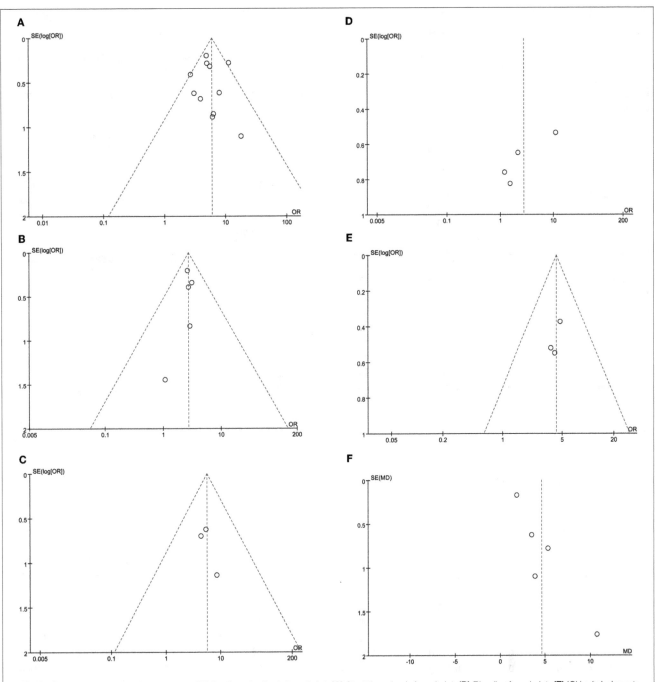

FIGURE 9 | (A) In-hospital mortality funnel plot. **(B)** Cardiogenic shock funnel plot. **(C)** Stent thrombosis funnel plot. **(D)** Bleeding funnel plot. **(E)** ICU admission rate funnel plot. **(F)** Length of stay funnel plot.

TABLE 4 | Leave-one-out analysis.

Study name	Statistics with study excluded		
	Odds ratio or SMD	95% CI	P-value
D2B time			
Güler et al. (30)	12.66	2.96 to 22.35	0.01
Popovic et al. (18)	13.06	7.13 to 18.99	<0.0001
Little et al. (24)	12.01	4.16 to 19.86	0.003
Choudry et al. (28)	12.52	4.35 to 20.68	0.003
Marfella et al. (25)	13.1	4.66 to 21.54	0.002
Garcia et al. (22)	9.92	4.47 to 15.35	0.0004
Kite et al. (23)	12.15	6.47 to 17.82	<0.0001
CRP			
Blasco et al. (29)	0.82	0.43 to 1.21	<0.0001
Güler et al. (30)	0.83	0.40 to 1.26	0.0002
Koutsoukis et al. (21)	0.59	0.29 to 0.90	0.0001
Popovic et al. (18)	0.67	0.28 to 1.06	0.0007
Little et al. (24)	0.8	0.33 to 1.26	0.0007
Choudry et al. (28)	0.86	0.45 to 1.26	<0.0001
Kiris et al. (20)	0.73	0.27 to 1.20	0.002
WBC			
Blasco et al. (29)	0.35	0.04 to 0.67	0.03
Güler et al. (30)	0.5	0.25 to 0.76	<0.0001
Choudry et al. (28)	0.42	0.04 to 0.81	0.03
Marfella et al. (25)	0.26	0.08 to 0.44	0.004
Kiris et al. (20)	0.038	0.18 to 0.59	0.0002
D-Dimer			
Güler et al. (30)	0.89	0.01 to 1.78	0.05
Popovic et al. (18)	0.62	0.35 to 0.88	<0.0001
Choudry et al. (28)	1.00	0.38 to 1.62	0.002
Primary Angioplasty			
Koutsoukis et al. (21)	0.27	0.05 to 1.43	0.12
Popovic et al. (18)	0.28	0.07 to 1.15	0.08
Pellegrini et al. (26)	0.31	0.01 to 1.24	0.10
Choudry et al. (28)	0.23	0.06 to 0.94	0.04
Rodriguez-Leor et al. (27)	0.12	0.08 to 0.17	<0.0001
Garcia et al. (22)	0.36	0.09 to 1.49	0.16
Kiris et al. (20)	0.21	0.16 to 0.29	<0.0001
MINOCA			
Koutsoukis et al. (21)	7.63	1.44 to 40.43	0.02
Popovic et al. (18)	8.49	1.37 to 52.74	0.02
Pellegrini et al. (26)	9.81	1.84 to 52.38	0.01

(Continued)

TABLE 4 | Continued

Study name	Statistics with study excluded		
	Odds ratio or SMD	95% CI	P-value
Rodriguez-Leor (27)	18.62	8.73 to 39.72	<0.0001
Garcia et al. (22)	7.56	1.38 to 41.37	0.02
Stent Implantation			
Blasco et al. (29)	0.46	0.28 to 0.75	0.002
Koutsoukis et al. (21)	0.25	0.06 to 1.01	0.05
Popovic et al. (18)	0.25	0.07 to 0.90	0.03
Rodriguez-Leor et al. (27)	0.20	0.09 to 0.43	<0.0001
Modified Thrombus Grade			
Choudry et al. (28)	7.03	0.52 to 96.03	0.14
Marfella et al. (25)	2.72	1.25 to 5.94	0.01
Kiris et al. (20)	10.69	1.75 to 65.11	0.01
Gp2b3a inhibitor use			
Güler et al. (30)	2.90	1.70 to 4.93	<0.0001
Koutsoukis et al. (21)	2.93	1.75 to 4.90	<0.0001
Popovic et al. (18)	3.03	1.87 to 4.93	<0.0001
Little et al. (24)	3.02	1.72 to 5.30	0.0001
Pellegrini et al. (26)	2.99	1.79 to 5.01	<0.0001
Choudry et al. (28)	2.37	1.81 to 3.11	<0.0001
Rodriguez-Leor et al. (27)	2.93	2.19 to 3.92	<0.0001
Marfella et al. (25)	2.41	1.83 to 3.17	<0.0001
Kiris et al. (20)	3.01	2.25 to 4.03	<0.0001
Bleeding			
Pellegrini et al. (26)	3.30	0.77 to 14.07	0.11
Rodriguez-Leor et al. (27)	2.95	0.55 to 15.73	0.21
Kite et al. (23)	1.62	0.71 to 3.73	0.25
Kiris et al. (20)	3.62	0.92 to 14.23	0.07
Length of Stay			
Güler et al. (30)	5.11	2.17 to 8.06	0.0007
Little et al. (24)	4.84	2.41 to 7.27	< 0.0001
Marfella et al. (25)	5.42	3.24 to 7.26	< 0.0001
Garcia et al. (22)	3.56	1.85 to 5.27	< 0.0001
Kite et al. (23)	4.41	2.14 to 6.69	0.0001

REFERENCES

1. Mahmud E, Dauerman HL, Welt FGP, Messenger JC, Rao SV, Grines C, et al. Management of Acute myocardial infarction during the COVID-19 pandemic: a position statement from the society for cardiovascular angiography and interventions (SCAI), the American college of cardiology (acc), and the American college of emergency physicians (ACEP). *J Am Coll Cardiol.* (2020) 76:1375–84. doi: 10.1016/j.jacc.2020.04.039

2. Reed GW, Rossi JE, Cannon CP. Acute myocardial infarction. *Lancet.* (2017) 389:197–210. doi: 10.1016/S0140-6736(16)30677-8

3. Gulati A, Pomeranz C, Qamar Z, Thomas S, Frisch D, George G, et al. A comprehensive review of manifestations of novel coronaviruses in the context of deadly COVID-19 global pandemic. *Am J Med Sci.* (2020) 360:5–34. doi: 10.1016/j.amjms.2020.05.006

4. Wang D, Hu B, Hu C, Zhu F, Liu X, Zhang J, et al. Clinical characteristics of 138 hospitalized patients with 2019. Novel Coronavirus-Infected Pneumonia in Wuhan, China. *Jama.* (2020) 323:1061–9. doi: 10.1001/jama.2020.1585

5. Gupta A, Madhavan MV, Sehgal K, Nair N, Mahajan S, Sehrawat TS, et al. Extrapulmonary manifestations of COVID-19. *Nat Med.* (2020) 26:1017–32. doi: 10.1038/s41591-020-0968-3

6. Behzad S, Aghaghazvini L, Radmard AR, Gholamrezanezhad A. Extrapulmonary manifestations of COVID-19: Radiologic and clinical overview. *Clin Imaging.* (2020) 66:35–41. doi: 10.1016/j.clinimag.2020.05.013

7. Choudhury T, West NE, El-Omar M. ST elevation myocardial infarction. *Clin Med (Lond).* (2016) 16:277–82. doi: 10.7861/clinmedicine.16-3-277

8. Gale CP, Allan V, Cattle BA, Hall AS, West RM, Timmis A, et al. Trends in hospital treatments, including revascularisation, following acute myocardial infarction, 2003–2010: a multilevel and relative survival analysis for the National Institute for Cardiovascular Outcomes Research (NICOR). *Heart.* (2014) 100:582–9. doi: 10.1136/heartjnl-2013-304517

9. Townsend N, Wilson L, Bhatnagar P, Wickramasinghe K, Rayner M, Nichols M. Cardiovascular disease in Europe: epidemiological update 2016. *Eur Heart J.* (2016) 37:3232–45. doi: 10.1093/eurheartj/ehw334

10. Pedersen F, Butrymovich V, Kelbæk H, Wachtell K, Helqvist S, Kastrup J, et al. Short- and long-term cause of death in patients treated with primary PCI for STEMI. *J Am Coll Cardiol.* (2014) 64:2101–8. doi: 10.1016/j.jacc.2014.08.037

11. Baumhardt M, Dreyhaupt J, Winsauer C, Stuhler L, Thiessen K, Stephan T, et al. The effect of the lockdown on patients with myocardial infarction during the COVID-19 pandemic. *Dtsch Arztebl Int.* (2021) 118:447–53. doi: 10.3238/arztebl.m2021.0253

12. Xiang D, Xiang X, Zhang W, Yi S, Zhang J, Gu X, et al. Management and outcomes of patients with STEMI during the COVID-19 pandemic in China. *J Am Coll Cardiol.* (2020) 76:1318–24. doi: 10.1016/j.jacc.2020.06.039

13. Bikdeli B, Madhavan MV, Jimenez D, Chuich T, Dreyfus I, Driggin E, et al. COVID-19 and thrombotic or thromboembolic disease: implications for prevention, antithrombotic therapy, and follow-up: JACC state-of-the-art review. *J Am Coll Cardiol.* (2020) 75:2950–73. doi: 10.1016/j.jacc.2020.04.031

14. Pérez-Bermejo JA, Kang S, Rockwood SJ, Simoneau CR, Joy DA, Ramadoss GN, et al. SARS-CoV-2 infection of human iPSC-derived cardiac cells predicts novel cytopathic features in hearts of COVID-19 patients. *bioRxiv.* (2020) doi: 10.1101/2020.08.25.265561

15. Hayek SS, Brenner SK, Azam TU, Shadid HR, Anderson E, Berlin H, et al. In-hospital cardiac arrest in critically ill patients with covid-19: multicenter cohort study. *Bmj.* (2020) 371:m3513. doi: 10.1136/bmj.m3513

16. Bonow RO, Fonarow GC, O'Gara PT, Yancy CW. Association of coronavirus disease (2019). (COVID-19) with myocardial injury and mortality. *JAMA Cardiol.* (2020) 5:751–3. doi: 10.1001/jamacardio.2020.1105

17. McGrath S, Zhao XF, Steele R, Thombs BD, Benedetti A, Levis B, et al. Estimating the sample mean and standard deviation from commonly reported quantiles in meta-analysis. *Statistic Methods Med Res.* (2020) 29:2520–37. doi: 10.1177/0962280219889080

18. Popovic B, Varlot J, Metzdorf PA, Jeulin H, Goehringer F, Camenzind E. Changes in characteristics and management among patients with ST-elevation myocardial infarction due to COVID-19 infection. *Catheter Cardiovasc Interv.* (2021) 97:E319–e26. doi: 10.1002/ccd.29114

19. Siudak Z, Grygier M, Wojakowski W, Malinowski KP, Witkowski A, Gasior M, et al. Clinical and procedural characteristics of COVID-19 patients treated with percutaneous coronary interventions. *Catheter Cardiovasc Interv.* (2020) 96:E568–e75. doi: 10.1002/ccd.29134

20. Kiris T, Avci E, Ekin T, Akgün DE, Tiryaki M, Yidirim A, et al. Impact of COVID-19 outbreak on patients with ST-segment elevation myocardial infarction (STEMI) in Turkey: results from TURSER study (TURKISH St-segment elevation myocardial infarction registry). *J Thromb Thrombolysis.* (2021) 2021:1–14. doi: 10.1007/s11239-021-02487-3

21. Koutsoukis A, Delmas C, Roubille F, Bonello L, Schurtz G, Manzo-Silberman S, et al. Acute coronary syndrome in the era of sars-cov-2 infection: a registry of the french group of acute cardiac care. *CJC Open.* (2021) 3:311–7. doi: 10.1016/j.cjco.2020.11.003

22. Garcia S, Dehghani P, Grines C, Davidson L, Nayak KR, Saw J, et al. Initial findings from the North American COVID-19 myocardial infarction registry. *J Am Coll Cardiol.* (2021) 77:1994–2003. doi: 10.1016/j.jacc.2021.02.055

23. Kite TA, Ludman PF, Gale CP, Wu J, Caixeta A, Mansourati J, et al. International prospective registry of acute coronary syndromes in patients with COVID-19. *J Am Coll Cardiol.* (2021) 77:2466–76. doi: 10.1016/j.jacc.2021.03.309

24. Little CD, Kotecha T, Candilio L, Jabbour RJ, Collins GB, Ahmed A, et al. COVID-19 pandemic and STEMI: pathway activation and outcomes from the pan-London heart attack group. *Open Heart.* (2020) 7:2. doi: 10.1136/openhrt-2020-001432

25. Marfella R, Paolisso P, Sardu C, Palomba L, D'Onofrio N, Cesaro A, et al. SARS-COV-2 colonizes coronary thrombus and impairs heart microcirculation bed in asymptomatic SARS-CoV-2 positive subjects with acute myocardial infarction. *Crit Care.* (2021) 25:217. doi: 10.1186/s13054-021-03643-0

26. Pellegrini D, Fiocca L, Pescetelli I, Canova P, Vassileva A, Faggi L, et al. Effect of respiratory impairment on the outcomes of primary percutaneous coronary intervention in patients with ST-segment elevation myocardial infarction and coronavirus disease-2019 (COVID-19). *Circ J.* (2021) 85:1701–7. doi: 10.1253/circj.CJ-20-1166

27. Rodriguez-Leor O, Cid Alvarez AB, Pérez de Prado A, Rossello X, Ojeda S, Serrador A, et al. In-hospital outcomes of COVID-19 ST-elevation myocardial infarction patients. *EuroIntervention.* (2021) 16:1426–33. doi: 10.4244/EIJ-D-20-00935

28. Choudry FA, Hamshere SM, Rathod KS, Akhtar MM, Archbold RA, Guttmann OP, et al. High thrombus burden in patients with COVID-19 presenting with st-segment elevation myocardial infarction. *J Am Coll Cardiol.* (2020) 76:1168–76. doi: 10.1016/j.jacc.2020.07.022

29. Blasco A, Coronado MJ, Hernández-Terciado F, Martín P, Royuela A, Ramil E, et al. Assessment of neutrophil extracellular traps in coronary thrombus of a case series of patients with COVID-19 and myocardial infarction. *JAMA Cardiol.* (2020) 6:1–6. doi: 10.1001/jamacardio.2020.7308

30. Güler A, Gürbak I, Panç C, Güner A, Ertürk M. Frequency and predictors of no-reflow phenomenon in patients with COVID-19 presenting with ST-segment elevation myocardial infarction. *Acta Cardiol.* (2021) 2021:1–9. doi: 10.1080/00015385.2021.1931638

31. Gibson CM, de Lemos JA, Murphy SA, Marble SJ, McCabe CH, Cannon CP, et al. Combination therapy with abciximab reduces angiographically evident thrombus in acute myocardial infarction: a TIMI 14 substudy. *Circulation.* (2001) 103:2550–4. doi: 10.1161/01.CIR.103.21.2550

32. Sianos G, Papafakli MI, Daemen J, Vaina S, van Mieghem CA, van Domburg RT, et al. Angiographic stent thrombosis after routine use of drug-eluting stents in ST-segment elevation myocardial infarction: the importance of thrombus burden. *J Am Coll Cardiol.* (2007) 50:573–83. doi: 10.1016/j.jacc.2007.04.059

33. Ferlini M, Andreassi A, Carugo S, Cuccia C, Bianchini B, Castiglioni B, et al. Centralization of the ST elevation myocardial infarction care network in the Lombardy region during the COVID-19 outbreak. *Int J Cardiol.* (2020) 312:24–6. doi: 10.1016/j.ijcard.2020.04.062

34. Tam CF, Cheung KS, Lam S, Wong A, Yung A, Sze M, et al. Impact of coronavirus disease (COVID-19) outbreak on st-segment-elevation myocardial infarction care in Hong Kong, China. *Circ Cardiovasc Qual Outcomes.* (2020) 13:e006631. doi: 10.1161/CIRCOUTCOMES.120.006631

35. Carugo S, Ferlini M, Castini D, Andreassi A, Guagliumi G, Metra M, et al. Management of acute coronary syndromes during the COVID-19 outbreak

in Lombardy: The "macro-hub" experience. *Int J Cardiol Heart Vasc.* (2020) 31:100662. doi: 10.1016/j.ijcha.2020.100662

36. Han Y, Zeng H, Jiang H, Yang Y, Yuan Z, Cheng X, et al. CSC Expert consensus on principles of clinical management of patients with severe emergent cardiovascular diseases during the COVID-19 epidemic. *Circulation.* (2020) 141:e810–e6. doi: 10.1161/CIRCULATIONAHA.120.047011

37. Wood DA, Sathananthan J, Gin K, Mansour S, Ly HQ, Quraishi AU, et al. Precautions and procedures for coronary and structural cardiac interventions during the COVID-19 pandemic: guidance from canadian association of interventional cardiology. *Can J Cardiol.* (2020) 36:780–3. doi: 10.1016/j.cjca.2020.03.027

38. Rashid M, Wu J, Timmis A, Curzen N, Clarke S, Zaman A, et al. Outcomes of COVID-19-positive acute coronary syndrome patients: a multisource electronic healthcare records study from England. *J Intern Med.* (2021) 290:88–100. doi: 10.1111/joim.13246

39. Fan BE, Chong VCL, Chan SSW, Lim GH, Lim KGE, Tan GB, et al. Hematologic parameters in patients with COVID-19 infection. *Am J Hematol.* (2020) 95:E131–e4. doi: 10.1002/ajh.25774

40. Klok FA, Kruip M, van der Meer NJM, Arbous MS, Gommers D, Kant KM, et al. Incidence of thrombotic complications in critically ill ICU patients with COVID-19. *Thromb Res.* (2020) 191:145–7. doi: 10.1016/j.thromres.2020.04.013

41. Beyrouti R, Adams ME, Benjamin L, Cohen H, Farmer SF, Goh YY, et al. Characteristics of ischaemic stroke associated with COVID-19. *J Neurol Neurosurg Psychiatry.* (2020) 91:889–91. doi: 10.1136/jnnp-2020-323586

42. Ruan Q, Yang K, Wang W, Jiang L, Song J. Clinical predictors of mortality due to COVID-19 based on an analysis of data of 150 patients from Wuhan, China. *Intensive Care Med.* (2020) 46:846–8. doi: 10.1007/s00134-020-05991-x

43. Masi P, Hékimian G, Lejeune M, Chommeloux J, Desnos C, Pineton De Chambrun M, et al. Systemic inflammatory response syndrome is a major contributor to COVID-19-associated coagulopathy: insights from a prospective, single-center cohort study. *Circulation.* (2020) 142:611–4. doi: 10.1161/CIRCULATIONAHA.120.048925

44. Duman H, Çetin M, Durakoglugil ME, Degirmenci H, Hamur H, Bostan M, et al. Relation of angiographic thrombus burden with severity of coronary artery disease in patients with ST segment elevation myocardial infarction. *Med Sci Monit.* (2015) 21:3540–6. doi: 10.12659/MSM.895157

45. Ge J, Li J, Dong B, Ning X, Hou B. Determinants of angiographic thrombus burden and impact of thrombus aspiration on outcome in young patients with ST-segment elevation myocardial infarction. *Catheter Cardiovasc Interv.* (2019) 93:E269–e76. doi: 10.1002/ccd.27944

46. Karagiannidis E, Papazoglou AS, Sofidis G, Chatzinikolaou E, Keklikoglou K, Panteris E, et al. Micro-CT-Based quantification of extracted thrombus burden characteristics and association with angiographic outcomes in patients with ST-elevation myocardial infarction: the QUEST-STEMI study. *Front Cardiovasc Med.* (2021) 8:646064. doi: 10.3389/fcvm.2021.646064

47. Elian D, Guetta V. Glycoprotein 2b3a inhibitors for acute coronary syndromes: what the trials tell us. *Harefuah.* (2003) 142:350–498.

48. Scholz KH, Maier SKG, Maier LS, Lengenfelder B, Jacobshagen C, Jung J, et al. Impact of treatment delay on mortality in ST-segment elevation myocardial infarction (STEMI) patients presenting with and without haemodynamic instability: results from the German prospective, multicentre FITT-STEMI trial. *Eur Heart J.* (2018) 39:1065–74. doi: 10.1093/eurheartj/ehy004

49. Singh M, Berger PB, Ting HH, Rihal CS, Wilson SH, Lennon RJ, et al. Influence of coronary thrombus on outcome of percutaneous coronary angioplasty in the current era (the Mayo Clinic experience). *Am J Cardiol.* (2001) 88:1091–6. doi: 10.1016/S0002-9149(01)02040-9

50. Solano-López J, Zamorano JL, Pardo Sanz A, Amat-Santos I, Sarnago F, Gutiérrez Ibañes E, et al. Risk factors for in-hospital mortality in patients with acute myocardial infarction during the COVID-19 outbreak. *Rev Esp Cardiol (Engl Ed).* (2020) 73:985–93. doi: 10.1016/j.recesp.2020.07.023

51. Matsushita K, Hess S, Marchandot B, Sato C, Truong DP, Kim NT, et al. Clinical features of patients with acute coronary syndrome during the COVID-19 pandemic. *J Thromb Thrombolysis.* (2021) 52:95–104. doi: 10.1007/s11239-020-02340-z

52. Sedgwick P. Meta-analyses: what is heterogeneity? *Bmj-Br Med J.* (2015) 15:350. doi: 10.1136/bmj.h1435

53. Rattka M, Dreyhaupt J, Winsauer C, Stuhler L, Baumhardt M, Thiessen K, et al. Effect of the COVID-19 pandemic on mortality of patients with STEMI: a systematic review and meta-analysis. *Heart.* (2020) 20:360. doi: 10.1136/heartjnl-2020-318360

54. Kamarullah W, Sabrina AP, Rocky MA, Gozali DR. Investigating the implications of COVID-19 outbreak on systems of care and outcomes of STEMI patients: a systematic review and meta-analysis. *Indian Heart J.* (2021) 73:404–12. doi: 10.1016/j.ihj.2021.06.009

20

Cumulative Evidence for the Association of Thrombosis and the Prognosis of COVID-19

Dongqiong Xiao [1,2], Fajuan Tang [1,2]*, Lin Chen [1,2], Hu Gao [1,2] and Xihong Li [1,2]*

[1] Department of Emergency, West China Second University Hospital, Sichuan University, Chengdu, China, [2] Key Laboratory of Birth Defects and Related Diseases of Women and Children (Sichuan University), Ministry of Education, Chengdu, China

Correspondence:
Fajuan Tang
kftangfajuan@163.com
Xihong Li
lixihonghxey@163.com

Background: Although thrombosis events have been reported in patients with coronavirus disease 2019 (COVID-19), the association between thrombosis and COVID-19-related critical status or risk of mortality in COVID-19 has been inconsistent.

Objective: We conducted a meta-analysis of reports assessing the association between thrombosis and the prognosis of COVID-19.

Methods: The EMBASE, Ovid-MEDLINE, and Web of Science databases were searched up to December 9, 2021, and additional studies were retrieved *via* manual searching. Studies were included if they reported the risk of COVID-19-related critical status or COVID-19-related mortality in relation to thrombosis. The related data were extracted by two authors independently, and a random effects model was conducted to pool the odds ratios (ORs). In addition, stratified analyses were conducted to evaluate the association.

Results: Among 6,686 initially identified studies, we included 25 studies published in 2020 and 2021, with a total of 332,915 patients according to predefined inclusion criteria. The associations between thrombosis and COVID-19-related mortality and COVID-19-related critical status were significant, with ORs of 2.61 (95% CI, 1.91–3.55, $p < 0.05$) and 2.9 (95% CI, 1.6–5.24, $p < 0.05$), respectively. The results were statistically significant and consistent in stratified analyses.

Conclusions: Thrombosis is associated with an increased risk of mortality and critical status induced by COVID-19. Further prospective studies with large sample sizes are required to establish whether these associations are causal by considering more confounders and to clarify their mechanisms.

Observational studies cannot prove causality. However, autopsy studies show thrombosis events preceding COVID-19-related deaths. The results of this meta-analysis reported that thrombosis was associated with a 161% increased risk of mortality from COVID-19 and a 190% increased risk of COVID-19-related critical status. The type of thrombosis included in the original studies also seemed to be related to the results.

Keywords: thrombosis and COVID-19 thrombosis, SARS-CoV-2, COVID-19, 2019-nCoV, mortality

INTRODUCTION

Coronavirus disease 2019 (COVID-19), a novel infectious disease, is highly prevalent globally and has infected over 271 million patients to date (https://www.who.int/emergencies/diseases/novel-coronavirus-2019). COVID-19 is caused by severe acute respiratory syndrome coronavirus 2 (SARS-CoV-2), and progressive respiratory failure is the primary cause of death (1) during the COVID-19 pandemic. Over 5 million individuals globally have succumbed to COVID-19 (https://covid19.who.int/). However, little is known about the causes of death. Histologic autopsy of pulmonary vessels in patients with COVID-19 showed widespread thrombosis with microangiopathy (1–3). Luca Spiezia et al. (4) reported that severe hypercoagulability rather than consumptive coagulopathy station was observed in patients with COVID-19 with acute respiratory failure. Fibrin formation and polymerization may contribute to thrombosis and correlate with critical status and a worse outcome in patients with COVID-19 (4, 5). An increased risk of thrombosis, such as venous thromboembolism (VTE), brain stroke, cardiac ischemia, and pulmonary embolism (PE), in patients with COVID-19 admitted to the intensive care unit (ICU) has been reported (6–9). The magnitude of this public health challenge is increasing, a concerning trend given that COVID-19 imposes a significant public health burden and large demand on health care systems. The association between thrombosis and COVID-19 prognosis should be recognized by clinical doctors globally.

There were four types of thrombosis found in patients with COVID-19: pale thrombus, mixed thrombus (arterial and venous thrombosis), red thrombus, and hyaline thrombus (microvascular thrombosis). A hypercoagulable state in the critically ill patients with COVID-19 was found due to the following mechanisms: severe hypofibrinolysis (10), endothelial dysfunction (11, 12), platelet activation (12, 13), endothelial-derived von Willebrand factor (vWF) activation (14), elevated soluble (s) P-selectin (13, 15), gene expression (13, 16), inflammatory cytokine activation (17, 18), and mannose-binding lectin (MBL)-related complement activation (19, 20). Serious adverse events, such as thrombosis and thrombocytopenia syndrome, after COVID-19 vaccination are rare (21) and are associated with a high mortality rate (22). Campello et al. found that no hypercoagulable condition was found after COVID-19 (ChAdOx1 or BNT162b2) vaccination (23).

A number of primary studies (24–28) have evaluated the association between thrombosis and the risk of adverse outcomes of COVID-19, including mortality and severity of COVID-19, with inconsistent results. We, therefore, conducted a meta-analysis to evaluate the association between thrombosis and the prognosis of COVID-19.

Abbreviations: BMI, body mass index; COVID-19, coronavirus disease 2019; DVT, deep venous thrombosis; ICU, intensive care unit; PE, pulmonary embolism; SARS-CoV-2, severe acute respiratory syndrome coronavirus 2; VTE, venous thromboembolism.

METHODS

Retrieval of Studies

The reporting of this meta-analysis of observational studies was in accordance with the Meta-Analysis of Observational Studies in Epidemiology (MOOSE) and Preferred Reporting Items for Systematic Reviews and Meta-Analyses (PRISMA) guidelines. The Embase, Ovid-MEDLINE, and Web of Science databases were searched up to 9 December 2021. The search consisted of three terms: thrombosis, COVID-19, and study design. We used the following key words to search for the first term: "thrombosis" OR "embolism" OR "thrombotic" OR "thrombus" OR "thrombi" OR "thromboembol*" OR "emboli*" OR "embolus" OR "clot?" OR "DVT" OR "VTE" OR "PE." We used the following key words to search for the second term: "SARS-CoV-2" OR "COVID-19." The third term was associated with "risk," "mortality," and "cohort." Finally, we used "AND" to connect the three terms. For the search strategy, see **Supplementary Material**. The retrieved studies were first screened by reading the titles and abstracts. Two authors (Dongqiong Xiao and Hu Gao) independently read the full texts of the remaining studies. Fajuan Tang resolved any disagreements.

Definition

The critical status among patients with COVID-19 is with any of the following conditions—shock, respiratory failure requiring mechanical ventilation, and/or other organ dysfunction requiring admission to the intensive care unit (ICU) (24).

Study Selection

The inclusion criteria were as follows: (1) studies with participants who were investigated for the following outcomes: the incidence, prevalence, or risk or odds ratio (OR) of mortality and critical status in patients with COVID-19 with thrombosis relative to those without thrombosis; (2) studies that evaluated the association between thrombosis and prognosis of COVID-19 and reported unadjusted or adjusted ORs and their corresponding 95% confidence intervals (CIs) or the number of patients with COVID-19 with thrombosis relative to those without thrombosis; and (3) studies with case-control, cohort, or cross-sectional designs published in English.

The exclusion criteria were as follows: (1) studies that reported the results of few autopsy cases of COVID-19; (2) unrelated studies or studies in which the data overlapped with those of another study or studies that reported the association between the D-dimer level and COVID-19 without evidence of definite thrombosis; or (3) reviews, case reports, and meta-analyses.

Data Extraction

The data were independently extracted from the studies by Dongqiong Xiao and Hu Gao, and they were aggregated in a standardized form; the collected data included study author and year, study location and design, sample size, type of thrombosis, primary outcomes (presence or absence of critical status, COVID-19-related mortality), adjusted for confounding factors, and Newcastle-Ottawa Scale (NOS) scores for the included studies.

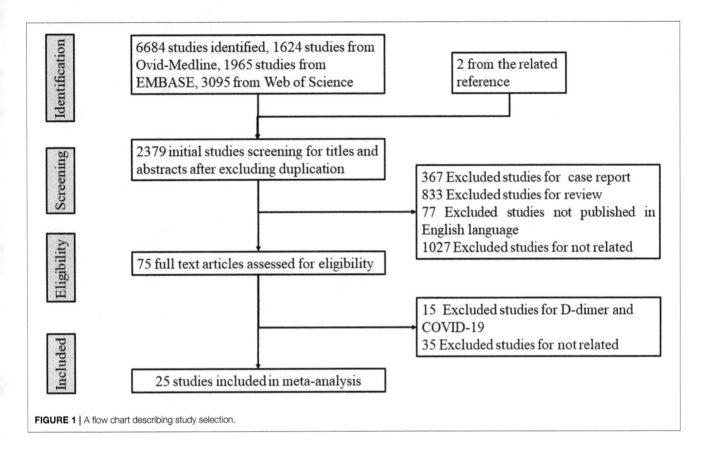

FIGURE 1 | A flow chart describing study selection.

Quality Evaluation

The methodological quality of all the included studies (**Supplementary Table 2**) was examined by Dongqiong Xiao and Hu Gao independently using the NOS (29), and Fajuan Tang resolved any disagreements. The reviewers assessed the quality scores (varying from 0 to 9) in three domains: selection of the study population, evaluation of exposure and outcomes, and comparability.

Statistical Analysis

The odds ratios (ORs) and 95% CIs were used as measures of the association between thrombosis and the prognosis of COVID-19 across studies. For original studies that compared the number of participants who developed critical status and death exposure to thrombosis compared with control groups, we calculated ORs and 95% CIs for each study (30). All data from the included studies were converted into log (ORs) and standard errors (SEs) (31). We pooled the log (ORs) and SEs of each study separately using the DerSimonian-Laird formula (random effects model) (32). We used the I^2 statistic to assess the statistical heterogeneity among the studies (33). High heterogeneity was indicated with values of $I^2 > 50\%$ and $p < 0.05$ (34).

We conducted stratified analyses based on the study location (Europe, the United States, and Asia), study design (cohort, cross-sectional), sample size ($\geq 1,000 < 1,000$), type of thrombosis (VTE, PE, DVT, and others), adjusted for confounding factors [not available (NA), adjusted ≤ 7 factors, adjusted ≥ 8 factors, ≤ 7 factors], adjusted for age (yes, no), adjusted for sex (yes, no), adjusted for body mass index (BMI) (yes, no), adjusted for diabetes (yes, no), and adjusted for comorbidities (yes, no).

We used Egger's tests, Begg's tests, and funnel plots in the meta-analysis to assess publication bias (33–36). We used Stata software, version 12.0 (StataCorp, College Station, TX) and Review Manager, version 5.3 to perform the statistical tests.

RESULTS

Literature Search

We identified 6,686 potential studies, including 1,624 from Ovid-MEDLINE, 1,965 from Embase, 3,095 from Web of Science, and 2 from the related references (**Supplementary Table 3**). After careful screening, 6,661 studies were excluded for the reasons listed in **Figure 1**, and 25 studies reporting the association between thrombosis and prognosis of COVID-19 met the inclusion criteria (see **Figure 1**). These 25 included studies are summarized in **Table 1**.

Characteristics and Quality of the Included Studies

Table 1 shows the characteristics of the 25 included studies. Among the included studies, 6 studies (24, 26, 37–40) were cross-sectional studies, and 19 studies (7, 25, 27, 28, 41–55) were cohort studies. The association between thrombosis and COVID-19-related mortality was the primary outcome of interest in 19

TABLE 1 | Characteristics of the included studies.

Study	Year	Study location	Sample size	Study design	Type of thrombosis	Outcomes	Adjusted for
Zhang	2020	China	143	CSS	VTE	Mortality and critical care status	NA
Yaghi, Shadi	2020	United States	3,556	Retrospective cohort	Brain stroke	Mortality	Age and NIHSS score
Stoneham, Simon M.	2020	UK	230	CSS	VTE	ICU hospitalization	NA
Middeldorp, S.	2020	Netherlands	198	Retrospective cohort	VTE	Mortality and critical care status	Age, sex, and ICU stay
Leonard-Lorant, Ian	2020	France	106	Retrospective cohort	PE	ICU hospitalization	NA
Klok, F. A.	2020	Netherlands	184	Retrospective cohort	Thrombotic complications	Mortality	NA
Jain, R.	2020	United States	3,218	Retrospective cohort	Brain stroke	Mortality	Age, BMI, and hypertension
Bhayana, R.	2020	United States	412	CSS	Abdominal ischaemia	ICU hospitalization	NA
Ren, B.	2020	China	48	CSS	VTE	Mortality	NA
Galloway, James B	2020	UK	1,157	Retrospective cohort	Cardiac ischaemia	Mortality and critical care status	>8 factors, age, sex, and with comorbidities (such as hypertension and diabetes mellitus)
Corrado Lodigiani	2020	Italy	338	Retrospective cohort	VTE	ICU hospitalization	NA
Avruscio	2020	Italy	85	Observational cohort	VTE	ICU hospitalization	NA
Contou	2020	France	92	CSS	PE	Mortality	NA
Abizaid	2021	Brazil	152	Prospective study	MI	Mortality	Age, prior coronary disease, and myocardial blush
Alharthy	2021	Saudi Arabia	352	Retrospective study	PE	Mortality	Age, ICU length of stay, SpO₂/FiO₂ ratio, WBCs, lymphocytes, D-dimer, lactate, and active smoking
Alwafi	2021	Saudi Arabia	706	CSS	VTE	Mortality	Age, sex, and comorbidities (diabetes mellitus, hypertension, coronary artery disease, end-stage renal disease, asthma, congestive heart failure, cerebrovascular accident, chronic obstructive pulmonary disease, chronic liver disease, and cancer)
Anderson	2021	UK	312,378	Cohort	VTE	Mortality Critical status	Comorbid cardiovascular disease (myocardial infarction, heart failure, angina, stroke, transient ischaemic attack, atrial fibrillation/flutter, and valve disease) and prevalent diabetes mellitus; use of exogenous oestrogens in women only
Arribalzaga	2021	Spain	5,966	Cohort	VTE	Mortality	Age, sex, follow-up (days), and time from admission to VTE diagnosis
Fournier	2021	France	531	Cohort	Arterial thrombotic events	Mortality	Age, sex, and comorbidities (cancer, HIV infection, inflammatory disorders, high blood pressure, smoking, and diabetes)
Purroy	2021	Spain	1,737	Cohort	Thromboembolism	Mortality	Age, diabetes, chronic obstructive pulmonary disease, ICU care, systolic blood pressure, and oxygen saturation
Riyahi	2021	USA	413	Retrospective cohort	PE	Mortality	NA

(Continued)

TABLE 1 | Continued

Study	Year	Study location	Sample size	Study design	Type of thrombosis	Outcomes	Adjusted for
Scudiero	2021	Italy	224	Retrospective cohort	PE	Mortality	Age, sex, and comorbidities
Violi	2021	Italy	373	Prospective multicentre study	Thrombotic events	Mortality	Age, sex, COPD, diabetes, and D-dimer
Wang	2021	China	88	Retrospective	DVT	Critical status	NA
Paz Rios	2021	USA	184	Retrospective observational study	VTE	Mortality	Age, sex, race, comorbidities (diabetes, hypertension, COPD, CKD, heart failure, cancer, and atrial fibrillation)

CSS, cross-sectional study; COPD, chronic obstructive pulmonary disease; CKD, chronic kidney disease; DVT, deep venous thrombosis; HIV, human immunodeficiency virus; ICU, intensive care unit; MI, myocardial infarction; NA, not available; PE, pulmonary embolism; USA, United States of America; VTE, venous thromboembolism; WBC, white blood cell.

studies, and the association between thrombosis and COVID-19-related critical status was the primary outcome in 10 studies.

The related studies were published in 2020 and 2021, and the sample size ranged from 48 to 312,378, for a total of 332,915 participants across studies.

Five studies (25, 38, 42, 51, 55) were conducted in the United States, 5 studies (24, 26, 39, 46, 54) were conducted in Asia, 14 studies (7, 27, 28, 37, 40, 41, 43, 44, 47–50, 52, 53) were conducted in Europe, and one study (45) was conducted in Brazil. All the included studies included both adult men and women.

Among the included studies, 13 studies (25–27, 39, 42, 45, 46, 48–50, 52, 53, 55) adjusted for age, 7 studies (27, 39, 48, 49, 52, 53, 55) adjusted for sex, one study (42) adjusted for BMI, 8 studies (26, 39, 47, 49, 50, 52, 53, 55) adjusted for diabetes mellitus, and 7 studies (39, 43, 46, 47, 49, 52, 55) adjusted for 8 or more confounding factors.

The quality scores of the included studies ranged from 6 to 8 (**Supplementary Table 1**), and they were considered high.

Quantitative Results (Meta-Analysis)

Among the 25 selected studies, 19 studies revealed the association between thrombosis and COVID-19-related mortality, and 10 studies investigated the association between thrombosis and COVID-19-related critical status. Among the included studies, 5 studies (26, 43, 47, 48, 51) found a non-significant association between thrombosis and COVID-19-related mortality, while the other 14 studies (24, 25, 27, 28, 39, 40, 42, 45, 46, 49, 50, 52, 53, 55) revealed that thrombosis would increase the risk of mortality from COVID-19. All 19 studies reported risks as ORs, ranging from 0.79 to 40.27. Any type of thrombosis was associated with an increased risk of mortality from COVID-19 compared with the control, with a pooled OR of 2.61 (95% CI, 1.91, 3.55). High heterogeneity was found in these studies ($I^2 = 84\%$, $p < 0.05$) (**Figure 2**).

Additionally, among the included studies, 4 studies (7, 37, 38, 43) found a non-significant association between thrombosis and COVID-19-related critical status, while the other 6 studies (24, 27, 41, 44, 47, 54) revealed that thrombosis would increase the risk of COVID-19-related critical status. All seven studies reported risks as ORs, ranging from 0.8 to 9.3. Any type of

thrombosis was associated with an increased risk of COVID-19-related critical status compared with the control, with a pooled OR of 2.9 (95% CI, 1.6, 5.24). High heterogeneity was reported in the studies ($I^2 = 80\%$, $p < 0.05$) (**Figure 2**).

Stratified Analyses

Thrombosis and COVID-19-Related Mortality

Among the 25 selected studies, 19 studies revealed the association between thrombosis and COVID-19-related mortality. Stratified analyses of clinical factors and study characteristics were conducted to evaluate possible sources of heterogeneity in the included studies (**Table 2**). The association between thrombosis and COVID-19-related mortality was significant at 2.61 (95% CI, 1.91, 3.55), and this association was consistent in all of the stratified analyses (**Table 2**). Stronger associations between thrombosis and the COVID-19-related mortality were found in cross-sectional studies (OR: 4.86, 95% CI, 1.99, 11.83) when compared to that in cohort studies (OR: 2.39, 95% CI, 1.72, 3.33) in studies with small sample sizes (< 1,000) (OR: 2.95, 95% CI, 2.28, 3.82) when compared to studies with large sample sizes (≥ 1,000) (OR: 1.99, 95% CI, 1.1, 3.58), and in studies that were conducted in the United States compared with studies conducted in Europe and Asia (**Table 2**).

The type of thrombosis included in the original reports also seemed to be related to the results. For example, studies demonstrated a weaker association between thrombosis and the COVID-19-related mortality if the thrombosis was VTE (OR: 2.48, 95% CI, 1.17, 5.25) when compared to other types of thrombosis (OR: 3.17, 95% CI, 1.95, 5.16).

The association between thrombosis and the COVID-19-related mortality was strong when the studies were not adjusted for sex, diabetes, comorbidities, or <8 confounding factors (**Table 2**).

Thrombosis and COVID-19-Related Critical Status

Among the 25 selected studies, 10 studies investigated the association between thrombosis and COVID-19-related critical

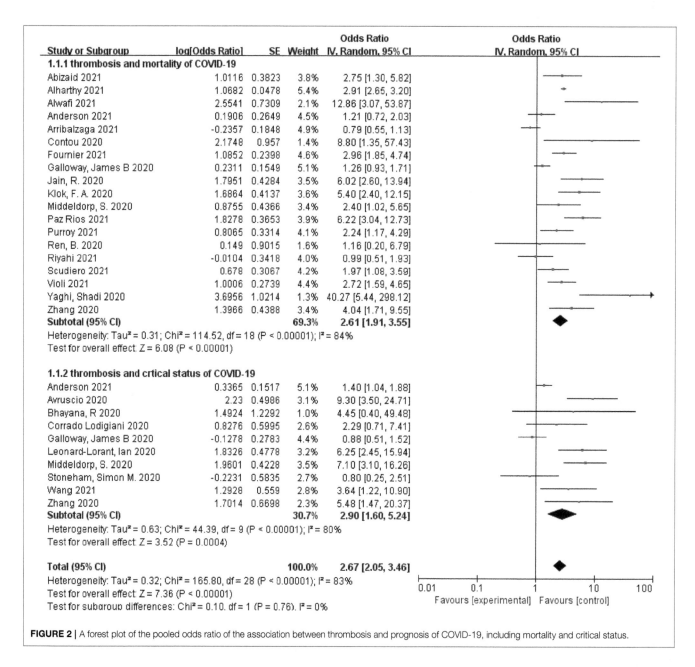

FIGURE 2 | A forest plot of the pooled odds ratio of the association between thrombosis and prognosis of COVID-19, including mortality and critical status.

status. The same stratified analyses were conducted (**Table 2**). The association between thrombosis and COVID-19-related critical status was significant (OR: 2.9, 95% CI, 1.6, 5.24), and it was consistent in all of the stratified analyses (**Table 2**). Sample size, study location, type of thrombosis, adjusted for more than 8 confounding factors, diabetes, and comorbidities seemed to be correlated with the results. For example, stronger associations between thrombosis and COVID-19-related critical status were found in studies that were conducted in Asia (OR: 4.31, 95% CI, 1.86, 9.99) when compared to those in studies that were conducted in Europe (OR: 2.58, 95% CI, 1.28, 5.19) and in studies with a small sample size (< 1,000) (OR: 4.17, 95% CI, 2.37, 7.35) when compared to those in studies with a large sample size (≥ 1,000) (OR: 1.18, 95% CI, 0.76, 1.83) (**Table 2**).

The association between thrombosis and COVID-19-related critical status was strong when the studies were not adjusted for diabetes, comorbidities, or <8 confounding factors (**Table 2**).

Publication Bias

Potential publication bias was revealed by asymmetrical funnel plots (**Figure 3**). The publication bias test for the association between thrombosis and COVID-19-related mortality was not significant (Begg's test with $p = 0.069$, $z = 1.82$), and publication bias was also not statistically significant for the association between thrombosis and COVID-19-related critical status with Begg's test ($p = 0.858$, $z = 0.18$) (**Supplementary Table 4**).

TABLE 2 | Stratified analysis of the associations between thrombosis and mortality and COVID-19-related critical status.

Variables	Thrombosis and mortality				Thrombosis and critical status			
	Studies	OR (95% CI)	I² (P-value)	P	Studies	OR (95% CI)	I² (P-value)	P
Total	19	2.61 (1.91, 3.55)	84% (<0.05)		10	2.9 (1.6, 5.24)	83% (<0.05)	
Study location				<0.05				<0.05
Europe	10	2.01 (1.37, 2.95)	79% (<0.05)		7	2.58 (1.28, 5.19)	85% (<0.05)	
Unites States-Brazil	5	4.24 (1.67, 10.76)	83% (<0.05)		1	4.45 (0.4, 49.48)	NA	
Asia	4	3.51 (1.95, 6.3)	47% (0.13)		2	4.31 (1.86, 9.99)	0 (0.64)	
Study design				<0.05				>0.05
Cohort	15	2.39 (1.72, 3.33)	87% (<0.05)		7	3.11 (0.55, 6.2)	85% (<0.05)	
Cross-sectional	4	4.86 (1.99, 11.83)	35% (0.18)		3	2.38 (0.58, 9.76)	61% (0.08)	
Sample size				>0.05				<0.05
≥1,000	6	1.99 (1.1, 3.58)	85% (<0.05)		2	1.18 (0.76, 1.83)	53% (0.14)	
<1,000	13	2.95 (2.28, 3.82)	53% (0.01)		8	4.17 (2.37, 7.35)	50% (0.05)	
Type of thrombosis				<0.05				<0.05
VTE	7	2.48 (1.17, 5.25)	86% (<0.05)		6	2.67 (1.28, 5.59)	75% (<0.05)	
PE	4	2.16 (1.18, 3.93)	76% (<0.05)		1	6.25 (2.45, 15.94)	NA	
DVT	0	NA	NA		1	3.64 (1.22, 10.90)	NA	
Other	8	3.17 (1.95, 5.16)	79% (<0.05)		2	1.27 (0.34, 4.38)	39%(0.2)	
Adjusted for confounding factors				<0.05				<0.05
NA	5	2.81 (1.16, 6.78)	72% (<0.05)		7	3.74 (1.95, 7.16)	52% (0.05)	
Adjusted (≤7 factors)	6	3.06 (1.35, 6.95)	88% (<0.05)		1	7.1 (3.1, 16.26)	NA	
Adjusted (≥8 factors)	8	2.25 (1.54, 3.31)	86% (<0.05)		2	1.18 (0.76, 1.83)	53% (0.14)	
Adjusted for age				>0.05				>0.05
Yes	12	2.8 (1.91, 4.1)	88% (<0.05)		2	2.44 (0.32, 18.87)	94% (<0.05)	
No	7	2.29 (1.26, 4.17)	68% (<0.05)		8	3.1 (1.59, 6.06)	74% (<0.05)	
Adjusted for sex				>0.05				>0.05
Yes	8	2.39 (1.43, 3.97)	87% (<0.05)		2	2.44 (0.32, 18.87)	94% (<0.05)	
No	11	2.84 (1.92, 4.18)	72% (<0.05)		8	3.1 (1.59, 6.06)	74% (<0.05)	
Adjusted for BMI				<0.05				NA
Yes	1	6.02 (2.6, 13.64)	NA		0	NA	NA	
No	18	2.49 (1.82, 3.42)	85% (<0.05)		10	2.9 (1.6, 5.24)	83% (<0.05)	
Adjusted for diabetes				>0.05				<0.05
Yes	7	2.59 (1.56, 4.31)	81% (<0.05)		2	1.18 (0.76, 1.83)	53% (0.14)	
No	12	2.69 (1.74, 4.16)	81% (<0.05)		8	4.17 (2.37, 7.35)	78% (<0.05)	
Adjusted for comorbidities				>0.05				<0.05
yes	6	2.53 (1.44, 4.44)	84% (<0.05)		2	1.18 (0.76, 1.83)	53% (0.14)	
no	13	2.71 (1.81,4.07)	83% (<0.05)		8	4.17 (2.37, 7.35)	78% (<0.05)	

BMI, body mass index; DVT, deep venous thrombosis; NA, not available; PE, pulmonary embolism; VTE, venous thromboembolism. Significantly different (p < 0.05).

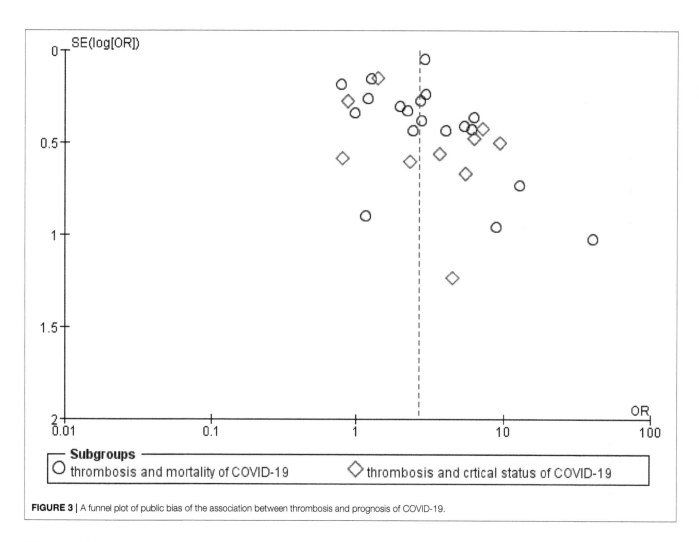

FIGURE 3 | A funnel plot of public bias of the association between thrombosis and prognosis of COVID-19.

DISCUSSION

To the best of our knowledge, this study tried to evaluate the association between thrombosis and the prognosis of COVID-19, which is often neglected by clinical physicians. The results of this meta-analysis, which included 25 studies, revealed that thrombosis was associated with a 161 and 190% increased risk of COVID-19-related mortality and COVID-19-related critical status, respectively. The association persisted and remained statistically significant in all of the stratified analyses.

Observational studies cannot prove causality. However, the following issues may explain the causation. First, there was an appropriate temporal relationship: thrombosis preceded COVID-19-related mortality in all studies. Second, there is theoretical biological plausibility for causality in that thrombosis may lead to organ dysfunction or prolong hypoxia, critical status, and death. The high rate of death-causing pulmonary embolism at autopsy is one of the strongest prognostic markers of a poor outcome (2). Additionally, the lungs of patients with COVID-19 displayed severe endothelial injury and diffuse thrombosis with microangiopathy (1, 56, 57). The association between deep venous thrombosis (DVT) and COVID-19 is uncertain, and the mechanisms may be related to the following

factors: the coagulation system may be activated by SARS-CoV-2, viral infection-induced release of cytokine, which is also thrombogenic, the plausible role of angiotensin-converting enzyme receptors induced severe endothelial injury, a pro-coagulatory state by tissue factor pathway activation (2, 4, 8, 58). Third, the findings revealed stronger associations for other thromboses, such as brain stroke and PE, relative to VTE. Hypoxia of important organs may lead to critical status and death (59). Fourth, there was consistency of this association across the included studies, as shown by the forest plot (**Figure 2**).

Conversely, there are also possible non-causal explanations for this association. Thrombosis is often associated with other confounding factors, including lack of physical activity, obesity, diabetes, hypertension, older age, sex, and chronic organ diseases (60, 61). Some of these factors were adjusted for the studies included in our meta-analysis, but the extent to which these potential intervening factors were controlled for in the individual studies was generally limited. The lack of adjustment for age (only 13 studies adjusted for age), sex (only 9 studies), BMI, diabetes, and comorbidities (only 7 studies) could contribute to a non-causal association between thrombosis and the COVID-19-related critical status and COVID-19-related mortality.

Our meta-analysis reports a stronger association between thrombosis and mortality without adjusting for sex relative to adjusting for sex. In our meta-analysis, two studies reported an association adjusted for sex. Xie et al. (62) may explain that age and sex are related to the COVID-19-related mortality. The authors reported that ACE2 concentration decreased almost 67% in older female rats and 78% in older male rats relative to younger groups. Additionally, evidence shows that sex hormones may modulate the expression of ACE2 (63). Kuba et al. (64) identified that ACE2 protects against acute lung injury, and decreased ACE2 may be related to the adverse outcome of COVID-19. The risk of severe infection and mortality increase with male sex (65). Sex was a strong factor in the COVID-19-related mortality, and several studies support this result (66, 67).

Our meta-analysis has many limitations. First, the sample size of the included studies was small, and the results of this meta-analysis should be interpreted with caution. Second, some of the included studies reported the association among thrombosis and mortality and critical status without adjustment for confounding factors, such as crude ORs or number of participants, which may have led to high heterogeneity and an overestimation of the results of the meta-analysis. Third, some related studies may be omitted by the study selection. Fourth, potential publication bias existed because studies published in English and articles were included. Fifth, there was no analysis of the association between different types of thrombosis and different statuses of COVID-19 based on the original studies. Furthermore, quantitative synthesis could not eliminate the bias inherent to observational studies.

There are a few merits of this meta-analysis. First, this study evaluated the association among thrombosis and mortality and the COVID-19-related critical status globally. Considering the consistent finding of increased mortality and critical status associated with thrombosis, we recommend that further prospective cohort studies considering additional adjusted confounding factors should be performed to test this hypothesis. Second, this study demonstrated that study location, study design, sample size, type of thrombosis, and adjusted confounding factors were all sources of heterogeneity.

CONCLUSIONS

In conclusion, our pooled analyses provide evidence that participants with thrombosis were associated with an increased risk of COVID-19-related mortality and COVID-19-related critical status. Further prospective studies with large sample sizes are required to establish whether this association is causal by considering more confounders and to clarify its mechanisms.

AUTHOR CONTRIBUTIONS

DX, HG, and FT: conceptualization. HG, FT, LC, and DX: methodology. DX, HG, FT, LC, and XL: software, validation, formal analysis, investigation, resources, data curation, and visualization. DX and FT: writing—original draft preparation. DX and XL: writing—review and editing and supervision. All authors read and approved the final manuscript.

ACKNOWLEDGMENTS

The manuscript was edited by AJE (American Journal Experts, https://www.aje.cn/) with certificated number (QPXLN8RC).

REFERENCES

1. Ackermann M, Verleden SE, Kuehnel M, Haverich A, Welte T, Laenger F, et al. Pulmonary vascular endothelialitis, thrombosis, and angiogenesis in Covid-19. N Engl J Med. (2020) 383:120–8. doi: 10.1056/NEJMoa2015432

2. Wichmann D, Sperhake J-P, Lutgehetmann M, Steurer S, Edler C, Heinemann A, et al. Autopsy findings and venous thromboembolism in patients with COVID-19. Ann Intern Med. (2020) 173:268–77. doi: 10.7326/M20-2003

3. Ciceri F, Beretta L, Scandroglio AM, Colombo S, Landoni G, Ruggeri A, et al. Microvascular COVID-19 lung vessels obstructive thromboinflammatory syndrome (MicroCLOTS): an atypical acute respiratory distress syndrome working hypothesis. Crit Care Resusc. (2020) 22:95–7. doi: 10.51893/2020.2.pov2

4. Spiezia L, Boscolo A, Poletto F, Cerruti L, Tiberio I, Campello E, et al. COVID-19-related severe hypercoagulability in patients admitted to intensive care unit for acute respiratory failure. Thromb Haemost. (2020) 120:998–1000. doi: 10.1055/s-0040-1710018

5. Spiezia L, Campello E, Cola M, Poletto F, Cerruti L, Poretto A, et al. More severe hypercoagulable state in acute COVID-19 pneumonia as compared with other pneumonia. Mayo Clin Proc Innov Qual Outcomes. (2020) 4:696–702. doi: 10.1016/j.mayocpiqo.2020.09.002

6. Demelo-Rodriguez P, Cervilla-Munoz E, Ordieres-Ortega L, Parra-Virto A, Toledano-Macias M, Toledo-Samaniego N, et al. Incidence of asymptomatic deep vein thrombosis in patients with COVID-19 pneumonia and elevated D-dimer levels. Thromb Res. (2020) 192:23–6. doi: 10.1016/j.thromres.2020.05.018

7. Lodigiani C, Iapichino G, Carenzo L, Cecconi M, Ferrazzi P, Sebastian T, et al. Venous and arterial thromboembolic complications in COVID-19 patients admitted to an academic hospital in Milan, Italy. Thromb Res. (2020) 191:9–14. doi: 10.1016/j.thromres.2020.04.024

8. Thomas W, Varley J, Johnston A, Symington E, Robinson M, Sheares K, et al. Thrombotic complications of patients admitted to intensive care with COVID-19 at a teaching hospital in the United Kingdom. Thromb Res. (2020) 191:76–7. doi: 10.1016/j.thromres.2020.04.028

9. Llitjos J-F, Leclerc M, Chochois C, Monsallier J-M, Ramakers M, Auvray M, et al. High incidence of venous thromboembolic events in anticoagulated severe COVID-19 patients. J Thromb Haemost. (2020) 18:1743–6. doi: 10.1111/jth.14869

10. Kruse JM, Magomedov A, Kurreck A, Münch FH, Koerner R, Kamhieh-Milz J, et al. Thromboembolic complications in critically ill COVID-19 patients are associated with impaired fibrinolysis. Crit Care. (2020) 24:676. doi: 10.1186/s13054-020-03401-8

11. Aid M, Busman-Sahay K, Vidal SJ, Maliga Z, Bondoc S, Starke C, et al. Vascular disease and thrombosis in SARS-CoV-2-infected rhesus macaques. Cell. (2020) 183:1354–66.e13. doi: 10.1016/j.cell.2020.10.005

12. Goshua G, Pine AB, Meizlish ML, Chang CH, Zhang H, Bahel P, et al. Endotheliopathy in COVID-19-associated coagulopathy: evidence from

a single-centre, cross-sectional study. *Lancet Haematol.* (2020) 7:e575–82. doi: 10.1016/S2352-3026(20)30216-7

13. Yatim N, Boussier J, Chocron R, Hadjadj J, Philippe A, Gendron N, et al. Platelet activation in critically ill COVID-19 patients. *Ann Intensive Care.* (2021) 11:113. doi: 10.1186/s13613-021-00899-1

14. Mei ZW, X.M.R. van Wijk, Pham HP, Marin MJ. Role of von Willebrand factor in COVID-19 associated coagulopathy. *J Appl Lab Med.* (2021) 6:1305–15. doi: 10.1093/jalm/jfab042

15. Agrati C, Bordoni V, Sacchi A, Petrosillo N, Nicastri E, Del Nonno F, et al. Elevated P-Selectin in severe Covid-19: considerations for therapeutic options. *Mediterr J Hematol Infect Dis.* (2021) 13:e2021016. doi: 10.4084/mjhid.2021.016

16. Calabrese C, Annunziata A, Coppola A, Pafundi PC, Guarino S, Di Spirito V, et al. ACE Gene I/D polymorphism and acute pulmonary embolism in COVID19 pneumonia: a potential predisposing role. *Front Med.* (2020) 7:631148. doi: 10.3389/fmed.2020.631148

17. Chen Y, Wang J, Liu C, Su L, Zhang D, Fan J, et al. IP-10 and MCP-1 as biomarkers associated with disease severity of COVID-19. *Mol Med.* (2020) 26:97. doi: 10.1186/s10020-020-00230-x

18. Conti P, Caraffa A, Gallenga CE, Ross R, Kritas SK, Frydas I, et al. IL-1 induces throboxane-A2 (TxA2) in COVID-19 causing inflammation and micro-thrombi: inhibitory effect of the IL-1 receptor antagonist (IL-1Ra). *J Biol Regul Homeost Agents.* (2020) 34:1623–7. doi: 10.23812/20-34-4EDIT-65

19. Ma L, Sahu SK, Cano M, Kuppuswamy V, Bajwa J, McPhatter J, et al. Increased complement activation is a distinctive feature of severe SARS-CoV-2 infection. *Sci Immunol.* (2021) 6:eabh2259. doi: 10.1126/sciimmunol.abh2259

20. Eriksson O, Hultström M, Persson B, Lipcsey M, Ekdahl KN, Nilsson B, et al. Mannose-binding lectin is associated with thrombosis and coagulopathy in critically ill COVID-19 patients. *Thromb Haemost.* (2020) 120:1720–4. doi: 10.1055/s-0040-1715835

21. Taquet M, Husain M, Geddes JR, Luciano S, Harrison PJ. Cerebral venous thrombosis and portal vein thrombosis: a retrospective cohort study of 537,913 COVID-19 cases. *EClinicalMedicine.* (2021) 39:101061. doi: 10.1016/j.eclinm.2021.101061

22. Wiedmann M, Skattør T, Stray-Pedersen A, Romundstad L, Antal EA, Marthinsen PB, et al. Vaccine induced immune thrombotic thrombocytopenia causing a severe form of cerebral venous thrombosis with high fatality rate: a case series. *Front Neurol.* (2021) 12:721146. doi: 10.3389/fneur.2021.721146

23. Campello E, Simion C, Bulato C, Radu CM, Gavasso S, Sartorello F, et al. Absence of hypercoagulability after nCoV-19 vaccination: an observational pilot study. *Thromb Res.* (2021) 205:24–8. doi: 10.1016/j.thromres.2021.06.016

24. Zhang L, Feng X, Zhang D, Jiang C, Mei H, Wang J, et al. Deep vein thrombosis in hospitalized patients with coronavirus disease 2019 (COVID-19) in Wuhan, China: prevalence, risk factors, and outcome. *Circulation.* (2020) 142:114–28. doi: 10.1161/CIRCULATIONAHA.120.046702

25. Yaghi S, Ishida K, Torres J, Mac Grory B, Raz E, Humbert K, et al. SARS2-CoV-2 and stroke in a New York healthcare system. *Stroke.* (2020) 51:2002–11. doi: 10.1161/STROKEAHA.120.030335

26. Ren B, Yan F, Deng Z, Zhang S, Xiao L, Wu M, et al. Extremely high incidence of lower extremity deep venous thrombosis in 48 patients with severe COVID-19 in Wuhan. *Circulation.* (2020) 142:181–3. doi: 10.1161/CIRCULATIONAHA.120.047407

27. Middeldorp S, Coppens M, van Haaps TF, Foppen M, Vlaar AP, Müller MCA, et al. Incidence of venous thromboembolism in hospitalized patients with COVID-19. *J Thromb Haemost.* (2020) 18:1995–2002. doi: 10.20944/preprints202004.0345.v1

28. Klok FA, Kruip MJHA, van der Meer NJM, Arbous MS, Gommers D, Kant KM, et al. Confirmation of the high cumulative incidence of thrombotic complications in critically ill ICU patients with COVID-19: An updated analysis. *Thromb Res.* (2020) 191:148–50. doi: 10.1016/j.thromres.2020.04.041

29. Gou X, Pan L, Tang F, Gao H, Xiao D. The association between vitamin D status and tuberculosis in children: a meta-analysis. *Medicine.* (2018) 97:e12179. doi: 10.1097/MD.0000000000012179

30. Xiao D, Zhang X, Ying J, Zhou Y, Li X, Mu D, et al. Association between vitamin D status and sepsis in children: a meta-analysis of observational studies. *Clin Nutr.* (2019) 39:1735–41. doi: 10.1016/j.clnu.2019.08.010

31. Willi C, Bodenmann P, Ghali WA, Faris PD, Cornuz J. Active smoking and the risk of type 2 diabetes: a systematic review and meta-analysis. *JAMA.* (2007) 298:2654–64. doi: 10.1001/jama.298.22.2654

32. Hartzel J, Agresti A, Caffo B. Multinomial logit random effects models. *Stat Model.* (2001) 1:81–102. doi: 10.1177/1471082X0100100201

33. Xiao D, Qu Y, Huang L, Wang Y, Li X, Mu D. Association between maternal overweight or obesity and cerebral palsy in children: a meta-analysis. *PLoS One.* (2018) 13:e0205733. doi: 10.1371/journal.pone.0205733

34. Wu YW, Colford JM Jr. Chorioamnionitis as a risk factor for cerebral palsy: a meta-analysis. *JAMA.* (2000) 284:1417–24. doi: 10.1001/jama.284.11.1417

35. Zeng Y, Tang Y, Tang J, Shi J, Zhang L, Zhu T, et al. Association between the different duration of breastfeeding and attention deficit/hyperactivity disorder in children: a systematic review and meta-analysis. *Nutr Neurosci.* (2018) 23:811–23. doi: 10.1080/1028415X.2018.1560905

36. Gou X, Yang L, Pan L, Xiao D. Association between bronchopulmonary dysplasia and cerebral palsy in children: a meta-analysis. *BMJ Open.* (2018) 8:e020735. doi: 10.1136/bmjopen-2017-020735

37. Stoneham SM, Milne KM, Nuttal E, Frew GH, Sturrock BR, Sivaloganathan H, et al. Thrombotic risk in COVID-19: a case series and case-control study. *Clin Med.* (2020) 20:e76–81. doi: 10.7861/clinmed.2020-0228

38. Bhayana R, Som A, Li MD, Carey DE, Anderson MA, Blake MA, et al. Abdominal imaging findings in COVID-19: preliminary observations. *Radiology.* (2020) 297:E207–15. doi: 10.1148/radiol.2020201908

39. Alwafi H, Naser AY, Qanash S, Brinji AS, Ghazawi MA, Alotaibi B, et al. Predictors of length of hospital stay, mortality, and outcomes among hospitalised COVID-19 patients in Saudi Arabia: a cross-sectional study. *J Multidiscip Healthc.* (2021) 14:839–52. doi: 10.2147/JMDH.S304788

40. Contou D, Pajot O, Cally R, Logre E, Fraissé M, Mentec H, et al. Pulmonary embolism or thrombosis in ARDS COVID-19 patients: A French monocenter retrospective study. *PLoS One.* (2020) 15:e0238413. doi: 10.1371/journal.pone.0238413

41. Leonard-Lorant I, Delabranche X, Severac F, Helms J, Pauzet C, Collange O, et al. Acute pulmonary embolism in COVID-19 patients on CT angiography and relationship to D-Dimer levels. *Radiology.* (2020) 296:E189–91. doi: 10.1148/radiol.2020201561

42. Jain R, Young M, Dogra S, Kennedy H, Nguyen V, Jones S, et al. COVID-19 related neuroimaging findings: a signal of thromboembolic complications and a strong prognostic marker of poor patient outcome. *J Neurol Sci.* (2020) 414:116923. doi: 10.1016/j.jns.2020.116923

43. Galloway JB, Norton S, Barker RD, Brookes A, Carey I, Clarke BD, et al. A clinical risk score to identify patients with COVID-19 at high risk of critical care admission or death: an observational cohort study. *J Infect.* (2020) 81:282–8. doi: 10.2139/ssrn.3590486

44. Avruscio G, Camporese G, Campello E, Bernardi E, Persona P, Passarella C, et al. COVID-19 and venous thromboembolism in intensive care or medical ward. *Clin Transl Sci.* (2020) 13:1108–14. doi: 10.1111/cts.12907

45. Abizaid A, Campos CM, Guimarães PO, Costa JR Jr, Falcão BAA, Cavalcante R, et al. Patients with COVID-19 who experience a myocardial infarction have complex coronary morphology and high in-hospital mortality: primary results of a nationwide angiographic study. *Catheter Cardiovasc Interv.* (2021) 98:E370–e8. doi: 10.1002/ccd.29709

46. Alharthy A, Aletreby W, Faqihi F, Balhamar A, Alaklobi F, Alanezi K, et al. Clinical characteristics and predictors of 28-day mortality in 352 critically ill patients with COVID-19: a retrospective study. *J Epidemiol Glob Health.* (2021) 11:98–104. doi: 10.2991/jegh.k.200928.001

47. Anderson JJ, Ho FK, Niedzwiedz CL, Katikireddi SV, Celis-Morales C, Iliodromiti S, et al. Remote history of VTE is associated with severe COVID-19 in middle and older age: UK Biobank cohort study. *J Thromb Haemost.* (2021) 19:2533–8. doi: 10.1111/jth.15452

48. Arribalzaga K, Martínez-Alfonzo I, Díaz-Aizpún C, Gutiérrez-Jomarrón I, Rodríguez M, Castro Quismondo N, et al. Incidence and clinical profile of venous thromboembolism in hospitalized COVID-19 patients from Madrid region. *Thromb Res.* (2021) 203:93–100. doi: 10.1016/j.thromres.2021.05.001

49. Fournier M, Faille D, Dossier A, Mageau A, Nicaise Roland P, Ajzenberg N, et al. Arterial Thrombotic events in adult inpatients with COVID-19. *Mayo Clin Proc.* (2021) 96:295–303. doi: 10.1016/j.mayocp.2020.11.018

50. Purroy F, Arqué G. Influence of thromboembolic events in the prognosis of COVID-19 hospitalized patients. results from a cross sectional study. *PLoS One.* (2021) 16:e0252351. doi: 10.1371/journal.pone.025 2351

51. Riyahi S, Dev H, Behzadi A, Kim J, Attari H, Raza SI, et al. Pulmonary embolism in hospitalized patients with COVID-19: a multicenter study. *Radiology.* (2021) 301:E426–33. doi: 10.1148/radiol.20212 10777

52. Scudiero F, Silverio A, Di Maio M, Russo V, Citro R, Personeni D, et al. Pulmonary embolism in COVID-19 patients: prevalence, predictors and clinical outcome. *Thromb Res.* (2021) 198:34–9. doi: 10.1016/j.thromres.2020.11.017

53. Violi F, Ceccarelli G, Cangemi R, Cipollone F, D'Ardes D, Oliva A, et al. Arterial and venous thrombosis in coronavirus 2019 disease (Covid-19): relationship with mortality. *Intern Emerg Med.* (2021) 16:1231–7. doi: 10.1007/s11739-020-02621-8

54. Wang W, Sun Q, Bao Y, Liang M, Meng Q, Chen H, et al. Analysis of risk factors for thromboembolic events in 88 patients with COVID-19 pneumonia in Wuhan, China: a retrospective descriptive report. *Med Sci Monit.* (2021) 27:e929708. doi: 10.12659/MSM.929708

55. Paz Rios LH, Minga I, Kwak E, Najib A, Aller A, Lees E, et al. Prognostic value of venous thromboembolism risk assessment models in patients with severe COVID-19. *TH Open.* (2021) 5:e211–9. doi: 10.1055/s-0041-17 30293

56. Duarte-Neto AN, Monteiro RAA, da Silva LFF, Malheiros DMAC, de Oliveira EP, Theodoro-Filho J, et al. Pulmonary and systemic involvement of COVID-19 assessed by ultrasound-guided minimally invasive autopsy. *Histopathology.* (2020) 77:186–97. doi: 10.1111/his.14160

57. Dolhnikoff M, Duarte-Neto AN, de Almeida Monteiro RA, da Silva LFF, de Oliveira EP, Saldiva PHN, et al. Pathological evidence of pulmonary thrombotic phenomena in severe COVID-19. *J Thromb Haemost.* (2020) 18:1517–9. doi: 10.1111/jth.14844

58. Giannis D, Ziogas IA, Gianni P. Coagulation disorders in coronavirus infected patients: COVID-19, SARS-CoV-1, MERS-CoV and lessons from the past. *J Clin Virol.* (2020) 127:104362. doi: 10.1016/j.jcv.2020.104362

59. Helms J, Tacquard C, Severac F, Leonard-Lorant I, Ohana M, Delabranche X, et al. High risk of thrombosis in patients with severe SARS-CoV-2 infection: a multicenter prospective cohort study. *Intensive Care Med.* (2020) 46:1089–98. doi: 10.1007/s00134-020-06062-x

60. Amasamy R, Milne KM, Stoneham SM, Chevassut TJ. Molecular mechanisms for thrombosis risk in black people: a role in excess mortality from Covid-19. *Br J Haematol.* (2020) 190:e78–80. doi: 10.1111/bjh.16869

61. Wu J, Zhang J, Sun X, Wang L, Xu Y, Zhang Y, et al. Influence of diabetes mellitus on the severity and fatality of SARS-CoV-2 infection. *Diabetes Obes Metab.* (2020) 22:1907–14. doi: 10.1111/dom.14105

62. Xie XD, Chen JZ, Wang XX, Zhang FR, Liu YR. Age- and gender-related difference of ACE2 expression in rat lung. *Life Sci.* (2006) 78:2166–71. doi: 10.1016/j.lfs.2005.09.038

63. La Vignera S, Cannarella R, Condorelli RA, Torre F, Aversa A, Calogero AE. Sex-specific SARS-CoV-2 mortality: among hormone-modulated ACE2 expression, risk of venous thromboembolism and hypovitaminosis D. *Int J Mol Sci.* (2020) 21:2948. doi: 10.3390/ijms21082948

64. Kuba K, Imai Y, Penninger JM. Angiotensin-converting enzyme 2 in lung diseases. *Curr Opin Pharmacol.* (2006) 6:271–6. doi: 10.1016/j.coph.2006.03.001

65. Guzik TJ, Mohiddin SA, Dimarco A, Patel V, Savvatis K, Marelli-Berg FM, et al. COVID-19 and the cardiovascular system: implications for risk assessment, diagnosis, treatment options. *Cardiovasc Res.* (2020) 116:1666–87. doi: 10.1093/cvr/cvaa106

66. Gemmati D, Bramanti B, Serino ML, Secchiero P, Zauli G, Tisato V. COVID-19 and individual genetic susceptibility/receptivity: role of ACE1/ACE2 genes, immunity, inflammation and coagulation. might the double X-chromosome in females be protective against SARS-CoV-2 compared to the single X-Chromosome in males? *Int J Mol Sci.* (2020) 21:3474. doi: 10.3390/ijms21103474

67. Albini A, Di Guardo G, Noonan DM, Lombardo M. The SARS-CoV-2 receptor, ACE-2, is expressed on many different cell types: implications for ACE-inhibitor- and angiotensin II receptor blocker-based cardiovascular therapies. *Intern Emerg Med.* (2020) 15:759–66. doi: 10.1007/s11739-020-02364-6

21

Mechanisms of Cardiovascular System Injury Induced by COVID-19 in Elderly Patients with Cardiovascular History

Yaliu Yang and Mengwen Yan*

Department of Cardiology, China-Japan Friendship Hospital, Beijing, China

Correspondence:
Mengwen Yan
ariel_ymw@163.com

The coronavirus disease-2019 (COVID-19) pandemic, caused by severe acute respiratory syndrome coronavirus (SARS-CoV-2), represents a great threat to healthcare and socioeconomics worldwide. In addition to respiratory manifestations, COVID-19 promotes cardiac injuries, particularly in elderly patients with cardiovascular history, leading to a higher risk of progression to critical conditions. The SARS-CoV-2 infection is initiated as virus binding to angiotensin-converting enzyme 2 (ACE2), which is highly expressed in the heart, resulting in direct infection and dysregulation of the renin-angiotensin system (RAS). Meanwhile, immune response and hyper-inflammation, as well as endothelial dysfunction and thrombosis implicate in COVID-19 infection. Herein, we provide an overview of the proposed mechanisms of cardiovascular injuries in COVID-19, particularly in elderly patients with pre-existing cardiovascular diseases, aiming to set appropriate management and improve their clinical outcomes.

Keywords: COVID-19, cardiovascular system injuries, renin-angiotensin system (RAS), inflammation, immune dysregulation, endothelial injury

INTRODUCTION

In December 2019, pneumonia of unknown cause was reported in Wuhan, China (1). By early January 2020, sequencing analysis indicated the pathogen as a novel coronavirus, severe acute respiratory syndrome coronavirus 2 (SARS-CoV-2), and the related clinical syndrome was named coronavirus disease-2019 (COVID-19) (2). It had spread rapidly throughout the world and on 11 March, 2020, the World Health Organization (WHO) declared COVID-19 a global pandemic. This infection has brought a great threat to healthcare and socioeconomics worldwide.

Whereas COVID-19 is characterized by respiratory symptoms, Huang et al. reported that 12% of patients present acute cardiac injury, defined as an ejection fraction decline and troponin I elevation (3), with a wide spectrum of clinical manifestations ranging from an acute coronary syndrome, myocarditis, arrhythmia, to cardiac dysfunction. Accumulating evidence reveals that acute cardiovascular injury is associated with increased severity and mortality of COVID-19 (4). Recent literature on long-term sequelae of COVID-19 shows prolonged cardiovascular damage in a large proportion of post-COVID-19 patients (5), for example, parasympathetic overtone and increased heart rate variability (6).

People with underlying cardiovascular diseases are prone to develop severe conditions, even in pediatric patients. The COVID-19-infected children with congenital heart disease represent worse clinical courses when compared to healthy control (7). Likewise, the elderly people with pre-existing cardiovascular comorbidities, who are more susceptible to cardiac injuries of COVID-19, are at a higher risk of poorer prognosis. In this review, we emphasize the pathogenesis of COVID-19-induced cardiovascular injury, particularly in elderly patients with underlying cardiovascular diseases.

THE ANGIOTENSIN-CONVERTING ENZYME 2 RECEPTOR AND RENIN-ANGIOTENSIN SYSTEM

As with SARS-CoV, ACE2 has been established as the dominant route of entry for SAR-CoV-2 upon binding of the viral spike protein (S protein) (8). In the process, furin, a proprotein convertase, cleaves S protein into two activated subunits, namely, S1 and S2. The S1 domain binds the ACE2 receptor through its receptor-binding domain (RBD), while the S2 subunit is necessary for virus-cell fusion after further processed by transmembrane serine protease 2 (TMPRSS2) (9). Compared to SARS-CoV, SARS-CoV-2 exhibits potent binding to ACE2 and immune evasion because of greater affinity of RBD, protease pre-activation of the spike, and hidden RBD, all of which in turn results in higher transmissibility of SARS-CoV-2 (9, 10). Until now, SARS-CoV-2 has undergone substantial evolution, for instance, SARS-CoV-2 Delta variant, one of the predominant circulating strains, exhibits higher infectivity, on a basis of increased ACE2 interaction owing to more RBD-up states and Delta T478K substitution (11). The virus-ACE2 binding actuates the virus-cell fusion, virus replication, and ACE2 loss at the same time.

Angiotensin-converting enzyme 2, a type I integral membrane protein, acts as a transmembrane protein or a soluble catalytic ectodomain *in vivo* (12). The transmembrane ACE2 can be measured as ACE2 expression, and studies indicate that the transmembrane ACE2 is abundant in lungs, heart, and endothelial cells (ECs) (13, 14). Chen et al. delineate ACE2 expression in cardiac resident cells, particularly in pericytes, a type of perivascular mural cells. Pericytes support capillary EC function and are associated with myocardial microcirculation (15). Pathology analysis of COVID-19 infections reveals direct viral infection and diffuses inflammation of the ECs, which may attribute to coronary plaque disruption and thrombosis (16). In this regard, direct viral infection of cardiac tissue implicates the cardiac complications of COVID-19 infection. A disintegrin and metalloproteinase domain-containing protein 17 (ADAM17) mediates cleavage and shedding of the soluble ACE2 ectodomain. ACE2 ectodomain, also known as soluble ACE2, can be detected as plasma ACE2 activity (12). The soluble ACE2 has been recently recognized to help in controlling SARS-CoV-2 infection *via* inhibiting their interaction with cell-bound ACE2 (17). The circulating ACE2 has been shown to correlate with cardiac remodeling, endothelial dysfunction, and is a predictor of major adverse cardiovascular events (18).

Beyond the host receptor in SAR-CoV-2 infection, ACE2 is an important component of the RAS. The circulating RAS system is finely controlled by complex feedback to maintain blood volume. Commonly, the action of Angiotensin (Ang) II on

Ang II type 1 receptor (AT_1R) stimulates aldosterone secretion regulated by renin in response to homeostatic demand. On the other hand, tissue angiotensin system has been identified since prorenin expression was found in many organs, tissues, such as heart, lungs, and brain. Thereafter, other biological effects of RAS have been recognized. Prorenin, firstly activated through proteolytic enzymes or unfolded by binding with (pro)renin receptor, converts the substrate angiotensinogen (AGT) to Ang I (10, 17). Ang I is cleaved to Ang II, the most active agent in RAS by ACE or chymase, the major catalytic enzyme in the heart (19). Ang II acts on two G-protein coupled receptors, AT_1R and type 2 receptor (AT_2R). Ang II/AT_1R binding exerts vasoconstriction, pro-inflammatory, pro-fibrotic, and proliferative effects through various intracellular protein signaling pathways, such as tyrosine kinases, serine/threonine kinases, mitogen-activated protein kinase (MAPK) family, and various protein kinase C isoforms, while Ang II/AT_2R interaction, with a much less affinity when compared to Ang II/AT_1R action, activates various protein phosphatases, the nitric oxide (NO)/cyclic GMP system, and phospholipase A_2, counteracting AT_1R actions (20–22). ACE2 mediates Ang (1–7) generation from Ang II. Ang (1–7) acts *via* AT_2R, Mas receptor (MasR), and Mas-related G protein-coupled receptor D (MgrD) and performs protective actions of anti-inflammation, vasodilation, and anti-fibrotic effects (10, 23). As such, Ang II degradation and Ang 1–7 generation accelerate cardiovascular protection. Previous animal studies showed that ACE2 inactivation was correlated with reduced cardiac contractility, coronary vasoconstriction, microvascular dysfunction, and less myocardial blood flow (24, 25).

Virus-ACE2 internalization in COVID-19 infection leads to ACE2 destruction. The ACE2 deficiency modulates the imbalance of Ang II/Ang (1–7) and thus amplifies Ang II/AT_1R actions (**Figure 1A**). Moreover, aging-related RAS alteration contributes to cardiac dysfunction in COVID-19 infection. A previous study discovers increased cardiac Ang II formation in a chymase-driven manner in aged rats (26). Ang II level *per se* mediates ACE and ACE2 expression, with higher ACE and lower ACE2 production, which in turn leads to outweighed Ang II/AT_1R interaction (27). In addition, animal studies display upregulation of AT_1R in both the aging heart and vasculature. On the other hand, AT_2R was highly expressed in fetal tissues but dropped to a comparatively low level in adulthood. The altered ratio of AT_1R and AT_2R might increase blood pressure and induce inflammation (22). Elderly patients with pre-existing cardiovascular diseases reported the increased ACE2 expression, promoting vulnerabilities to COVID-19 and direct viral damage. Noteworthy, RAS inhibitors, frequently medicated to older patients with cardiovascular diseases, are safe, despite increased membrane-bound ACE2 expression (28).

IMMUNITY AND INFLAMMATION

After initial infection with the virus, the innate immune signaling activates as the first-line defense, mediating virus recognition, killing virus-infected cells, stimulating inflammation, and adaptive immunity. The adaptive immune system, consisting of

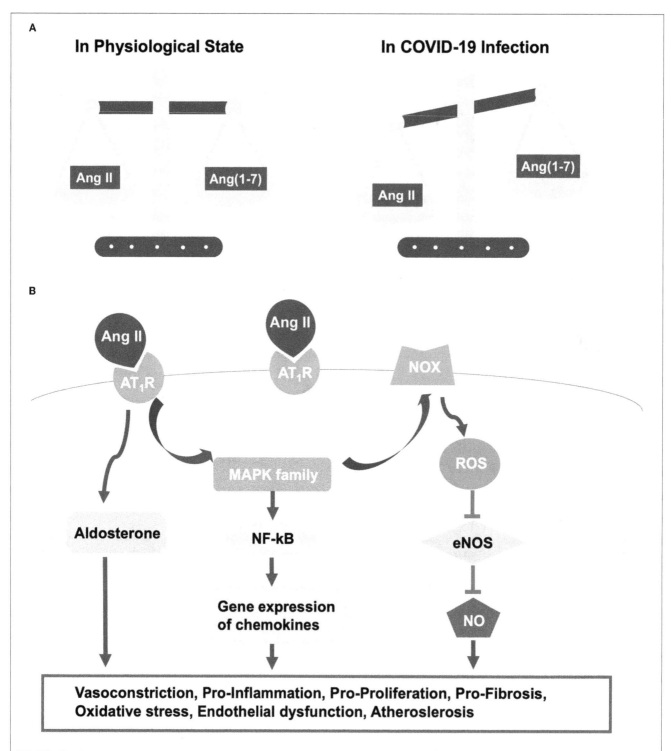

FIGURE 1 | RAS dysfunction in COVID-19 infection. **(A)** Outlines imbalance between Ang II/AT$_1$R and Ang(1-7)/Mas action. **(B)** Elucidates intracellular pathways upon Ang II/AT$_1$R interaction, which ultimately result in various cardiac and vascular injuries.

T and B cells, neutralizes viral particles, clears the virus, and sets long-term immunity.

Upon COVID-19 infection, pattern recognition receptors (PRRs) of antigen-presenting cells (APCs) detect pathogen-associated molecular patterns (PAMPs), namely, viral RNA and spike proteins as the main PAMPs in the case of SARS-CoV-2. Interaction of PAMPs with PRRs, such as membrane-bound Toll-like Receptors (TLRs), or cytosolic RIG-I-Like Receptors (RLRs), alongside the recruitment of cytoplasmic molecular adapters, such as MyD88, stimulates a variety of signaling cascades, mediating cytoplasmic transcription factors, such as nuclear factor kappa B (NF-KB), interferon regulatory transcription factor 3 (IRF3) translocating toward nuclear (29, 30). NF-KB facilitates the expression of genes in innate and adaptive immune response, as well as the development of cytokine storm (31, 32).

Subsequently, the immune cells produce cytokines, such as interferons (IFNs), interleukins (ILs), chemokine, and tumor necrosis factor (TNF), exerting broad antiviral effects (33). Type 1 IFNs, produced at the early stage of SARS-CoV-2 infection, exhibit pivotal antiviral effects by promoting apoptosis of virus-infected cells and antigen presentation to T cells *via* the induced expression of major histocompatibility complex class I (MHC I) (34, 35). However, SARS-CoV-2 produces multiple interferon antagonists and impairs IFN actions, resulting in viral replication, inflammation, and hypercytokinemia, which are considered the main causes of COVID-19 severity (32).

The adaptive immune response also plays a pivotal role in virus defense. B cells release virus-specific antibodies with the help of CD4+ T cells while CD8+ T cells mediate direct apoptosis of virus-infected cells (36). In the process, antigen presentation by APCs is essential for the adaptive immune response of T and B lymphocytes. However, COVID-19 infection is characterized by lymphopenia (37). Probably, SARS-CoV-2 exerts immune evasion through impaired maturation of dendritic cells, leading to hampered dendritic cells (DCs) homing to lymph nodes and failure of T lymphocytes activation (38).

In addition to direct viral infection, exacerbated inflammatory drivers and dysregulated cell-mediated response contribute to cardiovascular injuries in COVID-19 infection. Noteworthy, the elderly population are vulnerable to cardiovascular injuries and poor prognosis, partly attributed to the age-related changes of the immune system. Aging is well-characterized by chronic inflammatory responses in the absence of infection, also called inflammaging (39). Proper inflammation is necessary for pathogen clearance and tissue repair, whereas inflammaging is associated with tissue damage and disease. Meanwhile, with age, there is a decline in both the count and functionalities of immune cells. The DCs from aged mice and humans are less efficient to migrate, secret cytokines, and prime T cells in viral defense (40, 41). Less production of new lymphocytes was observed in the aged population (42). Sex hormones participate in immune activities directly, through the expression of estrogen or testosterone receptors on immune cells, such as lymphocytes and macrophages (17). The hormonal changes with aging may, to some extent, elucidate the age-related changes of the immune response.

ENDOTHELIOPATHY AND COAGULOPATHY

Endothelial dysfunction and coagulopathy are hallmarks of COVID-19 infection. The increased levels of von Willebrand factor (VWF) antigen, D-dimers, and tissue plasminogen activator are reported in the COVID-19 group, substantiating endothelial damage and pro coagulation in COVID-19 infection

(43, 44). Autopsy cases identify lymphocytic endotheliitis, frequent microthrombi as well as venous and arterial thromboembolism (16, 45, 46). A recent study indicates persistent endothelial damage in post-COVID-19 patients; on the other hand, Charfeddine et al. demonstrate that the lasting endothelial dysfunction is an independent risk factor of long COVID-19 syndrome (47, 48).

The wide distribution of ACE2 on ECs makes it a direct target for SARS-CoV-2 entry (49). Virus-cell binding downregulates membrane ACE2, resulting in reduced degradation of Ang II and decreased production of Ang (1–7). Subsequently, the mounting Ang II/AT$_1$R interaction exhibits pro-inflammatory cytokines secretion and pro-thrombotic actions by limiting NO and prostacyclin release. Otherwise, ACE2 regulates the kinin-kallikrein systems and participates in the inactivation of circulating bradykinin (BK). In this regard, ACE2 loss in COVID-19 infection leads to an increased level of BK, which induces EC activation and dysfunction, together with increased vascular permeability (50, 51). Exposure to SARS-CoV-2 spike protein *in vitro* stimulates caspase and apoptosis in ECs, whereby the loss of endothelial integrity triggers hypercoagulation (51).

The vascular endothelium participates in immune response and inflammation. Cytokines, such as IL-6, activate ECs, and in turn, the activated ECs express plenty of adhesion molecules, i.e., intercellular adhesion molecule-1 (ICAM-1) and vascular cell adhesion molecule-1 (VCAM-1), resulting in the recruitment of leukocytes and platelets. In addition, ECs express different TLRs, mediating PAMPs recognition and antigen presenting to T cells (52). Regulated EC activation helps in limiting pathogen invasion, whereas the hyperinflammatory profile, often seen in the severe COVID-19 cases, promotes profound endothelial dysfunction and damage, contributing to multiple organ failure (46).

Resting ECs also participate in the dynamic interplay between coagulation and fibrinolysis. Direct SAR-CoV-2 infection induces endothelium injury and apoptosis, decreasing its antithrombotic activity. In addition, in the setting of inflammation, inflammatory molecules or injured ECs stimulate coagulation by increasing tissue factor (TF) expression by monocytes and ECs *in vitro* (53). TF and its downstream activated factors ultimately stimulate the coagulation cascade and produce clots (54). In addition, SARS-CoV-2 infection, together with SARS and Middle East respiratory syndrome (MERS), is correlated with thrombocytopenia (55). One explanation is that platelets are hyper-activated in these viral-infected patients, probably owing to hypoxia, immune responses, and endothelial dysfunction in the case of COVID-19 (16, 55). The activated platelets interact with leukocytes, contributing to the leukocyte cytokine release, such as CC-chemokine ligand 2 (CCL2), CCL3, IL-1β, and the release of neutrophil extracellular traps (NETs) wrapped with TFs, which in turn activates the extrinsic coagulation cascade resulting in thrombin formation (56, 57). Terminal complement components, such as the C5b-9 (membrane attack complex) and the C4d, have been discovered in the microvasculature, suggesting the association of complement system with microvascular injury in COIVID-19 (58).

Indeed, cardiovascular complications of COVID-19 are highly prevalent and contain acute cardiac injury, myocarditis, and a hypercoagulable state, all of which may be influenced by endotheliopathy and coagulopathy. Age is the main risk factor for COVID-19-related death and intensive care unit (ICU) admission. Age-associated EC dysfunction might be the reason for the poor prognosis in the elderly, leading to vascular pathologies and cardiovascular diseases. Abundant evidence demonstrates that the impaired endothelium-dependent NO-mediated vasodilation is associated with cardiovascular events, and the findings that endothelial nitric oxide synthase (eNOS)-deficient mice display a premature cardiac aging phenotype together with early mortality indicate the critical role of endothelium-derived NO on cardiovascular protection in aging (59, 60). The reduced bioavailability of NO contributes to age-associated impairment of angiogenesis, leading to ischemic tissue injury, such as myocardial ischemia and infarction (61). Csiszar et al. (62) show with advancing age, coronary arteries undergo pro-inflammatory alterations, age-related decline in NO bioavailability as well as upregulation of TNFα and caspase 9, promoting endothelial apoptosis.

COVID-19-RELATED CARDIOVASCULAR COMPLICATIONS IN ELDERLY

A variety of cardiovascular complications are documented in COVID-19, ranging from myocardial injury, myocarditis, arrhythmia, to cardiac dysfunction and heart failure. The crosstalk between RAS, hyper-inflammation, endotheliopathy, and coagulopathy accounts for the mechanism of cardiovascular involvement in COVID-19 (**Figure 2**).

- Direct viral infection induces myocardial injury, whereas virus-ACE2 binding brings overactive Ang II/AT1R actions, resulting in vasoconstriction and increased blood pressure because of its role as an endocrine regulator. Additionally, activated Ang II/AT$_1$R interacts with multiple intracellular signaling, for example, the MAPK family (63), and regulates the inflammatory process. In this sense, AT$_1$R triggers NF-kB activation, which promotes the gene expression of chemokines, cytokines, and adhesion molecules (64). The immune response and hyper-inflammation concerning SARS-CoV-2 infection, partly owing to Ang II/AT$_1$R action, lead to cardiac and vascular remodeling, as well as atherosclerotic plaque growth and rupture (63, 65) (**Figure 1B**).

  - Likewise, Ang II promotes oxidative stress and endothelial dysfunction *via* action on AT$_1$R and the downstream phagocytic nicotinamide adenine dinucleotide phosphate (NADPH) oxidase (NOX) and reactive oxygen species (ROS) signaling (66), promoting lipid oxidation, macrophage uptake of lipids, and monocyte recruitment, leading to vascular inflammation and atherosclerosis (43, 67) (**Figure 1B**).

- In turn, previous studies show that the recruitment of immune cells, i.e., monocytes and macrophages, into the vascular wall strengthens the Ang II-induced endothelial dysfunction and

inflammation (68, 69). At the same time, ECs participate in the SARS-CoV-2-induced immune response and hyper-inflammation, which in turn trigger endothelial injury as we discussed above.

- In addition, vascular smooth muscle cells (VSMCs), responsible for vascular homeostasis, also play a key role in disease progressions, such as hypertension and atherosclerosis. In the process, phenotypic switching of VSMCs has been considered of fundamental importance, transforming the contractile VSMCs to synthetic phenotypes, i.e., macrophage-like genotypes. Activated EC-VSMC interaction *via* inflammatory cytokines promotes the transition of VSMCs to macrophage-like phenotypes. Macrophage-like VSMCs acquire inefficient phagocytic functions and express different scavenger receptors, for example, low-density lipoprotein receptor-related protein 1, facilitating the influx of low-density lipoprotein, thus attributing to the formation of VSMC-derived foam cells and subsequent atherosclerotic plaque growth (70). Meanwhile, Ang II/AT1R action mediates proliferation and migration of VSMCs through phosphatidylinositol 3-kinase (PI3K)/Akt and MAPKs, affecting atherogenesis (71, 72). Therefore, we are assuming that VSMCs modulate COVID-19 progression and the relevant cardiovascular complications. To support that, more investigations are needed.

Aging is associated with dysregulated RAS, inflammaging, and endothelial dysfunction as we described above. Therefore, we speculate that RAS activation, immune and hyper-inflammatory actions, endotheliopathy, and coagulopathy, all of which mutually reinforce each other, together with the pre-existing aging-related dysregulations, unfold the underlying mechanisms of COVID-19 infection, and the contaminant cardiovascular complications in the elderly.

The incidence of COVID-19-related stroke, one of the most important primary cardiovascular outcomes, ranges from 1 to 6% in hospitalized patients with COVID-19 (73). Concerningly, stroke in patients with COVID-19 is associated with a poorer prognosis when compared to COVID-19 negative stroke patients (74). Moreover, COVID-19-related stroke is more often in the elderly population, particularly those with pre-existing disorders, such as hypertension, atherosclerosis, and atrial fibrillation (75). The pathogenesis of ischemic stroke, the dominant subtype of strokes, is multifactorial and similar to other arterial thromboses, it is developed in COVID-19. In this regard, the interplay of inflammation, coagulopathy, endotheliopathy, and platelet activation, together with cardioembolism, contribute to COVID-19-related ischemic stroke (73).

COMORBIDITIES

The elderly people often have to deal with various comorbidities, i.e., diabetes mellitus (DM), chronic kidney disease (CKD), dyslipidemia, all of which are risk factors of cardiovascular disease. In the case of COVID-19 infection, the interplay between the viral infection and the concomitant comorbidities might exacerbate COVID-19 outcomes, such as cardiovascular injuries.

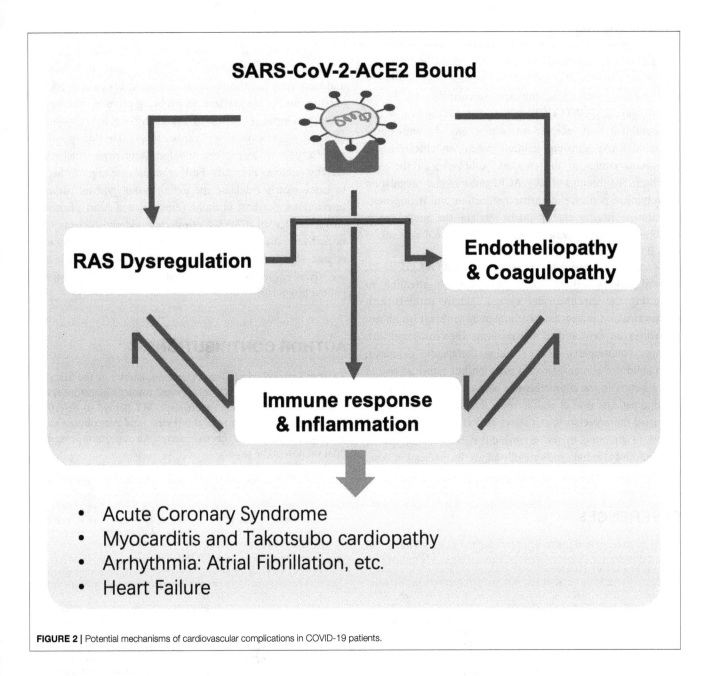

FIGURE 2 | Potential mechanisms of cardiovascular complications in COVID-19 patients.

Diabetes mellitus increases the risk of hospitalization, mortality, and need for critical care in COVID-19. The DM group with pre-existing systemic endothelial and microvascular dysfunction undergoes extra endothelial and microvascular impairment in COVID-19 infection and the "double-killing" results in worse prognosis and multiple organ failure (76).

The incidence of CKD increases with age, and 38% of the patients with CKD are more than 65 years old (77). Cardiovascular causes are recognized as the leading cause of death, accounting for 50%of the mortality in the CKD population (78). Therefore, it is of great importance to investigate the cardiovascular injuries in the elderly with CKD induced by the pandemic COVID-19 infection. A comprehensive review reveals

the effect of CKD on increased hospitalization and mortality of COVID-19, perhaps owing to immune dysfunction and increased susceptibility to infections (77, 79).

Accumulating studies demonstrate that lipid disorders are associated with an increased risk of COVID-19 progression by 39% (80, 81). Although Petrilli et al. (82) show no correlation between dyslipidemia and prognosis of COVID-19. Cholesterol is an essential factor in lipid rafts, which are involved in the entry of SARS-CoV-2. Therefore, increased cholesterol level increases susceptibility to SARS-CoV-2 (83). On the other hand, COVID-19 alters lipid metabolism, characterized by a decrease in total cholesterol, high-density lipoprotein, low-density lipoprotein, and an increase in triglycerides (83).

CONCLUSION

The COVID-19 pandemic has swept the world and brought significant loss of health, life, and livelihoods, especially in the aged and those with underlying cardiovascular diseases. To our current knowledge, the COVID-19 is initiated as the viral-ACE2, the dominant host receptor interaction, and the subsequent effects on RAAS signaling, immune system, endothelium, and thrombosis confer to the complex pathologies in the viral infection. The findings of ACE/ACE2 imbalance, dysregulation of immune responses, endothelial dysfunction, and angiogenesis impairment in the elderly might explain the more severe conditions and cardiovascular involved in the old patients of COVID-19 infection.

Consequently, during the course of treatment for COVID-19, medical experts/clinicians must pay particular attention to protecting the cardiovascular system. Elderly patients with cardiovascular disease will be encountered significant healthcare disparities that exist in their management, when compared with younger counterparts. While making therapeutic decisions, age should not be considered in isolation but rather as one of many factors in the comprehensive assessment model, keeping in mind patients' overall health, frailty, cognition, quality of life, estimated life expectancy, and above all preferences. We should pay close attention to the comorbidities, balance the risk of ischemia and bleeding, and carefully adjust the medication dose.

Overall, elderly patients with a history of cardiovascular disease remain undertreated with evidence-based therapies, experience worse outcomes, and represent an opportunity for enhancing and mitigating healthcare disparities. Scientists have developed vaccines for the coronavirus, which bring promise to tackle the global pandemic of COVID-19, especially for elderly patients. In addition, close monitoring of cardiac function in elderly patients with COVID-19 can prevent, or at least limit, myocardial injury, thereby reducing mortality. Further studies are urgently needed to more clearly elucidate the pathophysiology, host/pathogen interactions, the host immune response, and heart phenotype characteristics of COVID-19-infected elderly patients. The underlying mechanisms of myocardial injury, diagnosis, related effective medical treatment strategies, and follow-up are required to advance targeted treatments and improve patient prognosis.

AUTHOR CONTRIBUTIONS

YY searched and selected the references, and wrote the first draft of the review. YY and MY contributed towards literature review and interpretation of the manuscript. MY helped to determine the content and structure of the review, and contributed to the writing and revision of the manuscript. All authors approved the final version of the paper.

REFERENCES

1. Zhu N, Zhang D, Wang W, Li X, Yang B, Song J, et al. A novel coronavirus from patients with pneumonia in China, 2019. *N Engl J Med.* (2020) 382:727–33. doi: 10.1056/NEJMoa2001017

2. Sun J, He WT, Wang L, Lai A, Ji X, Zhai X, et al. COVID-19: epidemiology, evolution, and cross-disciplinary perspectives. *Trends Mol Med.* (2020) 26:483–95. doi: 10.1016/j.molmed.2020.02.008

3. Huang C, Wang Y, Li X, Ren L, Zhao J, Hu Y, et al. Clinical features of patients infected with 2019 novel coronavirus in Wuhan, China. *Lancet.* (2020) 395:497–506. doi: 10.1016/S0140-6736(20)30183-5

4. Guo T, Fan Y, Chen M, Wu X, Zhang L, He T, et al. Cardiovascular implications of fatal outcomes of patients with coronavirus disease 2019 (COVID-19). *JAMA Cardiol.* (2020) 5:811–8. doi: 10.1001/jamacardio.2020.1017

5. Serviente C, Decker ST, Layec G. From heart to muscle: pathophysiological mechanisms underlying long-term physical sequelae from SARS-CoV-2 infection. *J Appl Physiol.* (2022) 132:581–92. doi: 10.1152/japplphysiol.00734.2021

6. Asarcikli LD, Hayiroglu MI, Osken A, Keskin K, Kolak Z, Aksu T. Heart rate variability and cardiac autonomic functions in post-COVID period. *J Interv Card Electrophysiol.* (2022) 1:1–7. doi: 10.1007/s10840-022-01138-8

7. Zareef RO, Younis NK, Bitar F, Eid AH, Arabi M. COVID-19 in pediatric patients: a focus on CHD patients. *Front Cardiovasc Med.* (2020) 7:612460. doi: 10.3389/fcvm.2020.612460

8. Lan J, Ge J, Yu J, Shan S, Zhou H, Fan S, et al. Structure of the SARS-CoV-2 spike receptor-binding domain bound to the ACE2 receptor. *Nature.* (2020) 581:215–20. doi: 10.1038/s41586-020-2180-5

9. Shang J, Wan Y, Luo C, Ye G, Geng Q, Auerbach A, et al. Cell entry mechanisms of SARS-CoV-2. *Proc Natl Acad Sci USA.* (2020) 117:11727–34. doi: 10.1073/pnas.2003138117

10. Lumbers ER, Head R, Smith GR, Delforce SJ, Jarrott B. H Martin J, Pringle KG. The interacting physiology of COVID-19 and the renin-angiotensin-aldosterone system: Key agents for treatment. *Pharmacol Res Perspect.* (2022) 10:e00917. doi: 10.1002/prp2.917

11. Wang Y, Liu C, Zhang C, Wang Y, Hong Q, Xu S, et al. Structural basis for SARS-CoV-2 Delta variant recognition of ACE2 receptor and broadly neutralizing antibodies. *Nat Commun.* (2022) 13:871. doi: 10.1038/s41467-022-28528-w

12. García-Escobar A, Vera-Vera S, Jurado-Román A, Jiménez-Valero S, Galeote G, Moreno R. Calcium signaling pathway is involved in the shedding of ACE2 catalytic ectodomain: new insights for clinical and therapeutic applications of ACE2 for COVID-19. *Biomolecules.* (2022) 12:76. doi: 10.3390/biom12010076

13. Bertram S, Heurich A, Lavender H, Gierer S, Danisch S, Perin P, et al. Influenza and SARS-coronavirus activating proteases TMPRSS2 and HAT are expressed at multiple sites in human respiratory and gastrointestinal tracts. *PLoS ONE.* (2012) 7:e35876. doi: 10.1371/journal.pone.0035876

14. Batta Y, King C, Johnson J, Haddad N, Boueri M, Haddad G. Sequelae and Comorbidities of COVID-19 manifestations on the cardiac and the vascular systems. *Front Physiol.* (2022) 12:748972. doi: 10.3389/fphys.2021.748972

15. Chen L, Li X, Chen M, Feng Y, Xiong C. The ACE2 expression in human heart indicates new potential mechanism of heart injury among patients infected with SARS-CoV-2. *Cardiovasc Res.* (2020) 116:1097–100. doi: 10.1093/cvr/cvaa078

16. Varga Z, Flammer AJ, Steiger P, Haberecker M, Andermatt R, Zinkernagel AS, et al. Endothelial cell infection and endotheliitis in COVID-19. *Lancet.* (2020) 395:1417–8. doi: 10.1016/S0140-6736(20)30937-5

17. Wehbe Z, Hammoud SH, Yassine HM, Fardoun M, El-Yazbi AF, Eid AH. Molecular and biological mechanisms underlying gender differences in COVID-19 severity and mortality. *Front Immunol.* (2021) 12:659339. doi: 10.3389/fimmu.2021.659339

18. Epelman S, Shrestha K, Troughton RW, Francis GS, Sen S, Klein AL, et al. Soluble angiotensin-converting enzyme 2 in human heart failure: relation with myocardial function and clinical outcomes. *J Card Fail.* (2009) 15:565–71. doi: 10.1016/j.cardfail.2009.01.014

19. Urata H, Kinoshita A, Misono KS, Bumpus FM, Husain A. Identification of a highly specific chymase as the major angiotensin II-forming enzyme in the human heart. *J Biol Chem.* (1990) 265:22348–57. doi: 10.1016/S0021-9258(18)45712-2

20. Ferrario CM, Trask AJ, Jessup JA. Advances in biochemical and functional roles of angiotensin-converting enzyme 2 and angiotensin-(1-7) in regulation of cardiovascular function. *Am J Physiol Heart Circ Physiol.* (2005) 289:H2281–90. doi: 10.1152/ajpheart.00618.2005

21. Tikellis C, Thomas MC. Angiotensin-converting enzyme 2 (ACE2) is a key modulator of the renin angiotensin system in health and disease. *Int J Pept.* (2012) 2012:256294. doi: 10.1155/2012/256294

22. Abadir PM. The frail renin-angiotensin system. *Clin Geriatr Med.* (2011) 27:53–65. doi: 10.1016/j.cger.2010.08.004

23. Chappell MC. Emerging evidence for a functional angiotensin-converting enzyme 2-angiotensin-(1-7)-MAS receptor axis: more than regulation of blood pressure? *Hypertension.* (2007) 50:596–9. doi: 10.1161/HYPERTENSIONAHA.106.076216

24. Patel VB, Mori J, McLean BA, Basu R, Das SK, Ramprasath T, et al. ACE2 deficiency worsens epicardial adipose tissue inflammation and cardiac dysfunction in response to diet-induced obesity. *Diabetes.* (2016) 65:85–95. doi: 10.2337/db15-0399

25. Oudit GY, Crackower MA, Backx PH, Penninger JM. The role of ACE2 in cardiovascular physiology. *Trends Cardiovasc Med.* (2003) 13:93–101. doi: 10.1016/S1050-1738(02)00233-5

26. Froogh G, Pinto JT, Le Y, Kandhi S, Aleligne Y, Huang A, et al. Chymase-dependent production of angiotensin II: an old enzyme in old hearts. *Am J Physiol Heart Circ Physiol.* (2017) 312:H223–31. doi: 10.1152/ajpheart.00534.2016

27. Gonzalez AA, Gallardo M, Cespedes C, Vio CP. Potassium intake prevents the induction of the renin-angiotensin system and increases medullary ACE2 and COX-2 in the kidneys of angiotensin II-dependent hypertensive rats. *Front Pharmacol.* (2019) 10:1212. doi: 10.3389/fphar.2019.01212

28. Simko F, Baka T. Commentary: Effect of angiotensin-converting-enzyme inhibitor and angiotensin II receptor antagonist treatment on ACE2 expression and SARS-CoV-2 replication in primary airway epithelial cells. *Front Pharmacol.* (2022) 13:842512. doi: 10.3389/fphar.2022.842512

29. Akira S, Uematsu S, Takeuchi O. Pathogen recognition and innate immunity. *Cell.* (2006) 124:783–801. doi: 10.1016/j.cell.2006.02.015

30. McGettrick AF, O'Neill LA. The expanding family of MyD88-like adaptors in Toll-like receptor signal transduction. *Mol Immunol.* (2004) 41:577–82. doi: 10.1016/j.molimm.2004.04.006

31. Tang Y, Liu J, Zhang D, Xu Z, Ji J, Wen C. Cytokine storm in COVID-19: the current evidence and treatment strategies. *Front Immunol.* (2020) 11:1708. doi: 10.3389/fimmu.2020.01708

32. Lauro R, Irrera N, Eid AH, Bitto A. Could antigen presenting cells represent a protective element during SARS-CoV-2 infection in children? *Pathogens.* (2021) 10:476. doi: 10.3390/pathogens10040476

33. Perico L, Benigni A, Casiraghi F, Ng LFP, Renia L, Remuzzi G. Immunity, endothelial injury and complement-induced coagulopathy in COVID-19. *Nat Rev Nephrol.* (2021) 17:46–64. doi: 10.1038/s41581-020-00357-4

34. Stegelmeier AA, Darzianiazizi M, Hanada K, Sharif S, Wootton SK, Bridle BW, et al. Type I interferon-mediated regulation of antiviral capabilities of neutrophils. *Int J Mol Sci.* (2021) 22:4726. doi: 10.3390/ijms22094726

35. Hadjadj J, Yatim N, Barnabei L, Corneau A, Boussier J, Smith N, et al. Impaired type I interferon activity and inflammatory responses in severe COVID-19 patients. *Science.* (2020) 369:718–24. doi: 10.1126/science.abc6027

36. Mortaz E, Tabarsi P, Varahram M, Folkerts G, Adcock IM. The immune response and immunopathology of COVID-19. *Front Immunol.* (2020) 11:2037. doi: 10.3389/fimmu.2020.02037

37. Rydyznski Moderbacher C, Ramirez SI, Dan JM, Grifoni A, Hastie KM, Weiskopf D, et al. Antigen-specific adaptive immunity to SARS-CoV-2 in acute COVID-19 and associations with age and disease severity. *Cell.* (2020) 183:996–1012.e19. doi: 10.1016/j.cell.2020.09.038

38. Borcherding L, Teksen AS, Grosser B, Schaller T, Hirschbühl K, Claus R, et al. Impaired dendritic cell homing in COVID-19. *Front Med.* (2021) 8:761372. doi: 10.3389/fmed.2021.761372

39. Gubbels Bupp MR, Potluri T, Fink AL, Klein SL. The confluence of sex hormones and aging on immunity. *Front Immunol.* (2018) 9:1269. doi: 10.3389/fimmu.2018.01269

40. Wong CP, Magnusson KR, Ho E. Aging is associated with altered dendritic cells subset distribution and impaired proinflammatory cytokine production. *Exp Gerontol.* (2010) 45:163–9. doi: 10.1016/j.exger.2009.11.005

41. Panda A, Qian F, Mohanty S, van Duin D, Newman FK, Zhang L, et al. Age-associated decrease in TLR function in primary human dendritic cells predicts influenza vaccine response. *J Immunol.* (2010) 184:2518–27. doi: 10.4049/jimmunol.0901022

42. Min H, Montecino-Rodriguez E, Dorshkind K. Effects of aging on early B- and T-cell development. *Immunol Rev.* (2005) 205:7–17. doi: 10.1111/j.0105-2896.2005.00263.x

43. Kelliher S, Weiss L, Cullivan S, O'Rourke E, Murphy CA, et al. Non-severe COVID-19 is associated with endothelial damage and hypercoagulability despite pharmacological thromboprophylaxis. *J Thromb Haemost.* (2022) 20:1008–14. doi: 10.1111/jth.15660

44. Grasselli G, Zangrillo A, Zanella A, Antonelli M, Cabrini L, Castelli A, et al. Baseline characteristics and outcomes of 1591 patients infected with SARS-CoV-2 admitted to ICUs of the Lombardy Region, Italy. *JAMA.* (2020) 323:1574–81. doi: 10.1001/jama.2020.5394

45. Roshdy A, Zaher S, Fayed H, Coghlan JG. COVID-19 and the heart: a systematic review of cardiac autopsies. *Front Cardiovasc Med.* (2021) 7:626975. doi: 10.3389/fcvm.2020.626975

46. Otifi HM, Adiga BK. Endothelial dysfunction in Covid-19. *Am J Med Sci.* (2022) 27:S0002-9629(22)00026-X. doi: 10.1016/j.amjms.2021.12.010

47. Poyatos P, Luque N, Eizaguirre S, Sabater G, Sebastián L, Francisco-Albesa Í, et al. Post-COVID-19 patients show an increased endothelial progenitor cell production. *Transl Res.* (2022) 24:S1931-5244(22)00017-2. doi: 10.1016/j.trsl.2022.01.004

48. Charfeddine S, Ibn Hadj Amor H, Jdidi J, Torjmen S, Kraiem S, Hammami R, et al. Long COVID 19 syndrome: is it related to microcirculation and endothelial dysfunction? insights from TUN-EndCOV study. *Front Cardiovasc Med.* (2021) 8:745758. doi: 10.3389/fcvm.2021.745758

49. Hamming I, Timens W, Bulthuis ML, Lely AT, Navis G, van Goor H. Tissue distribution of ACE2 protein, the functional receptor for SARS coronavirus. A first step in understanding SARS pathogenesis. *J Pathol.* (2004) 203:631–7. doi: 10.1002/path.1570

50. Pober JS, Sessa WC. Evolving functions of endothelial cells in inflammation. *Nat Rev Immunol.* (2007) 7:803–15. doi: 10.1038/nri2171

51. Panigrahi S, Goswami T, Ferrari B, Antonelli CJ, Bazdar DA, Gilmore H, et al. SARS-CoV-2 spike protein destabilizes microvascular homeostasis. *Microbiol Spectr.* (2021) 9:e0073521. doi: 10.1128/Spectrum.00735-21

52. Heidemann J, Domschke W, Kucharzik T, Maaser C. Intestinal microvascular endothelium and innate immunity in inflammatory bowel disease: a second line of defense? *Infect Immun.* (2006) 74:5425–32. doi: 10.1128/IAI.00248-06

53. Franco RF, de Jonge E, Dekkers PE, Timmerman JJ, Spek CA, van Deventer SJ, et al. The in vivo kinetics of tissue factor messenger RNA expression during human endotoxemia: relationship with activation of coagulation. *Blood.* (2000) 96:554–9. doi: 10.1182/blood.V96.2.554.014k17_554_559

54. Schouten M, Wiersinga WJ, Levi M, van der Poll T. Inflammation, endothelium, and coagulation in sepsis. *J Leukoc Biol.* (2008) 83:536–45. doi: 10.1189/jlb.0607373

55. Gu SX, Tyagi T, Jain K, Gu VW, Lee SH, Hwa JM, et al. Thrombocytopathy and endotheliopathy: crucial contributors to COVID-19 thromboinflammation. *Nat Rev Cardiol.* (2021) 18:194–209. doi: 10.1038/s41569-020-00469-1

56. Chae WJ, Ehrlich AK, Chan PY, Teixeira AM, Henegariu O, Hao L, et al. The Wnt antagonist Dickkopf-1 promotes pathological type 2 cell-mediated inflammation. *Immunity.* (2016) 44:246–58. doi: 10.1016/j.immuni.2016.01.008

57. Skendros P, Mitsios A, Chrysanthopoulou A, Mastellos DC, Metallidis S, Rafailidis P, et al. Complement and tissue factor-enriched neutrophil extracellular traps are key drivers in COVID-19 immunothrombosis. *J Clin Invest.* (2020) 130:6151–7. doi: 10.1172/JCI141374

58. Magro C, Mulvey JJ, Berlin D, Nuovo G, Salvatore S, Harp J, et al. Complement associated microvascular injury and thrombosis in the pathogenesis of severe COVID-19 infection: a report of five cases. *Transl Res.* (2020) 220:1–13. doi: 10.1016/j.trsl.2020.04.007

59. Lerman A, Zeiher AM. Endothelial function: cardiac events. *Circulation.* (2005) 111:363–8. doi: 10.1161/01.CIR.0000153339.27064.14

60. Li W, Mital S, Ojaimi C, Csiszar A, Kaley G, Hintze TH. Premature death and age-related cardiac dysfunction in male eNOS-knockout mice. *J Mol Cell Cardiol.* (2004) 37:671–80. doi: 10.1016/j.yjmcc.2004.05.005

61. Ungvari Z, Tarantini S, Kiss T, Wren JD, Giles CB, Griffin CT, et al. Endothelial dysfunction and angiogenesis impairment in the ageing vasculature. *Nat Rev Cardiol.* (2018) 15:555–65. doi: 10.1038/s41569-018-0030-z

62. Csiszar A, Ungvari Z, Koller A, Edwards JG, Kaley G. Proinflammatory phenotype of coronary arteries promotes endothelial apoptosis in aging. *Physiol Genomics.* (2004) 17:21–30. doi: 10.1152/physiolgenomics.00136.2003

63. Wehbe Z, Hammoud S, Soudani N, Zaraket H, El-Yazbi A, Eid AH. Molecular insights into SARS COV-2 interaction with cardiovascular disease: role of RAAS and MAPK signaling. *Front Pharmacol.* (2020) 11:836. doi: 10.3389/fphar.2020.00836

64. Cantero-Navarro E, Fernández-Fernández B, Ramos AM, Rayego-Mateos S, Rodrigues-Diez RR, Sánchez-Niño MD, et al. Renin-angiotensin system and inflammation update. *Mol Cell Endocrinol.* (2021) 529:111254. doi: 10.1016/j.mce.2021.111254

65. Poznyak AV, Bezsonov EE, Eid AH, Popkova TV, Nedosugova LV, Starodubova AV, et al. ACE2 Is an adjacent element of atherosclerosis and COVID-19 pathogenesis. *Int J Mol Sci.* (2021) 22:4691. doi: 10.3390/ijms22094691

66. Birk M, Baum E, Zadeh JK, Manicam C, Pfeiffer N, Patzak A, et al. Angiotensin II induces oxidative stress and endothelial dysfunction in mouse ophthalmic arteries via involvement of AT1 receptors and NOX2. *Antioxidants.* (2021) 10:1238. doi: 10.3390/antiox10081238

67. Brasier AR, Recinos A. 3rd, Eledrisi MS. *Vascular inflammation and the renin-angiotensin system Arterioscler Thromb Vasc Biol.* (2002) 22:1257–66. doi: 10.1161/01.ATV.0000021412.56621.A2

68. Wenzel P, Knorr M, Kossmann S, Stratmann J, Hausding M, Schuhmacher S, et al. Lysozyme M-positive monocytes mediate angiotensin II-induced arterial hypertension and vascular dysfunction. *Circulation.* (2011) 124:1370–81. doi: 10.1161/CIRCULATIONAHA.111.034470

69. Kossmann S, Hu H, Steven S, Schönfelder T, Fraccarollo D, Mikhed Y, et al. Inflammatory monocytes determine endothelial nitric-oxide synthase uncoupling and nitro-oxidative stress induced by angiotensin II. *J Biol Chem.* (2014) 289:27540–50. doi: 10.1074/jbc.M114.604231

70. Sorokin V, Vickneson K, Kofidis T, Woo CC, Lin XY, Foo R, et al. Role of vascular smooth muscle cell plasticity and interactions in vessel wall inflammation. *Front Immunol.* (2020) 11:599415. doi: 10.3389/fimmu.2020.599415

71. Bennett MR, Sinha S, Owens GK. Vascular Smooth Muscle Cells in Atherosclerosis. *Circ Res.* (2016) 118:692–702. doi: 10.1161/CIRCRESAHA.115.306361

72. Zhang F, Ren X, Zhao M, Zhou B, Han Y. Angiotensin-(1-7) abrogates angiotensin II-induced proliferation, migration and inflammation in VSMCs through inactivation of ROS-mediated PI3K/Akt and MAPK/ERK signaling pathways. *Sci Rep.* (2016) 6:34621. doi: 10.1038/srep34621

73. Stein LK, Mayman NA, Dhamoon MS, Fifi JT. The emerging association between COVID-19 and acute stroke. *Trends Neurosci.* (2021) 44:527–37. doi: 10.1016/j.tins.2021.03.005

74. Strambo D, De Marchis GM, Bonati LH, Arnold M, Carrera E, Galletta S, et al. Ischemic stroke in COVID-19 patients: mechanisms, treatment, and outcomes in a consecutive Swiss Stroke Registry analysis. *Eur J Neurol.* (2022) 29:732–43. doi: 10.1111/ene.15199

75. Norouzi-Barough L, Asgari Khosroshahi A, Gorji A, Zafari F, Shahverdi Shahraki M, Shirian S. COVID-19-induced stroke and the potential of using mesenchymal stem cells-derived extracellular vesicles in the regulation of neuroinflammation. *Cell Mol Neurobiol.* (2022) 13:1–10. doi: 10.1007/s10571-021-01169-1

76. Basra R, Whyte M, Karalliedde J, Vas P. What is the impact of microvascular complications of diabetes on severe COVID-19? *Microvasc Res.* (2022) 140:104310. doi: 10.1016/j.mvr.2021.104310

77. Jdiaa SS, Mansour R, El Alayli A, Gautam A, Thomas P, Mustafa RA. COVID-19 and chronic kidney disease: an updated overview of reviews. *J Nephrol.* (2022) 35:69–85. doi: 10.1007/s40620-021-01206-8

78. de Jager DJ, Grootendorst DC, Jager KJ, van Dijk PC, Tomas LM, Ansell D, et al. Cardiovascular and noncardiovascular mortality among patients starting dialysis. *JAMA.* (2009) 302:1782–9. doi: 10.1001/jama.2009.1488

79. Kato S, Chmielewski M, Honda H, Pecoits-Filho R, Matsuo S, Yuzawa Y, et al. Aspects of immune dysfunction in end-stage renal disease. *Clin J Am Soc Nephrol.* (2008) 3:1526–33. doi: 10.2215/CJN.00950208

80. Atmosudigdo IS, Lim MA, Radi B, Henrina J, Yonas E, Vania R, et al. Dyslipidemia increases the risk of severe COVID-19: a systematic review, meta-analysis, and meta-regression. *Clin Med Insights Endocrinol Diabetes.* (2021) 14:1179551421990675. doi: 10.1177/1179551421990675

81. Hariyanto TI, Kurniawan A. Dyslipidemia is associated with severe coronavirus disease 2019 (COVID-19) infection. *Diabetes Metab Syndr.* (2020) 14:1463–5. doi: 10.1016/j.dsx.2020.07.054

82. Petrilli CM, Jones SA, Yang J, Rajagopalan H, O'Donnell L, Chernyak Y, et al. Factors associated with hospital admission and critical illness among 5279 people with coronavirus disease 2019 in New York City: prospective cohort study. *BMJ.* (2020) 369:m1966. doi: 10.1136/bmj.m1966

83. Surma S, Banach M, Lewek J. COVID-19 and lipids. The role of lipid disorders and statin use in the prognosis of patients with SARS-CoV-2 infection. *Lipids Health Dis.* (2021) 20:141. doi: 10.1186/s12944-021-01563-0

22

Co-occurrence of Myocarditis and Thrombotic Microangiopathy Limited to the Heart in a COVID-19 Patient

Thomas Menter[1], Nadine Cueni[2], Eva Caroline Gebhard[2] and Alexandar Tzankov[1]*

[1] *Department of Pathology, Institute of Medical Genetics and Pathology, University Hospital Basel, University of Basel, Basel, Switzerland,* [2] *Intensive Care Unit, University Hospital Basel, Basel, Switzerland*

*Correspondence:
Alexandar Tzankov
alexandar.tzankov@usb.ch

We report on an impressive case of a previously healthy 47-year-old female Caucasian SARS-CoV-2 positive patient who died within 48 h after initial cardiac symptoms. Autopsy revealed necrotizing myocarditis and extensive microthrombosis as the cause of death. The interesting feature of this case is the combination of both myocarditis and extensive localized microthrombosis of cardiac capillaries. Microthrombosis was not present in other organs, and the patient did not show typical features of diffuse alveolar damage in the lungs. Taken together, our morphologic findings illustrate the angiocentric, microangiopathic, thromboinflammatory disease with significant thrombotic diathesis prevalent in COVID-19, which has been previously described in the literature, likely warranting thromboprophylaxis even in oligosymptomatic circumstances. This case also delineates several potential etiologies for microthrombosis, i.e., inflammatory reactions and primary hypercoagulative states. Further systematic analyses on risk stratification for receipt of prophylactic anticoagulation in COVID-19 are urgently required.

Keywords: COVID-19, heart, myocarditis acute and fulminant, thrombus, thromboinflammation

INTRODUCTION

Based on early empiric evidence and autopsy observations (1–3), anticoagulation has emerged as an important topic in treatment of COVID-19 (4). It is now well-established that thromboses significantly contribute to disease burden in COVID-19 and thus warrant immediate attention by treating physicians regardless of disease severity (5, 6). Myocarditis is also rare but nevertheless an acknowledged comorbidity in COVID-19 (7). Few cases have been examined by histopathology so far, and they showed divergent features ranging from subtle inflammatory infiltrates not fulfilling diagnostic criteria for borderline myocarditis to overt necrotizing inflammation (8–10).

Here, we present a case of a previously healthy patient positive for SARS-CoV-2 who died of cardiac complications consisting of necrotizing myocarditis and extensive microthrombosis within 48 h after initial cardiac symptoms.

CASE

A 47-year-old female suffered from oligosymptomatic flu-like disease for a week before she was found unconscious and apneic at home. Advanced cardiac life support was promptly administered by paramedics. Upon hospital admission, electrocardiography (ECG) showed ST-segment

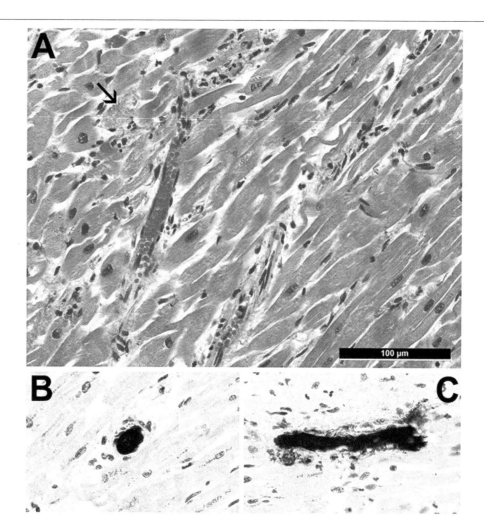

FIGURE 1 | Cardiopathological findings. **(A)** Morphology of the heart showing multifocal inflammatory infiltrates consisting of neutrophilic granulocytes, lymphocytes and histiocytes, capillarostasis, and perifocal single-cell necroses of cardiomyocytes (arrow) (H&E, ×400). **(B,C)** Immunohistochemical staining for fibrin demonstrating cross section and longitudinal section of capillaries with prominent microthrombi occluding the lumens (immunohistochemistry for fibrin, ×400).

depression in all the leads and elevations in augmented vector right (aVR). Subsequently performed coronary angiography revealed no relevant coronary stenosis. Echocardiography detected moderately reduced left ventricular function (left ventricular ejection fraction (LVEF) 30%) and normal right ventricular size and function. There was no evidence of left ventricular hypertrophy or dilatation. Computerized tomography excluded pulmonary thromboembolism but showed bilateral lower-lobe consolidations. High-sensitivity troponin T (hsTropT) was elevated (272 ng/l at admission; peak of 507 ng/l 10 h after admission), as were brain natriuretic peptide (>70,000 ng/l) and C-reactive protein (282 mg/l). The leucocyte count was within normal range. A nasopharyngeal swab was positive for SARS-CoV-2. Apart from mild thrombocytopenia (140 G/L) and mildly prolonged activated partial thromboplastin time (aPTT) (39 s) at the time of admission, all other coagulation parameters were within normal ranges. Despite exhaustive invasive intensive care interventions including continuous

adrenalin/noradrenaline infusion, prophylactic antibiotic therapy (piperacillin/tazobactam), and two further attempts of cardiac resuscitation, the patient died of cardio-respiratory failure within 48 h of admission. Her detailed clinical course is shown in the timeline section. Previous clinical history included episodes of depression, which had been treated with venlafaxine, and a cholecystectomy.

An autopsy was performed. No relevant comorbidities apart from obesity [body mass index (BMI) 31.6] were noticed. Major findings included moderate bilateral suppurative pneumonia with COVID-19-characteristic capillary stasis, yet without diffuse alveolar damage. Most notably, the heart presented as normotrophic and irregularly perfused with mild diffuse necrotizing myocarditis (**Figure 1A**) accompanied by extensive thrombotic microangiopathy of cardiac capillaries (**Figures 1B,C**; microthrombi in cardiac capillaries immunohistochemically stained for fibrin), which was determined as the cause of death. RT-qPCR of heart tissue was positive for SARS-CoV-2-*N*-gene (Ct 35.7). Immunohistochemistry for adenovirus was negative.

TIMELINE

Date	Event
1 week before admission to hospital	Flu-like symptoms with symptomatic treatment (SARS-CoV-2 test negative)
Day 1	Advanced cardiac life support due to asystole (after at least 10 min without basic life support measurements) with return of spontaneous circulation after 10 min
	Referral to the emergency department of a tertiary care center (SARS-CoV-2 test positive)
	Diagnostics: moderate left ventricular ejection dysfunction (LVEF 30%), lower pulmonary lobe opacities, no evidence of coronary artery disease or thrombosis, nor pulmonary embolisms or pneumothorax, normal electrolyte values
Day 2	Admission to intensive care unit requiring mechanical ventilation and with multiorgan failure
	One episode of ventricular fibrillation treated with defibrillation
	Extracorporeal membrane oxygenation not performed, as the time period between first reanimation attempts was prolonged, inducing severe hypoxic encephalopathy with extensively elevated neuron-specific enolase in the absence of hemolysis
Day 3	Death after renewed unsuccessful reanimation for 20 min

DISCUSSION

The interesting feature of this COVID-19 case study is the combination of both myocarditis and extensive microthrombosis of cardiac capillaries.

Our group, amongst others, has previously presented comprehensive autopsy cohorts of patients succumbing to COVID-19 describing microthrombosis predominantly in the lungs and further organs (2, 11, 12). Microthrombi in the pulmonary capillary bed and subsequently increased intravascular pressure in the pulmonary circulation have been attributed to heart failure in several studies. A recent report focusing on heart pathology described microthrombi in 12/15 COVID-19 cases (13); thrombi were also found in some control cases with influenza infection, metastatic carcinoma, or advanced severe bacterial pneumonia. In line with this case, we have previously investigated cardiopathological characteristics of patients succumbing to COVID-19 associated respiratory failure, similarly demonstrating a high incidence of capillary dilatation, stasis, and microthrombosis, especially in cases with detectable SARS-CoV-2 cardiac viral load (14).

It is well-acknowledged that COVID-19 predisposes to a procoagulatory state. The underlying pathophysiology for thromboinflammation is likely multifaceted, involving direct endothelial damage by SARS-CoV-2, secondary inflammatory endothelial damage, an overexpression of procoagulatory genes (e.g., *SERPINE* genes) in target organs, and generation of neutrophilic extracellular traps, and immunological, particularly antiphospholipid-mediated processes [rev. in (15)].

Myocarditis, in particular borderline myocarditis, in COVID-19 patients has been described (7). In a systematic review of 41 studies compiling 316 cases of COVID-19 autopsies, Roshdy et al. identified five cases (i.e., 1.5%) with inflammatory infiltrates fulfilling the Dallas criteria of myocarditis (8). In ≈10% of cases, mild focal inflammatory infiltrates in the myocardial interstitium had been noticed. In one study on endomyocardial biopsies taken for elucidating the cause of acute heart failure or in suspicion of myocarditis (16), isolated cases showed both presence of SARS-CoV-2 genomes and inflammatory infiltrates also affecting small vessels, while thrombi had not been described in this series.

In our case, the patient exclusively presented with localized cardiac microthrombi; other organs were not affected (also confirmed by immunohistochemistry). Microthrombi were partially associated with inflammatory infiltrates and single-cell cardiomyocyte necrosis, which we interpret as a sequela of the thrombotic microangiopathy. Acute heart failure, which is the non-disputable cause of death, can be attributed to both features—myocarditis and microthrombi—and our findings strongly support that both morphological features can be collectively interpreted as a rare but severe COVID-19-related thromboinflammatory cardiac complication. There was no evidence of a preexisting heart condition based on imaging and autopsy findings as well as the clinical history of the patient. Admittedly, it has to be considered that her intake of antidepressant (venlafaxine) might have contributed to cardiac pathology, yet the features described in single case reports and a review article of individuals treated with venlafaxine and cardiac problems were not evident in this case (17–19). Furthermore, there was no evidence of serotonin syndrome, mydriasis, or seizures.

Taken together, our morphologic findings and the preexisting literature illustrate that COVID-19 is an angiocentric, particularly microangiopathic, thromboinflammatory disease with significant thrombotic diathesis, in all likelihood warranting thromboprophylaxis even in oligosymptomatic circumstances. This case also delineates several potential etiologies for microthrombi: inflammatory reaction and primary hypercoagulative state. Further systematic analyses on risk stratification for receipt of prophylactic anticoagulation in COVID-19 are urgently required.

PATIENT PERSPECTIVE

Heart failure is a severe complication of COVID-19. As illustrated in this case, it can also arise in previously healthy patients and might develop independently of pulmonary findings. Myocarditis and microthrombosis of the cardiac capillaries are potentially treatable etiologies of heart failure in such instances, yet their diagnosis may be difficult without histological examination. Thorough investigation of both coagulation parameters and the myocardium might be therefore required in patients with unexplained or rapidly deteriorating heart failure in the setting of COVID-19. It remains to be determined if prophylactic anticoagulation even in oligosymptomatic COVID-19 patients is feasible.

AUTHOR CONTRIBUTIONS

AT performed the autopsy. AT and TM designed the study and

wrote the manuscript. NC and EG took care of the patient and provided clinical data. All authors contributed to the article and approved the submitted version.

ACKNOWLEDGMENTS

We thank Dr. med. J. D. Haslbauer for critically proofreading the manuscript.

REFERENCES

1. Wichmann D, Sperhake JP, Lutgehetmann M, Steurer S, Edler C, Heinemann A, et al. Autopsy findings and venous thromboembolism in patients with COVID-19: a prospective cohort study. *Ann Intern Med.* (2020) 173:268–77. doi: 10.7326/M20-2003

2. Menter T, Haslbauer JD, Nienhold R, Savic S, Hopfer H, Deigendesch N, et al. Postmortem examination of COVID-19 patients reveals diffuse alveolar damage with severe capillary congestion and variegated findings in lungs and other organs suggesting vascular dysfunction. *Histopathology.* (2020) 77:198–209. doi: 10.1111/his.14134

3. Lax SF, Skok K, Zechner P, Kessler HH, Kaufmann N, Koelblinger C, et al. Pulmonary arterial thrombosis in COVID-19 with fatal outcome : results from a prospective, single-center, clinicopathologic case series. *Ann Intern Med.* (2020) 173:350–61. doi: 10.7326/M20-2566

4. Bikdeli B, Madhavan MV, Jimenez D, Chuich T, Dreyfus I, Driggin E, et al. COVID-19 and thrombotic or thromboembolic disease: implications for prevention, antithrombotic therapy, and follow-up: JACC state-of-the-art review. *J Am Coll Cardiol.* (2020) 75:2950–73. doi: 10.1016/j.jacc.2020.04.031

5. Rentsch CT, Beckman JA, Tomlinson L, Gellad WF, Alcorn C, Kidwai-Khan F, et al. Early initiation of prophylactic anticoagulation for prevention of coronavirus disease 2019 mortality in patients admitted to hospital in the United States: cohort study. *BMJ.* (2021) 372:n311. doi: 10.1136/bmj.n311

6. Giannis D, Allen S, Tsang J, Flint S, Pinhasov T, Williams S, et al. Post-Discharge thromboembolic outcomes and mortality of hospitalized COVID-19 patients: the CORE-19 registry. *Blood.* (2021) 137:2838–47. doi: 10.1182/blood.2020010529

7. Mele D, Flamigni F, Rapezzi C, Ferrari R. Myocarditis in COVID-19 patients: current problems. *Intern Emerg Med.* (2021) 23:1–7. doi: 10.1007/s11739-021-02635-w

8. Roshdy A, Zaher S, Fayed H, Coghlan JG. COVID-19 and the heart: a systematic review of cardiac autopsies. *Front Cardiovasc Med.* (2020) 7:626975. doi: 10.3389/fcvm.2020.626975

9. Craver R, Huber S, Sandomirsky M, McKenna D, Schieffelin J, Finger L. Fatal eosinophilic myocarditis in a healthy 17-year-old male with severe acute respiratory syndrome coronavirus 2 (SARS-CoV-2c). *Fetal Pediatr Pathol.* (2020) 39:263–8. doi: 10.1080/15513815.2020.17 61491

10. Basso C, Leone O, Rizzo S, De Gaspari M, van der Wal AC, Aubry MC, et al. Pathological features of COVID-19-associated myocardial injury: a multicentre cardiovascular pathology study. *Eur Heart J.* (2020) 41:3827–35. doi: 10.1093/eurheartj/eha a664

11. Duarte-Neto AN, Monteiro RAA, da Silva LFF, Malheiros D, de Oliveira EP, Theodoro-Filho J, et al. Pulmonary and systemic involvement in COVID-19 patients assessed with ultrasound-guided minimally invasive autopsy. *Histopathology.* (2020) 77:186–97. doi: 10.1111/his.14160

12. Varga Z, Flammer AJ, Steiger P, Haberecker M, Andermatt R, Zinkernagel AS, et al. Endothelial cell infection and endotheliitis in COVID-19. *Lancet.* (2020) 395:1417–8. doi: 10.1016/S0140-6736(20)30937-5

13. Bois MC, Boire NA, Layman AJ, Aubry MC, Alexander MP, Roden AC, et al. COVID-19-associated nonocclusive fibrin microthrombi in the heart. *Circulation.* (2021) 143:230–43. doi: 10.1161/CIRCULATIONAHA.120.050754

14. Haslbauer JD, Tzankov A, Mertz KD, Schwab N, Nienhold R, Twerenbold R, et al. Characterisation of cardiac pathology in 23 autopsies of lethal COVID-19. *J Pathol Clin Res.* (2021) 7:326–37. doi: 10.1002/cjp2.212

15. Bosmuller H, Matter M, Fend F, Tzankov A. The pulmonary pathology of COVID-19. *Virchows Arch.* (2021) 478:137–50. doi: 10.1007/s00428-021-03053-1

16. Escher F, Pietsch H, Aleshcheva G, Bock T, Baumeier C, Elsaesser A, et al. Detection of viral SARS-CoV-2 genomes and histopathological changes in endomyocardial biopsies. *ESC Heart Fail.* (2020) 7:2440–7. doi: 10.1002/ehf2.12805

17. Vinetti M, Haufroid V, Capron A, Classen JF, Marchandise S, Hantson P. Severe acute cardiomyopathy associated with venlafaxine overdose and possible role of CYP2D6 and CYP2C19 polymorphisms. *Clin Toxicol.* (2011) 49:865–9. doi: 10.3109/15563650.2011.626421

18. Elikowski W, Malek-Elikowska M, Ganowicz-Kaatz T, Fertala N, Zawodna M, Baszko A, et al. Transient left ventricular hypertrophy in a 30-year-old female with chronic emotional stress and depression treated with venlafaxine. *Pol Merkur Lekarski.* (2019) 47:144–9.

19. Howell C, Wilson AD, Waring WS. Cardiovascular toxicity due to venlafaxine poisoning in adults: a review of 235 consecutive cases. *Br J Clin Pharmacol.* (2007) 64:192–7. doi: 10.1111/j.1365-2125.2007.02849.x

23

Outcomes of Hospitalized Patients with COVID-19 with Acute Kidney Injury and Acute Cardiac Injury

Justin Y. Lu[1†], Alexandra Buczek[1†], Roman Fleysher[1], Wouter S. Hoogenboom[1],
Wei Hou[2], Carlos J. Rodriguez[3], Molly C. Fisher[4] and Tim Q. Duong[1*]

[1] Department of Radiology, Montefiore Medical Center, Albert Einstein College of Medicine, Bronx, NY, United States,
[2] Department of Family, Population and Preventive Medicine, Stony Brook Medicine, New York, NY, United States,
[3] Cardiology Division, Department of Medicine, Montefiore Medical Center, Albert Einstein College of Medicine, Bronx, NY,
United States, [4] Nephrology Division, Department of Medicine, Montefiore Medical Center, Albert Einstein College of
Medicine, Bronx, NY, United States

*Correspondence:
Tim Q. Duong
tim.duong@einsteinmed.org

† These authors share first authorship

Purpose: This study investigated the incidence, disease course, risk factors, and mortality in COVID-19 patients who developed both acute kidney injury (AKI) and acute cardiac injury (ACI), and compared to those with AKI only, ACI only, and no injury (NI).

Methods: This retrospective study consisted of hospitalized COVID-19 patients at Montefiore Health System in Bronx, New York between March 11, 2020 and January 29, 2021. Demographics, comorbidities, vitals, and laboratory tests were collected during hospitalization. Predictive models were used to predict AKI, ACI, and AKI-ACI onset. Longitudinal laboratory tests were analyzed with time-lock to discharge alive or death.

Results: Of the 5,896 hospitalized COVID-19 patients, 44, 19, 9, and 28% had NI, AKI, ACI, and AKI-ACI, respectively. Most ACI presented very early (within a day or two) during hospitalization in contrast to AKI ($p < 0.05$). Patients with combined AKI-ACI were significantly older, more often men and had more comorbidities, and higher levels of cardiac, kidney, liver, inflammatory, and immunological markers compared to those of the AKI, ACI, and NI groups. The adjusted hospital-mortality odds ratios were 17.1 [95% CI = 13.6–21.7, $p < 0.001$], 7.2 [95% CI = 5.4–9.6, $p < 0.001$], and 4.7 [95% CI = 3.7–6.1, $p < 0.001$] for AKI-ACI, ACI, and AKI, respectively, relative to NI. A predictive model of AKI-ACI onset using top predictors yielded 97% accuracy. Longitudinal laboratory data predicted mortality of AKI-ACI patients up to 5 days prior to outcome, with an area-under-the-curve, ranging from 0.68 to 0.89.

Conclusions: COVID-19 patients with AKI-ACI had markedly worse outcomes compared to those only AKI, ACI and NI. Common laboratory variables accurately predicted AKI-ACI. The ability to identify patients at risk for AKI-ACI could lead to earlier intervention and improvement in clinical outcomes.

Keywords: SARS-CoV-2, cardiovascular sequelae, cardiac injury, predictive model, AKI

INTRODUCTION

Acute kidney injury (AKI) and acute cardiac injury (ACI) are well-recognized complications of coronavirus disease 2019 (COVID-19) caused by the severe acute respiratory syndrome coronavirus 2 (SARS-CoV-2) (1–3). AKI and ACI separately have been associated with increased risk of critical illness and mortality in COVID-19 patients (1–3). The mechanisms underlying the high incidence of AKI and ACI and their association with poor outcomes in COVID-19 are not well-understood and are likely multifactorial. SARS-CoV-2 uses the angiotensin-converting enzyme 2 (ACE2) as docking and entry receptor on host cells, and the transmembrane serine protease 2 (TMPRSS2) is also involved in its cellular entry (4, 5). Though unproven, it has been hypothesized that SARS-CoV2 may directly induce AKI and ACI as the kidney and heart have a high density of ACE2 receptors. Indirect effects of COVID-19 that contribute to AKI and ACI include hypoxia, hypotension, inflammation, thromboembolism, cytokine storm, and sepsis (1–3, 6, 7). Endothelial dysfunction has been reported in patients with severe COVID-19 (8) and also likely plays a role in AKI and ACI.

In addition to age, pre-existing hypertension, diabetes, and obesity are major risk factors for severe COVID-19 and increased mortality (9–11). Black and Hispanic patients have been disproportionately affected by COVID-19 and have increased mortality. This may be due to a higher prevalence of cardiovascular risk factors in this population or socioeconomic factors such as crowding, food insecurity and poverty (12–15).

Observational studies have characterized the risk factors and outcomes of AKI (16–21) and ACI (22–25) separately among hospitalized patients with COVID-19. However, there have been no systematic studies comparing outcomes of COVID-19 patients with AKI to COVID-19 patients with ACI or evaluating the incidence, risk factors and clinical outcomes of COVID-19 patients who develop both AKI and ACI during hospitalization. Understanding the clinical characteristics and risk factors that make COVID-19 patients susceptible to in-hospital AKI and ACI could lead to better patient management and clinical outcomes.

The purpose of this study was to investigate the demographics and the clinical variables of COVID-19 patients with combined injury (AKI-ACI), and to compare them with those with AKI only, ACI only, and no injury (NI). Our study population came from Montefiore Health System in the Bronx, New York, which serves a large, low-income, and diverse population and which was hit hard by the COVID-19 pandemic. Mathematical models were developed to predict AKI-ACI onset. In addition, we analyzed the temporal progression of different clinical variables with time-lock to outcome (discharged alive or in-hospital death) and use them to predict likelihood of mortality. To our knowledge this is the first systematic documentation of the longitudinal clinical variables associated with AKI-ACI, with comparison with AKI, ACI, and NI in COVID-19.

METHODS

Study Design, Population, and Data Source

This retrospective study was approved by the Einstein-Montefiore Institutional Review Board (#2020-11389). All patients in this study were seen in The Montefiore Health System (MHS) and tested for SARS-CoV-2 infection using real-time polymerase chain reaction test (RT-PCR) on a nasopharyngeal swab between January 1, 2020, and January 29, 2021. The Montefiore Health System is one of the largest healthcare systems in New York City with 15 hospitals located in the Bronx, the lower Hudson Valley, and Westchester County serving a large, low-income, and racially and ethnically diverse population that was hit hard by COVID-19 early in the pandemic (13, 26).

Health data were searched and extracted as described previously (13, 27). In short, de-identified data were made available for research by the Montefiore Einstein Center for Health Data Innovations after standardization to the Observational Medical Outcomes Partnership (OMOP) Common Data Model (CDM) version 6. OMOP CDM represents healthcare data from diverse sources, which are stored in standard vocabulary concepts (28), allowing for the systematic analysis of disparate observational databases, including data from the electronic medical record system, administrative claims, and disease classifications systems (e.g., ICD-10, SNOWMED, LOINC, etc.). ATLAS, a web-based tool developed by the Observational Health Data Sciences and Informatics (OHDSI) community that enables navigation of patient-level, observational data in the CDM format, was used to search vocabulary concepts and facilitate cohort building. Data were subsequently exported and queried as SQLite database files using the DB Browser for SQLite (version 3.12.0).

The primary study outcome was in-hospital mortality as extracted from electronic medical record. Demographic data included age, sex, ethnicity, and race. Chronic comorbidities included obesity, diabetes, congestive heart failure (CHF), chronic kidney disease (CKD), coronary artery disease (CAD), chronic obstructive pulmonary disease (COPD), and asthma. Longitudinal laboratory tests and vitals included creatinine (Cr), estimated glomerular filtration rate (eGFR), albumin, alanine aminotransferase (ALT), aspartate aminotransferase (AST), brain natriuretic peptide (BNP), C-reactive protein (CRP), D-dimer (DDIM), ferritin (FERR), lactate dehydrogenase (LDH), lymphocytes (LYMPH), troponin-T (TNT), white blood cells (WBC), fibrinogen, eosinophils, basophils, neutrophils, prothrombin time (PT), systolic blood pressure (SBP), body temperature, heart rate (HR), and pulse oximetry.

AKI and ACI Definitions

AKI was defined using the Kidney Disease Improving Global Outcomes criteria as either a 0.3 mg/dl increase in serum creatinine within 48 h or a 1.5x increase in serum creatinine within a 7-day iterative window. The baseline creatinine was determined as the mean of all serum creatinine values 8–365 days preceding hospitalization (20, 21, 29). For patients who did not have creatinine baseline values, the lowest creatinine value during hospitalization was used as the baseline creatinine (19, 30). Urine

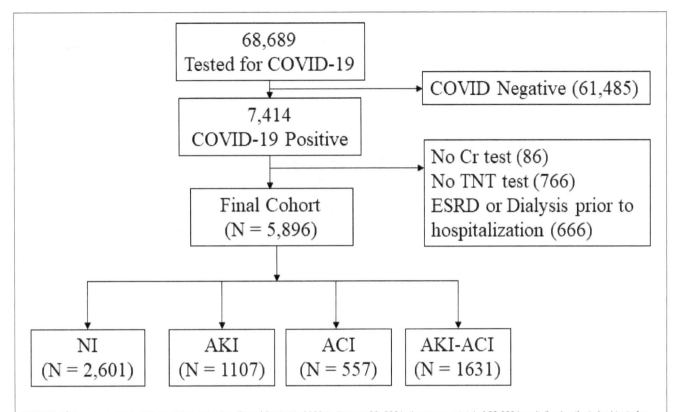

FIGURE 1 | Flowchart of hospitalized patient selection. From March 11, 2020 to January 29, 2021, there were a total of 68,689 hospitalized patients had tests for COVID-19 and 7,414 had a positive COVID-19 test. Cr, creatinine; TNT, troponin-T; NI, no injury; AKI, acute kidney injury; ACI, acute myocardial injury; ESRD, end-stage renal disease.

output was not used to define AKI due to significant missing data. ACI was defined using the 4th Universal Definition of Myocardial Infarction, with a high-sensitivity troponin T level above the 99th-percentile upper reference limit (0.0141 ng/mL) (31–33).

Patients without AKI or ACI were assigned to the no injury group. Note that we also evaluated isolated liver injury and found 713 patients had elevated liver enzymes [AST > 1ULN (>40U/L) and ALT > 1ULN (>35U/L)] (34).

From March 11, 2020 to January 29, 2021 (**Figure 1**), there were a total of 68,689 hospitalized patients were tested for COVID-19 and 7,414 had a positive COVID-19 test. Patients who were not hospitalized were excluded. Patients missing Cr or TNT data, and patients with ESKD on dialysis were excluded. This left 5,896 hospitalized COVID-19 patients for the final analysis. Of these, 2,601 had NI, 1,107 had AKI only, 557 had ACI only and 1,631 had AKI-ACI. There were no statistically significant differences in major baseline characteristics (i.e., age, gender, race, ethnicity, and comorbidities) between the included and excluded patients ($p > 0.05$).

Prediction of AKI, ACI, and AKI-ACI

Logistic regression models were used to rank the importance of clinical variables (demographics, comorbidities, vitals, and blood tests) and predict AKI, ACI, and AKI-ACI onsets using data at admission. Prediction of mortality was also performed using logistic regression. Performance was evaluated using the area

under the curve (AUC) of the receiver operating characteristic (ROC) curve with 5-fold cross validation. Note that Cr and TNT, which were used to define AKI and ACI onset respectively, were included in the predictive models because their quantitative values at different days could be predictive of outcomes.

Temporal Profiles of Clinical Variables

Clinical variables were collected 5 days prior to outcome (death or hospital discharge). Temporal progression of clinical data was time-locked to outcome and compared between groups stratified by survivors and non-survivors. Logistic regression models were used to rank the importance of clinical variables. Prediction performance was evaluated using ROC analysis for individual top variables for different days prior to outcome.

Statistical Analysis

Statistical analyses were performed using Python and Statistical Analysis System (SAS) software (Cary, NC, USA). Group differences in frequencies and percentages for categorical variables were tested using χ^2 or Fisher's exact tests. Group comparison of continuous used the non-parametric Kruskal Wallis/ Mann-Whitney U-test. Mortality odds ratios (aOR) were adjusted for age, gender, ethnicity, and comorbidities and provided. Differences among AKI-ACI, AKI, ACI, and NI groups for clinical variables in time-series graphs were analyzed *via* linear mixed models and least-squares means. $P < 0.05$ was

TABLE 1 | Demographics, comorbidities, and laboratory variables at admission of NI, AKI, ACI, and AKI-ACI groups.

	NI	AKI	ACI	AKI-ACI	ACI vs. AKI	AKI-ACI vs. AKI	AKI-ACI vs. ACI
N (%)	2,601 (44.11%)	1,107 (18.78%)	557 (9.45%)	1,631 (27.66%)			
Demographics							
Age in years, mean (SEM)	57.4 (0.4)	63.6 (0.5)	72.7 (0.7)	72.1 (0.4)	*	#	
Female sex, n (%)	1,394 (53.6%)	529 (47.7%)	231 (41.4%)	674 (41.3%)		#	
Race, n (%)							
White	210 (15.9%)	86 (12.7%)	66 (18.9)	157 (15.0%)			
Black/African American	719 (54.3%)	404 (59.8%)	193 (55.1%)	642 (61.5%)			
Asian	63 (4.8%)	26 (3.8%)	19 (5.4%)	45 (4.3%)			
Other	209 (15.8%)	87 (12.9%)	44 (12.6%)	115 (11.0%)			
Unknown	122 (9.2%)	73 (10.8%)	28 (8.0%)	85 (8.2%)			
Ethnicity, n (%)							
Hispanic	1,278 (49.1%)	431 (38.9%)	207 (37.2%)	587 (36.0%)			
Non-Hispanic	1,323 (50.9%)	676 (61.1%)	350 (62.8%)	1,044 (64.0%)			
Comorbidities, n (%)							
Hypertension	669 (21.5%)	343 (31.0%)	176 (31.5%)	643 (39.4%)		#	$
COPD and asthma	259 (10.0%)	91 (8.2%)	52 (9.3%)	136 (8.3%)			
Stroke	44 (1.7%)	28 (2.5%)	16 (2.9%)	79 (4.8%)		#	
Diabetes	587 (22.6%)	334 (30.1%)	136 (24.4%)	562 (34.4%)			$
Chronic kidney disease	189 (7.3%)	180 (16.3%)	134 (24.1%)	577 (35.4%)	*	#	$
Coronary artery disease	123 (4.7%)	59 (5.3%)	77 (13.8%)	192 (11.8%)	*	#	
Heart failure	50 (1.9%)	32 (2.9%)	44 (7.9%)	140 (8.6%)	*	#	
Liver disease	34 (1.3%)	21 (1.9%)	6 (1.0%)	36 (2.7%)			
Presenting laboratory values, mean, SEM							
Troponin, ng/mL	0.01 (0.00)	0.01 (0.00)	0.20 (0.04)	0.17 (0.03)	*	#	
Brain Natriuretic Peptide (pg/mL)	265 (28)	594 (71)	3,343 (288)	3,199 (171)	*	#	
Creatinine, mg/dL	0.9 (0.01)	1.4 (0.06)	2.3 (0.16)	3.7 (0.23)	*	#	$
eGFR, mg/mL	85 (0.8)	64 (2.3)	43 (2.3)	32 (1.6)	*	#	$
Alanine aminotransferase, U/L	35 (1.0)	35 (2.3)	48 (7.9)	74 (13.9)		#	$
Aspartate aminotransferase, U/L	39 (1.0)	50 (2.7)	73 (10.8)	102 (16.9)		#	$
C-reactive protein, mg/dL	6 (0.32)	11 (0.87)	13 (1.11)	16 (0.81)		#	
D-dimer, ug/mL	1.4 (0.10)	3.6 (0.44)	5.6 (0.60)	5.7 (0.43)	*	#	
Ferritin, ng/mL	554 (35)	1,062 (146)	1,446 (236)	2,137 (505)		#	
Lactate dehydrogenase, U/L	327 (6)	454 (17)	492 (36)	543 (25)		#	
White blood cell count, x10^9/L	6.9 (0.14)	8.8 (0.33)	9.5 (0.77)	10.4 (0.36)	*	#	
Lymphocytes, x10^9/L	1.5 (0.02)	1.2 (0.06)	1.5 (0.20)	1.3 (0.06)			
Basophil x10^9/L	0.02 (0.000)	0.02 (0.002)	0.03 (0.002)	0.03 (0.001)			
Neutrophils, x10^9/L	4.7 (0.08)	6.6 (0.28)	6.6 (0.26)	8.2 (0.27)		#	$
Eosinophil x10^9/L	0.07 (0.004)	0.04 (0.009)	0.05 (0.006)	0.03 (0.005)		#	
Prothrombin time, s	14 (0.11)	15 (0.26)	16 (0.32)	17 (0.23)	*	#	
Systolic Blood Pressure, mmHg	132 (0.5)	128 (1.5)	131 (2.1)	122 (1.6)			
Pulse Oximetry (%)	97 (0.08)	96 (0.24)	94 (0.66)	94 (0.46)	*	#	
Temperature, °F	99 (0.03)	99 (0.09)	99 (0.08)	99 (0.08)			
Heart Rate, bpm	90 (0.5)	91 (1.5)	90 (1.6)	97 (1.4)			
In-hospital mortality, n (%)	80 (3.1%)	190 (17.2%)	165 (29.6%)	710 (43.5%)	*	#	$

Group comparison of categorical variables in frequencies and percentages used chi-squared test or Fisher exact tests. Group comparison of continuous variables in means and SEMs (standard error of means) used the Kruskal Wallis/Mann-Whitney U-tests.
COPD, Chronic obstructive pulmonary disease.
All values are in n (%) unless otherwise specified. Note that all variables shown of all injury groups were significant compared to those of the NI group.
*, #, $ Denote significance in pairwise comparisons.

considered statistically significant and corrected for multiple comparison using the Bonferroni method.

RESULTS

Demographics and Comorbidities

The final hospitalized COVID-19 cohort (5,896) consisted of 2,602 (44%) NI patients, 1,107 (19%) AKI-only patients, 557 (9%) ACI-only patients, and 1,631 (28%) combined injury (AKI-ACI) patients. The AKI and ACI incidences were 46.4 and 37.1%, respectively. **Table 1** summarizes patient demographics, comorbidities, and laboratory values at admission for each group. The mean ages were 57, 64, 73, and 72 years old in the NI, AKI, ACI, and AKI-ACI groups, respectively ($p < 0.05$ across groups), with ACI or AKI-ACI patients being ~15 years older compared to NI patients ($p < 0.05$). Percentages of female were 54, 48, 41, and 41% in the NI, AKI, ACI, and AKI-ACI groups, respectively ($p < 0.05$ across groups), with ~13% more males in the ACI or AKI-ACI group compared to NI group ($p < 0.05$). There were no group differences across race ($p > 0.05$) and ethnicity ($p > 0.05$).

Patients with ACI-only had more comorbidities including CKD, CAD, and CHF compared to those with AKI-only ($p < 0.05$). Patients with AKI-ACI had a higher prevalence of hypertension, stroke, CKD, CAD, and CHF than those with AKI-only ($p < 0.05$) and had significantly more hypertension, diabetes, CKD than those with ACI-only ($p < 0.05$).

To assess the relative contribution of covariates on prediction of mortality, we performed a relative weight analysis (36) for the logistic regression. The relative weights of these organ injuries, age, CKD, and heart failure were 74.33, 19.24, 1.58, and 1.24, respectively. The relative weights of other comorbidities and demographics were all <1.

Markers of Organ Injury

At hospital admission, those with combined AKI-ACI had significantly worse levels of cardiac (TNT, BNP), kidney (Cr, eGFR), liver (ALT, AST), inflammatory/immunological (LDH, neutrophils and others) markers ($p < 0.05$) followed by those with ACI or AKI ($p < 0.05$) compared to those with NI. All laboratory values of the three injury groups were significantly different from NI group ($p < 0.05$), except pulse oximetry.

For between group comparisons, those with ACI had significantly higher levels of TNT, BNP, Cr, D-dimer, WBC, prothrombin time, and lower eGFR and pulse oximetry compared to those with AKI. Patients with AKI-ACI had significantly higher levels of TNT, BNP, Cr, eGFR, ALT, AST, CRP, D-dimer, ferritin, LDH, WBC, neutrophils, eosinophil, prothrombin time, and lower pulse oximetry than those with AKI alone and significantly higher levels of Cr, eGFR, ALT, AST, and neutrophil than those with ACI alone.

In-hospital Mortality

The unadjusted mortality rates of NI, AKI, ACI, and AKI-ACI were 3.1, 17.2, 29.6, and 43.5%, respectively. Odds ratios for in-hospital mortality with adjustment for sex, age and significantly different comorbidities are summarized in **Table 2**. AKI-ACI patients had 17-fold higher odds of in-hospital mortality

TABLE 2 | Adjusted odds ratios and 95% confidence intervals for in-hospital mortality by group.

	OR	95% CI	P
AKI-ACI (ref = NI)	17.1	13.6–21.7	<0.001
ACI (ref = NI)	7.17	5.35–9.64	<0.001
AKI (ref = NI)	4.74	3.66–6.13	<0.001
AKI-ACI (ref = ACI)	1.98	1.61–2.44	<0.001
AKI-ACI (ref = AKI)	3.68	3.05–4.44	<0.001
ACI (ref = AKI)	1.78	1.39–2.29	<0.001

Covariates used in logistic regression were age, gender, ethnicity and comorbidities that showed statistically significant differences between groups.
AKI, acute kidney injury; ACI, acute cardiac injury; ref, reference; NI, no injury.

[adjusted OR (aOR) = 17.11, 95% CI = 13.63–21.66, $p < 0.001$], ACI patients had 7-fold higher odds of in-hospital mortality (aOR = 7.17, 95% CI = 5.35–9.64, $p < 0.001$), and AKI patients had 4.7-fold higher odds of in-hospital mortality (aOR = 4.74, 95% CI = 3.66–6.13, $p < 0.001$) compared to the NI cohort.

Those with combined AKI-ACI had higher risk of death than ACI alone (aOR = 1.98, 95% CI = 1.61–2.44, $p < 0.001$) and AKI alone (aOR = 3.68, 95% CI = 3.05–4.44, $p < 0.001$). The ACI group had a higher mortality rate than the AKI group (aOR = 1.78, 95% CI = 1.39–2.29, $p < 0.001$).

AKI and ACI Onset

In the AKI-only group, AKI onset peaked 1 day after hospital admission, but a significant proportion of patients developed AKI throughout the hospitalization (**Figure 2**). In contrast, in the ACI only group, ACI onset peaked and was predominantly localized to 1 day after admission. In the AKI-ACI group, the onsets of AKI and ACI were similar to those in the AKI-only and ACI-only groups.

Prediction of AKI, ACI, and AKI-ACI

The top predictors of AKI were Cr, WBC, age, diabetes, and AST, and the predictive model yielded 73 ± 5% accuracy, 93 ± 3% sensitivity, and 27 ± 10% specificity **Table 3**. The top predictors of ACI were TNT, BNP, Cr, Age, PT, and the predictive model yielded 93 ± 1% accuracy, 96 ± 1% sensitivity, and 82 ± 4% specificity. The top predictors of AKI-ACI were TNT, Cr, DDIM, BNP, PT, and the predictive model yielded 89 ± 2% accuracy, 93 ± 2% sensitivity, and 83 ± 2% specificity.

Temporal Profiles of Clinical Variables

Figure 3 depicts the time series of clinical variables relative to death or discharge for NI, AKI, ACI, and AKI-ACI groups. Overall, laboratory tests at admission were more abnormal, progressively worsened among non-survivors compared to survivors.

For non-survivors, AKI-ACI cardiac (TNT, BNP) and kidney markers (Cr, eGFR) markers were markedly worse days prior compared to the other groups, and liver markers (ALT, AST) markers were markedly elevated and early on only in the AKI-ACI, but not in AKI and ACI group. Furthermore, cell death (LDH), and immunological markers (lymphocyte, WBC,

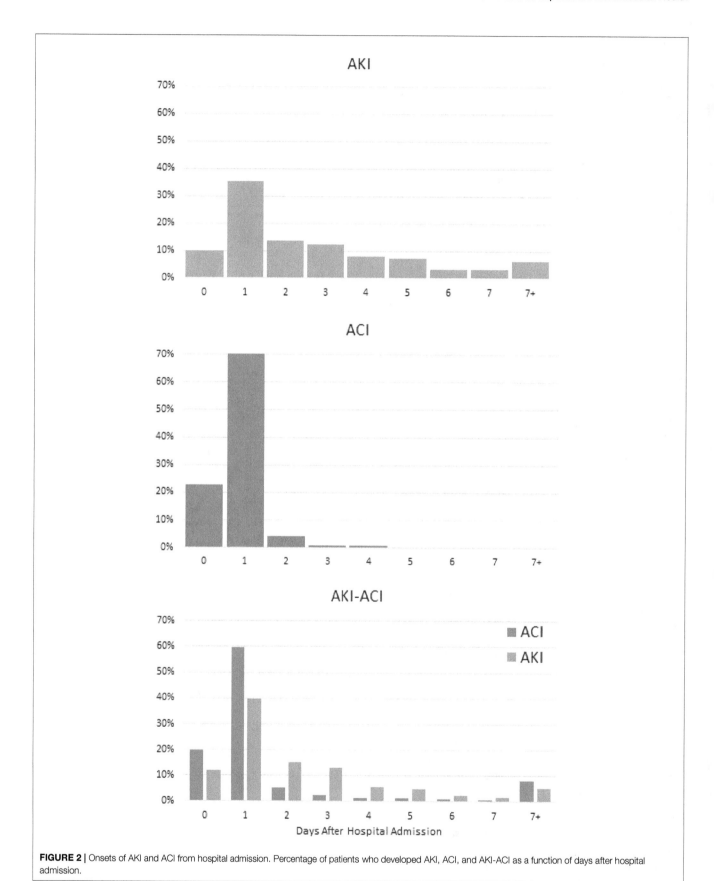

FIGURE 2 | Onsets of AKI and ACI from hospital admission. Percentage of patients who developed AKI, ACI, and AKI-ACI as a function of days after hospital admission.

TABLE 3 | Top predictors of AKI, ACI, and AKI+ACI and their performance metrics.

Cohorts	Top predictors	Accuracy	Sensitivity	Specificity
AKI	Cr, DDIM, LDH, CRP, Neutrophil	0.73 ± 0.05	0.93 ± 0.03	0.27 ± 0.10
ACI	TNT, BNP, Cr, Age, PT	0.93 ± 0.01	0.96 ± 0.01	0.82 ± 0.04
AKI-ACI	TNT, Cr, DDIM, BNP, PT	0.89 ± 0.02	0.93 ± 0.02	0.83 ± 0.02

Cr, creatine; DDIM, D-dimer; LDH, lactate dehydrogenase; CRP, C-reactive protein; TNT, troponin T; BNP, brain natriuretic peptide; PT, prothrombin time.

neutrophil, basophil, and eosinophil) were also worse days prior compared to the other groups, whereas inflammatory (CRP, D-dimer, and ferritin) and most vitals were similarly elevated in all groups.

Moreover, the temporal fluctuations of the most of these variables were markedly higher in the AKI-ACI compared to the AKI, ACI, and NI groups. These temporal fluctuations were most noticeable in the non-survivor group.

Predictors of Mortality

The top predictors of mortality in the AKI-ACI cohort were CRP, D-dimer, LDH, neutrophils, and WBC in AKI-ACI cohort. Prediction AUCs were high at days 0 and progressively decreased away from day of outcome, ranging from 0.68 to 0.89 (**Figure 4**).

DISCUSSION

This study investigated the clinical characteristics of COVID-19 patients who developed AKI and ACI during hospitalization. ACI onset occurred within a day of hospitalization in contrast to AKI onset which was more distributed across the hospitalization. Patients with AKI-ACI were significantly older, more often men and had significantly more comorbidities compared to those with AKI and NI. COVID-19 patients with AKI-ACI had more elevated levels of cardiac, kidney, liver, inflammatory and immunological markers, followed by those with ACI or AKI compared to those with NI. Patients with AKI-ACI, ACI, and AKI were, respectively, 17.1, 7.2, and 4.7 times more likely to die in the hospital compared to patients with NI. The top clinical predictors of AKI-ACI were TNT, age, Cr, WBC, BNP, and the predictive model yielded 97% accuracy, 94% sensitivity, and 72% specificity. Although physicians already know anecdotally that patients with AKI-ACI have worse outcomes, this study documented the incidence, likelihood of in-hospital mortality using odds ratio and the early clinical laboratory markers that predict which patient will develop AKI-ACI and die in the hospital.

Incidence of AKI and ACI

We observed a higher incidence of ACI (37.1%) among hospitalized COVID-19 patients compared to previously reported studies with incidences ranging from 16.1 to 23.8% (24). These differences may be explained due to differences in patient populations. Our cohort was minority-predominant and had a relatively high prevalence of cardiovascular comorbidities and lower socioeconomic status that may have been contributing factors to increased adverse cardiovascular outcomes in the

setting of COVID-19. We also observed a high incidence of AKI-ACI (28%), suggesting a strong association between AKI and ACI. This is consistent with a previous study that reported an association between AKI and cardiovascular events among COVID-19 patients in the American Heart Association COVID-19 Cardiovascular Disease Registry (37).

Risk Factors Contributing to AKI and ACI

Compared to those with NI, ACI, and AKI-ACI patients were ~15 years older and had 13% more men. Compared to AKI, ACI, and AKI-ACI patients were ~10 years older and had 6% more men, suggesting that older age and male sex are risk factors for AKI-ACI and ACI. Moreover, preexisting CKD, CAD, CHF, and stroke carried additional risks of developing ACI relative to AKI. The contributions of these additional preexisting cardiovascular comorbidities are not surprising (35, 38). Similarly, preexisting hypertension and diabetes carried additional risk of developing AKI-ACI. Notably, CKD prevalence was remarkably high (35.4%) in the AKI-ACI group compared to only 7.3% in NI, 16.3% in AKI, and 24.1% in ACI group, suggesting that having preexisting CKD markedly increases susceptibility to developing both AKI and ACI.

Having both AKI-ACI signaled a patient is 17.11 times more likely to die in the hospital compared to those without injury, whereas ACI COVID-19 patients were 7.2 times and AKI COVID-19 patients were 4.74 times more likely to die. These observations reflect the multiplicative nature of cardiac and kidney injury on risk of death and that the COVID-19 related cardiovascular event may be the driver of markedly higher mortality.

ACI develops early compared to other organ injuries. The heart may be more susceptible to early damage than other organs as heart muscle has a high density of ACE2 receptors (4, 39). The early ACI onset suggests that ACI is a primary effect of COVID-19, whereas AKI (20, 21) and acute liver injury (40) occur later in the COVID-19 clinical disease course and with more distributed onsets, suggesting that AKI and acute liver injury may arise from secondary effects of COVID-19 (i.e., systemic hypoxia, hypotension, shock, sepsis, and cytokine storm) and/or COVID-19 treatments (6, 7). These secondary effects could also contribute to sustained ACI (41–43). Cardiac injury could lead to AKI or liver injury. Our findings support consideration of pre-emptive and prophylactic treatment early in the disease course and careful monitoring of clinical variables for AKI development.

Longitudinal Characterization of Clinical Variables Associated With AKI and ACI

Patients with AKI-ACI had markedly worse cardiac, kidney and liver markers days prior to death compared to other groups, suggesting higher incidence of and more severe multi-organ injury. Furthermore, immunological markers were also worse days prior compared to the other groups, whereas inflammatory markers and most vitals were similarly elevated in all groups. These observations indicate AKI-ACI patients had differentially high levels of clinical markers that included more severe multiorgan injuries and overwhelming inflammation and immunological responses.

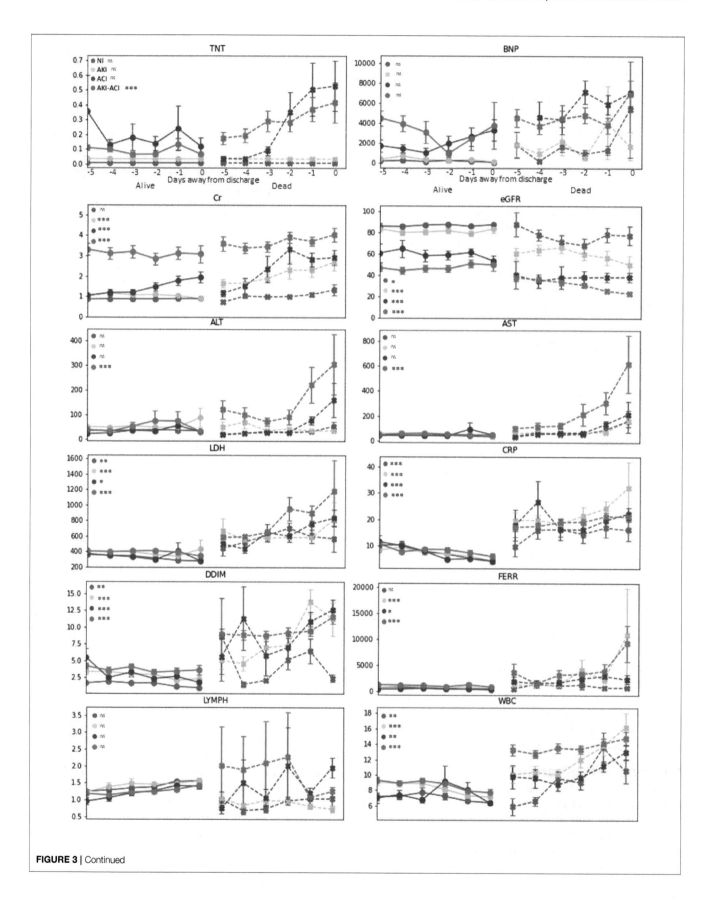

FIGURE 3 | Continued

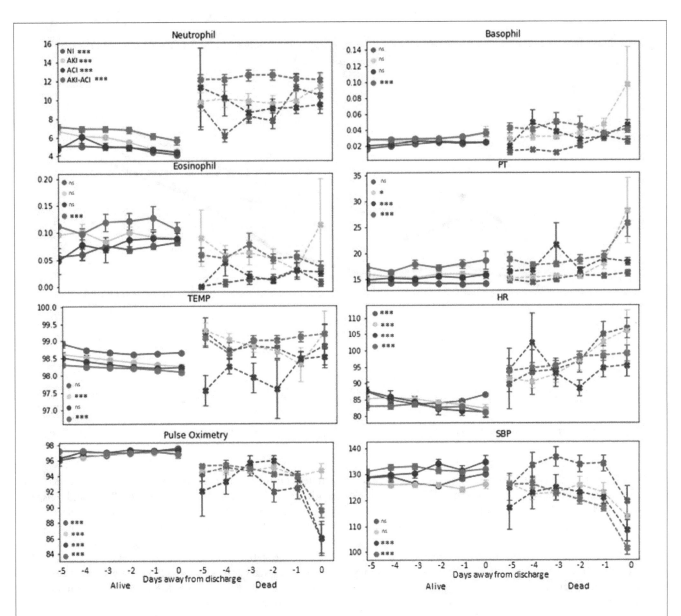

FIGURE 3 | Temporal progression of clinical variables days from outcome. Temporal progression of laboratory tests and vital signs with $t = 0$ representing day of death (for non-survivors) or day of discharge (for survivors). Error bars are SEM. *Indicates $p < 0.05$ between survivors and non-survivors. **Indicates $p < 0.01$ between survivors and non-survivors. ***Indicates $p < 0.001$ between survivors and non-survivors. ns, indicates no significant difference between survivors and non-survivors.

Significantly elevated TNT and BNP in both ACI and AKI-ACI non-survivor groups 2–3 days prior to death supports a hypothesis of heart attack or heart failure being a possible cause of death in these two groups. In contrast, TNT and BNP were not as elevated in the AKI and NI non-survivor groups. Elevated LDH and CRP seen in non-survivors in all groups are evidence of increased inflammation and immune response to infection. Similarly, elevated WBC in all non-survivors supports sepsis as a possible cause of death in all groups. The steep increase in both ALT and AST in the AKI-ACI non-survivor group points to liver damage close to death and lend evidence to multi-organ failure being a third possible cause of death.

Laboratory variables of the AKI-ACI group were temporally more unstable compared to those with AKI, ACI or NI, especially among non-survivors, suggesting these temporal profiles of clinical variables can also be used to predict mortality (44, 45).

Predicting of Mortality Associated With AKI and ACI

Understanding the temporal progression of these clinical markers allowed us to construct a prediction model. Longitudinal data accurately predicted mortality likelihood up to 5 days prior. These top predictors of mortality are consistent with a previous

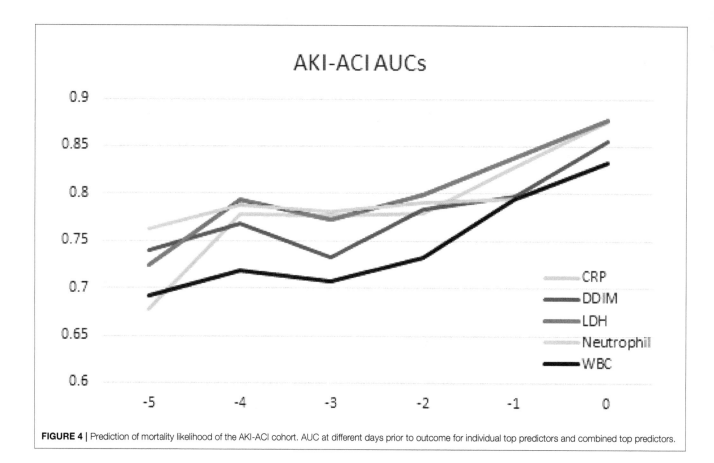

FIGURE 4 | Prediction of mortality likelihood of the AKI-ACI cohort. AUC at different days prior to outcome for individual top predictors and combined top predictors.

report (44) from a different hospital. Most published models used clinical data at admission, not longitudinal variables prior to outcomes (46–49). Prediction using the admission timepoint has relatively poor accuracy compared to a few days prior to outcome. While this finding is intuitively logical, this study provides evidence that our current model can yield a highly accurate prediction a few days prior to the outcome which may lead to earlier recognition, intervention and improvement in clinical outcomes.

Limitations
A strength of our study is that it addressed multiorgan injury with detailed clinical characteristics in a large diverse population. Our study has several limitations. This is a descriptive retrospective study that could not address the underlying cause of AKI and ACI among hospitalized patients with COVID-19. Missing certain laboratory variables could alter ranking of top predictors. We were unable to analyze how treatment of COVID-19 could have affected AKI and ACI. This study used TNT as indicator of ACI. We were unable to analyze other cardiovascular variables (such as EKGs and echocardiograms) because they would have required manual chart reviews of a large cohort of patients. We also did not study cardiac complications of atrial arrhythmias, ventricular arrhythmias, pericarditis, myocarditis, and heart failure, although this was found to be rare. Although ACI incidence and mortality among COVID-19 patients were generally higher than non-COVID-19 patients, comparison

studies controlling for age, race, and ethnicity are needed. This study came from a large population of Black and Hispanic patients and these findings may not be generalizable to other populations. Additional and prospective studies are needed. We did not investigate the effects of anticoagulants on organ injuries (50, 51), the status of the COVID-19 survivors at discharge (52, 53) and the longer-term outcomes (54). As with any retrospective study, there could be unintended patient selection bias and unaccounted confounders.

CONCLUSION

A significant number of patients hospitalized with COVID-19 developed combined AKI and ACI. These patients had additional pre-existing risk factors, worse clinical and laboratory variables, markedly worse disease courses, and increased in-hospital mortality. Predictive models using readily available laboratory variables accurately predict which patients are at risk of AKI-ACI and death. Our study has potential clinical implications for hospitalized patients with COVID-19. First, the high incidence of AKI-ACI suggest that AKI-ACI is an important marker of future adverse outcomes in COVID-19. Second, health providers should increase awareness for kidney-cardiovascular complications when AKI-ACI is detected as these complications may assume a lower priority in individuals admitted with COVID-19 given the high respiratory morbidity and mortality of this illness. Third, initiation of kidney and cardiovascular preventive therapies to mitigate kidney and cardiac damages in patients with COVID-19 may be warranted. The ability to identify patients at-risk of developing AKI-ACI early on could enable timely care.

AUTHOR CONTRIBUTIONS

JL: concept, design, collected data, analyzed data, created tables and figures, and drafted paper. AB: concept, design, collected data, analyzed data, and drafted paper. RF and WSH: concept, design, collected data, and edited paper. WH: analyzed data and drafted paper. MF and CR: concept, design, and edited paper. TD: concept, design, supervised, and edited paper. All authors contributed to the article and approved the submitted version.

REFERENCES

1. Huang C, Wang Y, Li X, Ren L, Zhao J, Hu Y, et al. Clinical features of patients infected with 2019 novel coronavirus in Wuhan, China. *Lancet.* (2020) 395:497–506. doi: 10.1016/S0140-6736(20)30183-5

2. Wang D, Hu B, Hu C, Zhu F, Liu X, Zhang J, et al. Clinical characteristics of 138 hospitalized patients with 2019 novel coronavirus-infected pneumonia in Wuhan, China. *J Am Med Assoc.* (2020) 323:1061–9. doi: 10.1001/jama.2020.1585

3. Guo T, Fan Y, Chen M, Wu X, Zhang L, He T, et al. Cardiovascular implications of fatal outcomes of patients with coronavirus disease 2019 (COVID-19). *J Am Med Assoc Cardiol.* (2020) 5:811–8. doi: 10.1001/jamacardio.2020.1017

4. Hoffmann M, Kleine-Weber H, Schroeder S, Kruger N, Herrler T, Erichsen S, et al. SARS-CoV-2 cell entry depends on ACE2 and TMPRSS2 and is blocked by a clinically proven protease inhibitor. *Cell.* (2020) 181:271–80 e278. doi: 10.1016/j.cell.2020.02.052

5. Matarese A, Gambardella J, Sardu C, Santulli G. miR-98 regulates TMPRSS2 expression in human endothelial cells: key implications for COVID-19. *Biomedicines.* (2020) 8:462. doi: 10.3390/biomedicines8110462

6. Lorenz G, Moog P, Bachmann Q, La Rosee P, Schneider H, Schlegl M, et al. Cytokine release syndrome is not usually caused by secondary hemophagocytic lymphohistiocytosis in a cohort of 19 critically ill COVID-19 patients. *Sci Rep.* (2020) 10:18277. doi: 10.1038/s41598-020-75260-w

7. Guo H, Sheng Y, Li W, Li F, Xie Z, Li J, et al. Coagulopathy as a prodrome of cytokine storm in COVID-19-infected patients. *Front Med.* (2020) 7:572989. doi: 10.3389/fmed.2020.572989

8. Quinaglia T, Shabani M, Breder I, Silber HA, Lima JAC, Sposito AC. Coronavirus disease-19: the multi-level, multi-faceted vasculopathy. *Atherosclerosis.* (2021) 322:39–50. doi: 10.1016/j.atherosclerosis.2021.02.009

9. Sardu C, Gambardella J, Morelli MB, Wang X, Marfella R, Santulli G. Hypertension, thrombosis, kidney failure, and diabetes: is COVID-19 an endothelial disease? A comprehensive evaluation of clinical and basic evidence. *J Clin Med.* (2020) 9:1417. doi: 10.3390/jcm9051417

10. Sardu C, Gargiulo G, Esposito G, Paolisso G, Marfella R. Impact of diabetes mellitus on clinical outcomes in patients affected by Covid-19. *Cardiovasc Diabetol.* (2020) 19:76. doi: 10.1186/s12933-020-01047-y

11. Sardu C, D'Onofrio N, Balestrieri ML, Barbieri M, Rizzo MR, Messina V, et al. Outcomes in patients with hyperglycemia affected by COVID-19: can we do more on glycemic control? *Diabetes Care.* (2020) 43:1408–15. doi: 10.2337/dc20-0723

12. Louis-Jean J, Cenat K, Njoku CV, Angelo J, Sanon D. Coronavirus (COVID-19) and racial disparities: a perspective analysis. *J Racial Ethn Health Disparities.* (2020) 7:1039–45. doi: 10.1007/s40615-020-00879-4

13. Hoogenboom WS, Pham A, Anand H, Fleysher R, Buczek A, Soby S, et al. Clinical characteristics of the first and second COVID-19 waves in the Bronx, New York: a retrospective cohort study. *Lancet Reg Health Am.* (2021) 3:100041. doi: 10.1016/j.lana.2021.100041

14. Wilder JM. The disproportionate impact of COVID-19 on racial and ethnic minorities in the United States. *Clin Infect Dis.* (2021) 72:707–9. doi: 10.1093/cid/ciaa959

15. Zalla LC, Martin CL, Edwards JK, Gartner DR, Noppert GA, A. Geography of risk: structural racism and coronavirus disease 2019 mortality in the United States. *Am J Epidemiol.* (2021) 190:1439–46. doi: 10.1093/aje/kwab059

16. Hamilton P, Hanumapura P, Castelino L, Henney R, Parker K, Kumar M, et al. Characteristics and outcomes of hospitalised patients with acute kidney injury and COVID-19. *PLoS ONE.* (2020) 15:e0241544. doi: 10.1371/journal.pone.0241544

17. Fisher M, Neugarten J, Bellin E, Yunes M, Stahl L, Johns TS, et al. AKI in hospitalized patients with and without COVID-19: a comparison study. *J Am Soc Nephrol.* (2020) 31:2145–57. doi: 10.1681/ASN.2020040509

18. Ouyang L, Gong Y, Zhu Y, Gong J. Association of acute kidney injury with the severity and mortality of SARS-CoV-2 infection: a meta-analysis. *Am J Emerg Med.* (2021) 43:149–57. doi: 10.1016/j.ajem.2020.08.089

19. Hirsch JS, Ng JH, Ross DW, Sharma P, Shah HH, Barnett RL, et al. Acute kidney injury in patients hospitalized with COVID-19. *Kidney Int.* (2020) 98:209–18. doi: 10.1016/j.kint.2020.05.006

20. Lu JY, Hou W, Duong TQ. Longitudinal prediction of hospital-acquired acute kidney injury in COVID-19: a two-center study. *Infection.* (2021) 2021:1–11. doi: 10.1007/s15010-021-01646-1

21. Lu JY, Babatsikos I, Fisher MC, Hou W, Duong TQ. Longitudinal clinical profiles of hospital vs. community-acquired acute kidney injury in COVID-19. *Front Med.* (2021) 8:647023. doi: 10.3389/fmed.2021.647023

22. Shi S, Qin M, Shen B, Cai Y, Liu T, Yang F, et al. Association of cardiac injury with mortality in hospitalized patients with COVID-19 in Wuhan, China. *J Am Med Assoc Cardiol.* (2020) 5:802–10. doi: 10.1001/jamacardio.2020.0950

23. Lala A, Johnson KW, Januzzi JL, Russak AJ, Paranjpe I, Richter F, et al. Prevalence and impact of myocardial injury in patients hospitalized with COVID-19 infection. *J Am Coll Cardiol.* (2020) 76:533–46. doi: 10.1016/j.jacc.2020.06.007

24. Prasitlumkum N, Chokesuwattanaskul R, Thongprayoon C, Bathini T, Vallabhajosyula S, Cheungpasitporn W. Incidence of myocardial injury in COVID-19-infected patients: a systematic review and meta-analysis. *Diseases.* (2020) 8:40. doi: 10.3390/diseases8040040

25. Zhao YH, Zhao L, Yang XC, Wang P. Cardiovascular complications of SARS-CoV-2 infection (COVID-19): a systematic review and meta-analysis. *Rev Cardiovasc Med.* (2021) 22:159–65. doi: 10.31083/j.rcm.2021.01.238

26. Wadhera RK, Wadhera P, Gaba P, Figueroa JF, Joynt Maddox KE, Yeh RW, et al. Variation in COVID-19 hospitalizations and deaths across New York City boroughs. *J Am Med Assoc.* (2020) 323:2192–5. doi: 10.1001/jama.2020.7197

27. Hoogenboom WS, Fleysher R, Soby S, Mirhaji P, Mitchell WB, Morrone KA, et al. Individuals with sickle cell disease and sickle cell trait demonstrate no increase in mortality or critical illness from COVID-19 - a fifteen hospital observational study in the Bronx, New York. *Haematologica.* (2021) 106:3014–6. doi: 10.3324/haematol.2021.279222

28. Hripcsak G, Duke JD, Shah NH, Reich CG, Huser V, Schuemie MJ, et al. Observational health data sciences and informatics (OHDSI): opportunities for observational researchers. *Stud Health Technol Inform.* (2015) 216:574–8.

29. Siew ED, Ikizler TA, Matheny ME, Shi Y, Schildcrout JS, Danciu I, et al. Estimating baseline kidney function in hospitalized patients with impaired kidney function. *Clin J Am Soc Nephrol.* (2012) 7:712–9. doi: 10.2215/CJN.10821011

30. Pelayo J, Lo KB, Bhargav R, Gul F, Peterson E, DeJoy Iii R, et al. Clinical characteristics and outcomes of community- and hospital-acquired acute kidney injury with COVID-19 in a US Inner City Hospital System. *Cardiorenal Med.* (2020) 10:223–31. doi: 10.1159/000509182

31. Reichlin T, Hochholzer W, Bassetti S, Steuer S, Stelzig C, Hartwiger S, et al. Early diagnosis of myocardial infarction with sensitive cardiac troponin assays. *N Engl J Med.* (2009) 361:858–67. doi: 10.1056/NEJMoa0900428

32. Calvo-Fernandez A, Izquierdo A, Subirana I, Farre N, Vila J, Duran X, et al. Markers of myocardial injury in the prediction of short-term COVID-19 prognosis. *Rev Esp Cardiol.* (2021) 74:576–83. doi: 10.1016/j.rec.2020.09.011

33. Thygesen K, Alpert JS, Jaffe AS, Chaitman BR, Bax JJ, Morrow DA, et al. Fourth universal definition of myocardial infarction (2018). *Circulation.* (2018) 138:e618–51. doi: 10.1161/CIR.0000000000000617

34. Frager SZ, Szymanski J, Schwartz JM, Massoumi HS, Kinkhabwala M, Wolkoff AW. Hepatic predictors of mortality in severe acute respiratory syndrome coronavirus 2: role of initial aspartate aminotransferase/alanine aminotransferase and preexisting cirrhosis. *Hepatol Commun.* (2021) 5:424–33. doi: 10.1002/hep4.1648

35. Maynard C, Lowy E, Rumsfeld J, Sales AE, Sun H, Kopjar B, et al. The prevalence and outcomes of in-hospital acute myocardial infarction in the Department of Veterans Affairs Health System. *Arch Intern Med.* (2006) 166:1410–6. doi: 10.1001/archinte.166.13.1410

36. Tonidandel S, LeBreton JM, Johnson JW. Determining the statistical significance of relative weights. *Psychol Methods.* (2009) 14:387–99. doi: 10.1037/a0017735

37. Rao A, Ranka S, Ayers C, Hendren N, Rosenblatt A, Alger HM, et al. Association of kidney disease with outcomes in COVID-19: results from the American Heart Association COVID-19 cardiovascular disease registry. *J Am Heart Assoc.* (2021) 10:e020910. doi: 10.1161/JAHA.121.020910

38. Bradley SM, Borgerding JA, Wood GB, Maynard C, Fihn SD. Incidence, risk factors, and outcomes associated with in-hospital acute myocardial infarction. *J Am Med Assoc Netw Open.* (2019) 2:e187348. doi: 10.1001/jamanetworkopen.2018.7348

39. Lam KW, Chow KW, Vo J, Hou W, Li H, Richman PS, et al. Continued in-hospital ACE inhibitor and ARB Use in hypertensive COVID-19 patients is associated with positive clinical outcomes. *J Infect Dis.* (2020) 222:1256–64. doi: 10.1093/infdis/jiaa447

40. Lu JY, Anand H, Frager SZ, Hou W, Duong TQ. Longitudinal progression of clinical variables associated with graded liver injury in COVID-19 patients. *Hepatol Int.* (2021). doi: 10.1007/s12072-021-10228-0

41. Oudit GY, Kassiri Z, Jiang C, Liu PP, Poutanen SM, Penninger JM, et al. SARS-coronavirus modulation of myocardial ACE2 expression and inflammation in patients with SARS. *Eur J Clin Invest.* (2009) 39:618–25. doi: 10.1111/j.1365-2362.2009.02153.x

42. Zhu N, Zhang D, Wang W, Li X, Yang B, Song J, et al. A novel coronavirus from patients with pneumonia in China, 2019. *N Engl J Med.* (2020) 382:727–33. doi: 10.1056/NEJMoa2001017

43. Xu X, Chen P, Wang J, Feng J, Zhou H, Li X, et al. Evolution of the novel coronavirus from the ongoing Wuhan outbreak and modeling of its spike protein for risk of human transmission. *Sci China Life Sci.* (2020) 63:457–60. doi: 10.1007/s11427-020-1637-5

44. Chen A, Zhao Z, Hou W, Singer AJ, Li H, Duong TQ. Time-to-death longitudinal characterization of clinical variables and longitudinal prediction of mortality in COVID-19 patients: a two-center study. *Front Med.* (2021) 8:661940. doi: 10.3389/fmed.2021.661940

45. Hou W, Zhao Z, Chen A, Li H, Duong TQ. Machining learning predicts the need for escalated care and mortality in COVID-19 patients from clinical variables. *Int J Med Sci.* (2021) 18:1739–45. doi: 10.7150/ijms.51235

46. Wynants L, Van Calster B, Collins GS, Riley RD, Heinze G, Schuit E, et al. Prediction models for diagnosis and prognosis of covid-19 infection: systematic review and critical appraisal. *BMJ.* (2020) 369:m1328. doi: 10.1101/2020.03.24.20041020

47. Zhu JS, Ge P, Jiang C, Zhang Y, Li X, Zhao Z, et al. Deep-learning artificial intelligence analysis of clinical variables predicts mortality in COVID-19 patients. *J Am Coll Emerg Physicians Open.* (2020) 1:1364–73. doi: 10.1002/emp2.12205

48. Li X, Ge P, Zhu J, Li H, Graham J, Singer A, et al. Deep learning prediction of likelihood of ICU admission and mortality in COVID-19 patients using clinical variables. *PeerJ.* (2020) 8:e10337. doi: 10.7717/peerj.10337

49. Zhao Z, Chen A, Hou W, Graham JM, Li H, Richman PS. Prediction model and risk scores of ICU admission and mortality in COVID-19. *PLoS ONE.* (2020) 15:e0236618. doi: 10.1371/journal.pone.0236618

50. Hoogenboom WS, Lu JQ, Musheyev B, Borg L, Janowicz R, Pamlayne S, et al. Prophylactic versus therapeutic dose anticoagulation effects on survival among critically ill patients with COVID-19. *PLoS ONE* (2022) 17:e0262811. doi: 10.1371/journal.pone.0262811

51. Sadeghipour P, Talasaz AH, Rashidi F, Sharif-Kashani B, Beigmohammadi MT, Farrokhpour M, et al. Effect of intermediate-dose vs standard-dose prophylactic anticoagulation on thrombotic events, extracorporeal membrane oxygenation treatment, or mortality among patients with COVID-19 admitted to the intensive care unit: the inspiration randomized clinical trial. *JAMA.* (2021) 325:1620–30. doi: 10.1001/jama.2021.4152

52. Musheyev B, Borg L, Janowicz R, Matarlo M, Boyle H, Singh G, et al. Functional status of mechanically ventilated COVID-19 survivors at ICU and hospital discharge. *J Intens Care.* (2021) 9:31. doi: 10.1186/s40560-021-00542-y

53. Musheyev B, Janowicz R, Borg L, Matarlo M, Boyle H, Hou W, et al. Characterizing non-critically ill COVID-19 survivors with and without in-hospital rehabilitation. *Sci Rep.* (2021) 11:21039. doi: 10.1038/s41598-021-00246-1

54. Lu JQ, Lu JY, Wang W, Liu Y, Buczek A, Flyeysher R, et al. Clinical predictors of acute cardiac injury and normalization of troponin after hospital discharge from COVID-19. *EBiomed.* (2022). doi: 10.1016/j.ebiom.2022.103821. [In Press].

24

Hospitalized Children with Familial Hypercholesterolemia and COVID-19: A Case for Preventive Anticoagulation

Alpo Vuorio [1,2*†], Frederick Raal [3†] and Petri T. Kovanen [4†]

[1] Mehiläinen Airport Health Centre, Vantaa, Finland, [2] Department of Forensic Medicine, University of Helsinki, Helsinki, Finland, [3] Faculty of Health Sciences, University of Witwatersrand, Johannesburg, South Africa, [4] Atherosclerosis Laboratory, Wihuri Research Institute, Helsinki, Finland

*Correspondence:
Alpo Vuorio
alpo.vuorio@gmail.com

†These authors have contributed equally to this work

Keywords: familial hypercholesterolemia, COVID-19, D-dimer, anticoagulation, endotheliitis

INTRODUCTION

Heterozygous familial hypercholesterolemia (HeFH) affects about one in 200 to 250 persons or over 30 million people worldwide, of whom about 20–25% are children and adolescents (1, 2). In those with HeFH, the level of serum low-density lipoprotein cholesterol (LDL-C) is elevated about two-fold from birth (3). If left untreated, the severe hypercholesterolemia causes pre-mature atherosclerosis. The standard treatment in HeFH children is statin therapy, which should start when the child is between 8 and 12 years of age (4). Homozygous familial hypercholesterolemia (HoFH) is the severe form of familial hypercholesterolemia (FH) affecting approximately 1 in 300,000 persons worldwide and causing four- to five-fold elevated levels of serum LDL-C (5). Despite the availability of multiple lipid-lowering therapies most HoFH patients do not achieve sufficiently low LDL-C levels, and accordingly are at high risk of symptomatic atherosclerotic cardiovascular disease already in childhood (6). In fact, there have been several case reports of sudden cardiac death due to fatal myocardial infarction in children with HoFH before the age of 10 years (7). Of note, the majority of the clinical studies performed on FH patients have included only the much more common form of FH, i.e., HeFH. Accordingly, when we refer to mere "FH," we refer to studies with HeFH patients, unless specified otherwise.

ENDOTHELIAL DYSFUNCTION IN FAMILIAL HYPERCHOLESTEROLEMIA

The significantly elevated serum LDL-C causes endothelial dysfunction already in young children with FH (8, 9). Additionally, many FH patients have raised serum levels of lipoprotein(a) [Lp(a)] (10). Thus, endothelial function in FH children can be severely compromised when both LDL-C and Lp(a) levels are increased (8). Moreover, compared with unaffected controls, FH children display a proinflammatory and prothrombotic phenotype which is associated with vascular dysfunction (11). Because Lp(a) is circulating in the blood, both proinflammatory and antifibrinolytic (i.e., prothrombotic) effects may extend from the macrovascular to the microvascular level, so affecting the entire circulatory system. Furthermore, because Lp(a) inhibits fibrinolysis, the risk of forming non-occluding or occluding thrombi is increased in FH children, in contrast to non-FH children with a primarily healthy endothelium (12).

COVID-19–AN ENDOTHELIAL DISEASE

COVID-19 is considered to be an endothelial disease (13). Thus, the effect of this disease on vessel wall endothelial linings should particularly affect FH patients with COVID-19, in whom the already dysfunctional endothelium is acutely exposed to additional damaging insults caused by the excessive immunoinflammatory response of the host (i.e., the cytokine storm) and because the coronavirus can damage the endothelial cells also directly thereby leading to "endotheliitis" (13, 14). When exposed to inflammatory and infectious signals, the normally anticoagulant, antithrombotic, and profibrinolytic endothelial cells become activated and locally promote the activation of the coagulation cascade and thrombus formation. The pro-coagulant/pro-aggregatory, pro-inflammatory, vasoconstrictor, pro-oxidant, and barrier function-impairing properties of such damaged endothelium then critically contribute to the multiorgan failure characteristic of advanced stages of COVID-19.

COVID-19 IS A PROTHROMBOTIC STATE

A recent autopsy study revealed that adult COVID-19 patients frequently have fibrin microthrombi in the heart without acute ischemic injury (15). The risk of developing such non-occluding or even occluding cardiac microthrombi is likely to be higher in children with FH. According to the results of a recent meta-analysis, among hospitalized adult patients with COVID-19, the prevalence of acute myocardial infarction was 3.3% (95% CI 0.3–8.5) (16). Therefore, the possibility that children with FH, particularly those with HoFH and COVID-19, are at increased risk of coronary thrombus formation and, despite their young age, may be at risk for an ischemic cardiac event (6).

Current data have demonstrated a COVID-19-induced prothrombotic state in children, as reflected by elevated D-dimer levels (17). This prothrombotic state can be further followed in the clinical setting by using a diagnostic disseminated intravascular coagulation (DIC) score, which has been established by The International Society on Thrombosis and Haemostasis (ISTH) (18, 19). The ISTH DIC score is taking into account several mechanisms related to the DIC syndrome which is characterized by widespread intravascular activation of coagulation. The pathophysiological mechanisms include, among others, cytokine-initiated inflammatory activation of coagulation and insufficient control of anticoagulant pathways, which together lead to endothelial dysfunction and microvascular thrombosis (19). The usefulness of the ISTH DIC score was shown in a retrospective large cohort study of 1,127 adult COVID-19 patients in Spain (20). In this study, the initial ISTH DIC score was significantly higher among the ultimately non-surviving patients.

Al-Ghafry et al. (21) recently published a case series of eight hospitalized COVID-19 pediatric patients, in which the coagulation profiles were determined. Six children had elevated D-dimer levels and required oxygen supplementation, and five children also required intensive care unit treatment. The authors carried out rotational thromboelastometry and found an increased blood clot firmness with a contribution from fibrinogen. Based on these laboratory findings, the children of whom the youngest were 8 years old received anticoagulation according to institutional adult anticoagulation guidelines, and no thromboembolic complications were observed in the treated children. Based on the above findings there is a potential need to expand and study the indication for prophylactic anticoagulation in hospitalized children with COVID-19 (22) to children with FH, provided there are no contraindications to anticoagulant therapy. Furthermore, in FH children, it is essential to continue effective statin therapy because statins not only improve endothelial function but also decrease serum D-dimer levels by about 15%, thus providing additional mild anticoagulation (23, 24). Moreover, because proprotein convertase subtilisin/kexin type 9 (PCSK9) inhibitors effectively lower serum LDL-C concentration, reduce the Lp(a) level by about 30%, and may also enhance the antiviral action of interferon in patients with hypercholesterolemia, the use of these inhibitors could be considered in hospitalized pediatric FH patients with COVID-19, particularly those with HoFH, if not already in use (25–27).

DISCUSSION

Results from controlled studies investigating the clinical effects of anticoagulation in hospitalized children with COVID-19 are lacking. Meanwhile, Loi et al. (22) have recommended that children with COVID-19 are eligible for anticoagulation. Based on the considerations presented here and on a recent expert consensus-based pediatric opinion (28), anticoagulant prophylaxis in children should be carried out (in the absence of any contraindications) by using low-dose low-molecular-weight heparin. Loi et al. also recommend that, in hospitalized children with COVID-19, it is important to trend the disseminated intravascular coagulation score with attention to the D-dimer level. Additionally, a pediatric risk assessment and consideration of prophylactic anticoagulation to prevent thrombosis should be performed at baseline and daily thereafter. When considering that FH is a prothrombotic condition by itself, the above recommendations would particularly apply to hospitalized FH children with COVID-19 (10, 29). This idea is supported by the above consensus-based clinical recommendation for anticoagulation in children hospitalized for COVID-19-related illnesses (28).

AUTHOR CONTRIBUTIONS

AV: writing the first draft. AV, FR, and PK: reviewing and editing to produce the final draft. All authors contributed to the article and approved the submitted version.

REFERENCES

1. Wiegman A, Gidding SS, Watts GF, Chapman MJ, Ginsberg HN, Cuchel M, et al. Familial hypercholesterolaemia in children and adolescents: gaining decades of life by optimizing detection and treatment. *Eur Heart J.* (2015) 36:2425–37. doi: 10.1093/eurheartj/ehv157

2. Representatives of the Global Familial Hypercholesterolemia Community, Wilemon KA, Patel J, Aguilar-Salinas C, Ahmed CD, Alkhnifsawi M, et al. Reducing the Clinical and Public Health Burden of Familial Hypercholesterolemia: A Global Call to Action. *JAMA Cardiol.* (2020) 5:217–229. doi: 10.1001/jamacardio.2019.5173

3. Vuorio AF, Turtola H, Kontula K. Neonatal diagnosis of familial hypercholesterolemia in newborns born to a parent with a molecularly defined heterozygous familial hypercholesterolemia. *Arterioscler Thromb Vasc Biol.* (1997) 17:3332–7. doi: 10.1161/01.ATV.17.11.3332

4. Vuorio A, Kuoppala J, Kovanen PT, Humphries SE, Tonstad S, Wiegman A, et al. Statins for children with familial hypercholesterolemia. *Cochrane Database Syst Rev.* (2019) 2019:CD006401. doi: 10.1002/14651858.CD006401.pub5

5. Sjouke B, Hovingh GK, Kastelein JJ, Stefanutti C. Homozygous autosomal dominant hypercholesterolaemia: prevalence, diagnosis, and current and future treatment perspectives. *Curr Opin Lipidol.* (2015) 26:200–9. doi: 10.1097/MOL.0000000000000179

6. Cuchel M, Bruckert E, Ginsberg HN, Raal FJ, Santos RD, Hegele RA. Homozygous familial hypercholesterolaemia: new insights and guidance for clinicians to improve detection and clinical management. A position paper from the Consensus Panel on Familial Hypercholesterolaemia of the european atherosclerosis society. *Eur Heart J.* (2014) 35:2146–57. doi: 10.1093/eurheartj/ehu274

7. Gautschi M, Pavlovic M, Nuoffer JM. Fatal myocardial infarction at 4.5 years in a case of homozygous familial hypercholesterolaemia. *JIMD Rep.* (2012) 2:45–50. doi: 10.1007/8904_2011_45

8. Sorensen KE, Celermajer DS, Georgakopoulos D, Hatcher G, Betteridge DJ, Deanfield JE. Impairment of endothelium-dependent dilation is an early event in children with familial hypercholesterolemia and is related to the lipoprotein(a) level. *J Clin Invest.* (1994) 93:50–5. doi: 10.1172/JCI116983

9. Nenseter MS, Bogsrud MP, Græsdal A, Narverud I, Halvorsen B, Ose L, et al. LDL-apheresis affects markers of endothelial function in patients with homozygous familial hypercholesterolemia. *Thromb Res.* (2012) 130:823–5. doi: 10.1016/j.thromres.2012.06.004

10. Vuorio A, Watts GF, Schneider WJ, Tsimikas S, Kovanen PT. Familial hypercholesterolemia and elevated lipoprotein(a): double heritable risk and new therapeutic opportunities. *J Intern Med.* (2020) 287:2–18. doi: 10.1111/joim.12981

11. Charakida M, Tousoulis D, Skoumas I, Pitsavos C, Vasiliadou C, Stefanadi E, et al. Inflammatory and thrombotic processes are associated with vascular dysfunction in children with familial hypercholesterolemia. *Atherosclerosis.* (2009) 204:532–7. doi: 10.1016/j.atherosclerosis.2008.09.025

12. Cyranoski D. Why healthy arteries may help lead to avoid Covid complications. *Nature.* (2020) 582:324–5. doi: 10.1038/d41586-020-01692-z

13. Libby P, Lüscher T. COVID-19 is, in the end, an endothelial disease. *Eur Heart J.* (2020) 41:3038–44. doi: 10.1093/eurheartj/ehaa623

14. Varga Z, Flammer AJ, Steiger P, Haberecker M, Andermatt R, Zinkernagel AS, et al. Endothelial cell infection and endotheliitis in COVID-19. *Lancet.* (2020) 395:1417–8. doi: 10.1016/S0140-6736(20)30937-5

15. Bois MC, Boire NA, Layman AJ, Aubry MC, Alexander MP, Roden AC, et al. COVID-19-associated non-occlusive fibrin microthrombi in the heart. *Circulation.* (2020) 143:230–4. doi: 10.1161/CIRCULATIONAHA.120.050754

16. Kunutsor SK, Laukkanen JA. Incidence of venous and arterial thromboembolic complications in COVID-19: a systematic review and meta-analysis. *Thromb Res.* (2020) 196:27–30. doi: 10.1016/j.thromres.2020.08.022

17. Hoang A, Chorath K, Moreira A, Evans M, Burmeister-Morton F, Burnmeister F, et al. COVID-19 in 7780 pediatric patients: a systematic review. *EClinicalMedicine.* (2020) 24:100433. doi: 10.1016/j.eclinm.2020.100433

18. Taylor FBJr, Toh CH, Hoots WK, Wada H, Levi M. Towards definition, clinical and laboratory criteria, and a scoring system for disseminated intravascular coagulation. *J Thromb Haemost.* (2001) 86:1327–30. doi: 10.1055/s-0037-1616068

19. Gando S, Levi M, Toh CH. Disseminated intravascular coagulation. *Nat Rev Dis Primers.* (2016) 2:16037. doi: 10.1007/978-3-319-28308-1_13

20. Muñoz-Rivas N, Abad-Motos A, Mestre-Gómez B, Sierra-Hidalgo F, Cortina-Camarero C, Lorente-Ramos RM, et al. Systemic thrombosis in a large cohort of COVID-19 patients despite thromboprophylaxis: a retrospective study. *Thromb Res.* (2021) 199:132–42. doi: 10.1016/j.thromres.2020.12.024

21. Al-Ghafry M, Aygun B, Appiah-Kubi A, Vlachos A, Ostovar G, Capone C, et al. Are children with SARS-CoV-2 infection at high risk for thrombosis? Viscoelastic testing and coagulation profiles in a case series of pediatric patients *Pediatr Blood Cancer.* (2020) 67:e28737. doi: 10.1002/pbc.28737

22. Loi M, Branchford B, Kim J, Self C, Nuss R. COVID-19 anticoagulation recommendations in children. *Pediatr Blood Cancer.* (2020) 67:e28485. doi: 10.1002/pbc.28485

23. Undas A, Brummel-Ziedins KE, Mann KG. Anticoagulant effects of statins and their clinical implications. *Thromb Haemost.* (2014) 111:392–400. doi: 10.1160/TH13-08-0720

24. Schol-Gelok S, van der Hulle T, Biedermann JS, van Gelder T, Leebeek FWG, Lijfering WM, et al. Clinical effects of antiplatelet drugs and statins on D-dimer levels. *Eur J Clin Invest.* (2018) 48:e12944. doi: 10.1111/eci.12944

25. Kastelein JJ, Ginsberg HN, Langslet G, Hovingh GK, Ceska R, Dufour R, et al. ODYSSEY FH I and FH II: 78 week results with alirocumab treatment in 735 patients with heterozygous familial hypercholesterolaemia. *Eur Heart J.* (2015) 36:2996–3003. doi: 10.1093/eurheartj/ehv370

26. Santos RD, Ruzza A, Hovingh GK, Wiegman A, Mach F, Kurtz CE. Evolocumab in pediatric heterozygous familial hypercholesterolemia. *N Engl J Med.* (2020) 383:1317–27. doi: 10.1056/NEJMoa2019910

27. Vuorio A, Kovanen PT. PCSK9 inhibitors for COVID-19: an opportunity to enhance the antiviral action of interferon in patients with hypercholesterolemia. *J Intern Med.* (2020). doi: 10.1111/joim.13210. [Epub ahead of print].

28. Goldenberg NA, Sochet A, Albisetti M, Biss T, Bonduel M, Jaffray J, et al. Consensus-based clinical recommendations and research priorities for anticoagulant thromboprophylaxis in children hospitalized for COVID-19-related illness. *J Thromb Haemost.* (2020) 18:3099–105. doi: 10.1111/jth.15073

29. Vuorio A, Kovanen PT. Prevention of endothelial dysfunction and thrombotic events in COVID-19 patients with familial hypercholesterolemia. *J Clin Lipidol.* (2020) 14:617–8. doi: 10.1016/j.jacl.2020.06.006

25

Mitochondria, a Missing Link in COVID-19 Heart Failure and Arrest?

Ralph Ryback[1]* and Alfonso Eirin[2]

[1] *Mindful Health Foundation, Naples, FL, United States,* [2] *Department of Internal Medicine, Division of Nephrology and Hypertension, Mayo Clinic, Rochester, MN, United States*

***Correspondence:**
Ralph Ryback
rsryback@gmail.com;
ralphrybackmd.com

Keywords: COVID-19, mitochondria, heart failure, cardiovascular disease, ATP

Over the last 2 years, we have all been trying to understand the interrelationships of COVID-19's numerous symptoms, clinical risk factors, and lethality. Autopsy cases of patients with COVID-19 revealed that the virus was present in the heart of more than 60% of patients, associated with evidence of active viral replication, suggesting direct viral cardiac infection (1). Contrarily, a recent study reported that the virus was detected in the heart of only one out of 30 patients who died after a prolonged hospital stay due to Sars-Cov-2 infection., associated with modest histological alterations (2). Macroscopic, histological, and immunohistochemical analysis revealed modest cardiac histological alterations, underscoring the lack of evidence to establish the contribution of a direct effect of SARS-CoV-2 on cardiac lesions. Mehra and Ruschitzka (3) noted in the elderly, especially with cardiovascular disease, mortality was associated with a very significant elevation of natriuretic peptides (NPs) with death attributed to cardiac failure and arrest in almost 25% of cases. They wondered whether cardiac inflammation or dysfunction suggested by elevated NP's might play a role in the respiratory hypoxic failure observed in COVID-19. NPs, hormones secreted from the heart, have many functions including promoting Na^+, excretion by the kidney. In addition, NPs are involved in important mitochondrial mediated processes including Ca^{2+} signaling, apoptosis, reactive oxygen species production, biogenesis, and fat oxidation, etc. (4). Cardiac followed by kidney cells have the highest mitochondrial content (high ATP energy needs) and thus their function is directly dependent on mitochondrial health (4). However, cardiac mitochondrial function extends well-beyond energy production and includes modulation of numerous cellular signaling pathways at molecular and biochemical levels (5). Thus, mitochondrial damage has a tremendous impact on overall cardiomyocyte function.

Evidence reveals the virus localizes to mitochondria which it attacks and disrupts (**Figure 1**), thereby taking energy away from the cells' battle with the virus including autophagy (6, 7). In this process, SARS-CoV-2 manipulates mitochondrial function by angiotensin-converting enzyme 2 (ACE2) regulation and open-reading frames (ORFs) to evade host cell immunity and facilitate virus replication. The virus-encoded protein Orf-96 localizes to mitochondria and triggers degradation of mitochondria-related genes, including DRP1, MAVS, TRAF3, and TRAF6 (8). ORFs, such as ORF3a, can target the mitochondrial deubiquitinase USP30, altering mitochondrial homeostasis (biogenesis, fusion, fission, and mitophagy) and function (9). Furthermore, the 3a protein of the virus promotes mitochondrial apoptosis (10). In cellular homeostasis, there is a balance between the BCL-2 family protein, which are neuroprotective and Bax proteins which can be transformed to set off a cell-death cascade. This can occur in response to extracellular stimulation by stress, viral infection, excessive immune cytokines secretions, etc. Bax exist in a relatively stable molecular form, but with viral infection it changes form and moves to the outer membrane of the mitochondria where it inserts itself, causing the release of the cytochrome c, initiating apoptosis (10) with the release of its DNA. In addition, the 3a protein promotes activation of truncated Bid (tBid) which form pores in the mitochondria, favoring the release of apoptogenic factors. The unique DNA of the degraded mitochondria is then released into the blood whose presence at high levels has now been reported (11) to predict poor COVID-19 outcomes.

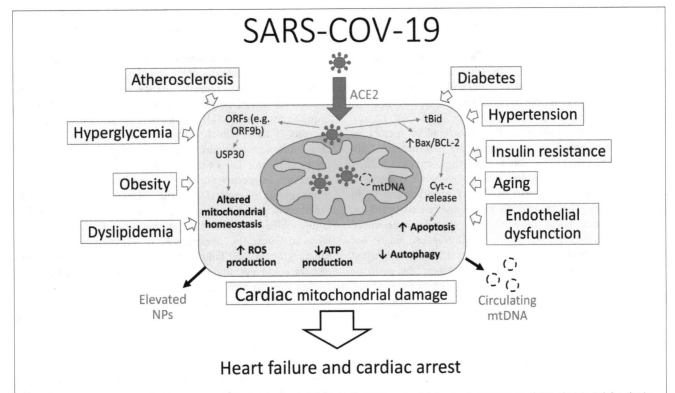

FIGURE 1 | Interplay of mechanisms of cardiac mitochondrial damage in COVID-19. Viral RNA and protein localize to mitochondria and manipulate their function by angiotensin-converting enzyme 2 (ACE2) regulation and open-reading frames (ORFs) to evade host cell immunity and facilitate virus replication. ORFs can target the mitochondrial deubiquitinase USP30, altering mitochondrial homeostasis and function. The virus promotes activation of truncated Bid (tBid) and alters Bax/BCL-2 ratio, favoring the release of apoptogenic factors. Concomitantly, several cardiovascular risk factors can compromise mitochondrial integrity and function by decreasing ATP levels and increasing reactive oxygen species (ROS) production. This in turn leads to cardiac mitochondrial damage and heart failure, associated with elevation of natriuretic peptides (NPs) and circulating mitochondrial DNA (mtDNA).

Importantly, pre-existent mitochondrial damage might exacerbate cardiomyocyte injury and dysfunction. It seems pertinent that all of the clinical risk factors (atherosclerosis, age, obesity, hypertension, and other conditions such as endothelial dysfunction) share impaired mitochondrial respiration, or a decrease in its ability to produce ATP. Hypertension, one of the main risk factors for SARS-COV and SARS-COV-19, is "prominently associated with the loss of cardiolipin" (12), a phospholipid uniquely found in the inner mitochondrial membrane and necessary for its proper formation and function. Furthermore, cardiolipin regulates mitochondrial dynamics and prevents the formation and opening of the mitochondrial permeability transition pore (mPTP), and release of cytochrome C to the cytosol. Hypertension is part of a process whereby a hole is opened in the "armored nuclear power plant" of the mitochondria that can be pierced and destroyed by SARS-COV-19.

Similarly, insulin resistance in skeletal muscle, a major hallmark of type 2 diabetes and obesity, has been linked to decreased muscle mitochondria reproduction and dysfunction (13). Endothelial cells exposed to high glucose concentrations exhibit augmented mitochondrial superoxide generation, which damages lipids, proteins, and mtDNA, and contributes to cellular oxidative stress (14). The uncoupled mitochondrial state is

necessary for ATP synthesis. Excessive mitochondrial coupling is a central expression of "dysfunction in obesity that may contribute to the development of metabolic pathologies such as insulin resistance and diabetes" (15). Cardiac mitochondria also deteriorate with age, losing respiratory activity, accumulating damage to their DNA (mtDNA), and producing excessive amounts of reactive oxygen species (ROS), ultimately increasing susceptibility to infections (16). Therefore, results from these studies are consistent with established mitochondrial injury that may aggravate cardiac damage and accelerate COVID-19-related mortality rates in patients with cardiovascular risk factors.

Recent evidence suggests that cardiac troponin I (cTnI), an important structural protein implicated in contraction and relaxation of cardiomyocytes, is a critical biomarker of myocardial injury in COVID-19 and is directly related to survival (17). Interestingly, mitochondrial structure and function are significantly impaired in cardiomyocytes with mutated cTnI, suggesting an important role of this protein in maintaining the structural and functional integrity of myocardial mitochondria (18). Thus, monitoring cTnI may be useful to assess cardiac mitochondrial damage and disease progression in patients with COVID-19.

Beyond mediating damage of infected cardiac cells, mitochondria are emerging as critical components of the innate immune response. It has been shown that the ATP needed for purinergic signaling (e.g., adenosine and ATP), T-cell regulation, and initial activation of neutrophils comes from mitochondria. ATP production and mitochondrial Ca^{2+} buffering are needed for antigen presentation and processing, and ROS are a part of the signaling pathway that activates inflammatory proteins (19). As mediators of immunity, mitochondria are consequently targeted by several viruses, including the SARS-CoV-2 virus. As noted, Orf-96 localizes on the mitochondrial membrane and suppresses type 1 interferon responses (20). Immune cells (and all cells) cannot function without their multiple healthy mitochondria. With aging, immune T cells don't respond as well to pathogens or vaccines as T cells' mitochondria begin to malfunction. This is reflected in the age related cognitive, cardiovascular, physical, metabolic, etc. changes, experienced and observed. Nevertheless, poor T cell response might not only be the result of aging but may be part of the cause of aging by releasing excessive inflammatory cytokines (the cytokine storm). When T cell mitochondria had been genetically modified (TFAM deficiency) to be energy production inefficient, it forced T cells from ATP into a less efficient mode of energy production. These mice rapidly aged with deterioration in their functions noted previously. "T cell metabolic failure induces the accumulation of circulating cytokines, characteristic of aging ('inflammaging'). This cytokine storm itself acts as a systemic inducer of senescence" (21).

A major immune defense against viral infection necessary for cellular viability, is autophagy. It delivers viral proteins and viruses to lysosomes for degradation. However, lysosomes are impaired by the loss of mitochondrial function (22) such as in SARS-COV, and COV-19 related impairments. "Inflammaging" and decreased autophagy accelerate the metabolic compromised state of people with known risk factors. It is no surprise that our young are more resilient since they usually generate sufficient ATP. However, when elevated blood mtDNA is found even in seemingly younger healthier patients and others, it reflects severe complications that can lead to ICU care and even death (11). All of the 97 adult subjects had COVID-19, but those that died had

higher cell free plasma levels of mtDNA and fragments derived from mitochondrial encoded gene cytochrome B (MT-CYTB). MT-CYTB levels were highly correlated with plasma SC5b-9, which is "a marker of complement activation and suggests the formation of a membrane attack complex" (11).

Many questions remain unanswered including, is the appearance of mtDNA just part of an "over exuberant innate immune response?" (11). Would viral infection trigger cellular necrosis if their mitochondria remained more intact? Does viral induced mitochondrial dysfunction underlie the myocardial injury observed? Does the appearance of plasma mtDNA and MT-CYTB fragments portend a possible cascade of negative immunologic responses? Are the extreme elevations in NPs observed in part a hormonal response to protect and stabilize failing cardiac mitochondrial respiration and/or an expression thereof? Given the importance of mitochondria in kidney function, could their failure be expressed as excess deaths from end-stage kidney failure early in the pandemic? (23). Could finding ways to protect cardiac mitochondrial function open a whole new field of prevention or even treatment?

Studies have demonstrated that normalizing tubular cell mitochondrial function and energy balance could be a preventative strategy in kidney disease (24). Moreover, targeting the regulation of mitochondrial biogenesis and/or correcting abnormal electron chain function, can improve renal disease outcome. Could acute IV infusion of beta-hydroxybutyrate, the body's primary ketone body, improve cardiac mitochondrial respiration? This is supported by studies in healthy, and heart failure patients showing improved hemodynamic and cardiac output (25). Undoubtedly, additional studies are needed to establish the exact role of cardiac mitochondrial damage in the setting of COVID-19 and heart failure.

AUTHOR CONTRIBUTIONS

RR and AE conceived the manuscript, revised the drafts, and approved the submitted version. Both authors contributed to the article and approved the submitted version.

REFERENCES

1. Lindner D, Fitzek A, Brauninger H, Aleshcheva G, Edler C, Meissner K, et al. Association of cardiac infection with SARS-CoV-2 in confirmed COVID-19 autopsy cases. JAMA Cardiol. (2020) 5:1281–5. doi: 10.1001/jamacardio.2020.3551
2. Ferrer-Gomez A, Pian-Arias H, Carretero-Barrio I, Navarro-Cantero A, Pestana D, de Pablo R, et al. Late cardiac pathology in severe covid-19. A postmortem series of 30 patients. Front Cardiovasc Med. (2021) 8:748396. doi: 10.3389/fcvm.2021.748396
3. Mehra MR, Ruschitzka F. COVID-19 illness and heart failure: a missing link? JACC Heart Fail. (2020) 8:512–4. doi: 10.1016/j.jchf.2020.03.004
4. Domondon M, Nikiforova AB, DeLeon-Pennell KY, Ilatovskaya DV. Regulation of mitochondria function by natriuretic peptides. Am J Physiol Renal Physiol. (2019) 317:F1164–8. doi: 10.1152/ajprenal.00384.2019
5. Marin-Garcia J, Goldenthal MJ. Heart mitochondria signaling pathways: appraisal of an emerging field. J Mol Med. (2004) 82:565–78. doi: 10.1007/s00109-004-0567-7
6. Wu KE, Fazal FM, Parker KR, Zou J, Chang HY. RNA-GPS predicts SARS-CoV-2 RNA residency to host mitochondria and nucleolus. Cell Syst. (2020) 11:102–8.e3. doi: 10.1016/j.cels.2020.06.008
7. Singh KK, Chaubey G, Chen JY, Suravajhala P. Decoding SARS-CoV-2 hijacking of host mitochondria in COVID-19 pathogenesis. Am J Physiol Cell Physiol. (2020) 319:C258–67. doi: 10.1152/ajpcell.00224.2020
8. Lane RK, Hilsabeck T, Rea SL. The role of mitochondrial dysfunction in age-related diseases. Biochim Biophys Acta. (2015) 1847:1387–400. doi: 10.1016/j.bbabio.2015.05.021
9. Pasquier C, Robichon A. Computational search of hybrid human/SARS-CoV-2 dsRNA reveals unique viral sequences that diverge from those of other coronavirus strains. Heliyon. (2021) 7:e07284. doi: 10.1016/j.heliyon.2021.e07284
10. Padhan K, Minakshi R, Towheed MAB, Jameel S. Severe acute respiratory syndrome coronavirus 3a protein activates the mitochondrial death pathway through p38 MAP kinase activation. J Gen Virol. (2008) 89:1960–9. doi: 10.1099/vir.0.83665-0
11. Scozzi D, Cano M, Ma L, Zhou D, Zhu JH, O'Halloran JA, et al. Circulating mitochondrial DNA is an early indicator of severe illness and mortality from COVID-19. JCI Insight. (2021) 6:e143299. doi: 10.1172/jci.insight.143299

12. Eirin A, Lerman A, Lerman LO. Mitochondrial injury and dysfunction in hypertension-induced cardiac damage. *Eur Heart J.* (2014) 35:3258–66. doi: 10.1093/eurheartj/ehu436

13. Hojlund K, Mogensen M, Sahlin K, Beck-Nielsen H. Mitochondrial dysfunction in type 2 diabetes and obesity. *Endocrinol Metab Clin North Am.* (2008) 37:713–31, x. doi: 10.1016/j.ecl.2008.06.006

14. Wautier MP, Chappey O, Corda S, Stern DM, Schmidt AM, Wautier JL. Activation of NADPH oxidase by AGE links oxidant stress to altered gene expression via RAGE. *Am J Physiol Endocrinol Metab.* (2001) 280:E685–94. doi: 10.1152/ajpendo.2001.280.5.E685

15. Arruda AP, Pers BM, Parlakgul G, Guney E, Inouye K, Hotamisligil GS. Chronic enrichment of hepatic endoplasmic reticulum-mitochondria contact leads to mitochondrial dysfunction in obesity. *Nat Med.* (2014) 20:1427–35. doi: 10.1038/nm.3735

16. Wang Y, Li Y, He C, Gou B, Song M. Mitochondrial regulation of cardiac aging. *Biochim Biophys Acta Mol Basis Dis.* (2019) 1865:1853–64. doi: 10.1016/j.bbadis.2018.12.008

17. Al Abbasi B, Torres P, Ramos-Tuarez F, Dewaswala N, Abdallah A, Chen K, et al. Cardiac troponin-I and COVID-19: a prognostic tool for in-hospital mortality. *Cardiol Res.* (2020) 11:398–404. doi: 10.14740/cr1159

18. Luo J, Zhao W, Gan Y, Pan B, Liu L, Liu Z, et al. Cardiac troponin I R193H mutation is associated with mitochondrial damage in cardiomyocytes. *DNA Cell Biol.* (2021) 40:184–91. doi: 10.1089/dna.2020.5828

19. Angajala A, Lim S, Phillips JB, Kim JH, Yates C, You Z, et al. Diverse roles of mitochondria in immune responses: novel insights into immuno-metabolism. *Front Immunol.* (2018) 9:1605. doi: 10.3389/fimmu.2018.01605

20. Jiang HW, Zhang HN, Meng QF, Xie J, Li Y, Chen H, et al. SARS-CoV-2 Orf9b suppresses type I interferon responses by targeting TOM70. *Cell Mol Immunol.* (2020) 17:998–1000. doi: 10.1038/s41423-020-0514-8

21. Desdin-Mico G, Soto-Heredero G, Aranda JF, Oller J, Carrasco E, Gabande-Rodriguez E, et al. T cells with dysfunctional mitochondria induce multimorbidity and premature senescence. *Science.* (2020) 368:1371–6. doi: 10.1126/science.aax0860

22. Baixauli F, Acin-Perez R, Villarroya-Beltri C, Mazzeo C, Nunez-Andrade N, Gabande-Rodriguez E, et al. Mitochondrial respiration controls lysosomal function during inflammatory T cell responses. *Cell Metab.* (2015) 22:485–98. doi: 10.1016/j.cmet.2015.07.020

23. Kuehn BM. Excess deaths from end-stage kidney disease early in pandemic. *JAMA.* (2021) 326:300. doi: 10.1001/jama.2021.11312

24. Eirin A, Lerman A, Lerman LO. Mitochondria: a pathogenic paradigm in hypertensive renal disease. *Hypertension.* (2015) 65:264–70. doi: 10.1161/HYPERTENSIONAHA.114.04598

25. Stubbs BJ, Koutnik AP, Volek JS, Newman JC. From bedside to battlefield: intersection of ketone body mechanisms in geroscience with military resilience. *Geroscience.* (2021) 43:1071–81. doi: 10.1007/s11357-020-00277-y

26

A Case Series of Myocarditis Following Third (Booster) Dose of COVID-19 Vaccination: Magnetic Resonance Imaging Study

*Arthur Shiyovich, Guy Witberg, Yaron Aviv, Ran Kornowski and Ashraf Hamdan**

Department of Cardiology, Rabin Medical Center, Tel Aviv University, Tel Aviv, Israel

Correspondence:
Ashraf Hamdan
hamdashraf@gmail.com

Background: Myocarditis has been reported following the first two doses of Pfizer-BNT162b2 messenger RNA (mRNA) COVID-19 vaccination. Administration of a third dose (booster) of the vaccine was initiated recently in Israel.

Objective: The aim of this study was to describe the characteristics of patients referred for cardiac magnetic resonance (CMR) imaging with myocarditis following the booster.

Methods: Patients referred for CMR imaging with a clinical diagnosis of myocarditis within 21 days following the booster, between July 13 and November 11, 2021, were analyzed.

Results: Overall, 4 patients were included, 3/4 (75%) were men, and the mean age was 27 ± 10 years. The time from booster administration to the onset of symptoms was 5.75 ± 4.8 days (range 2–14). Obstructive coronary artery disease was excluded in 3 of the patients (75%). CMR was performed 34 ± 15 days (range 8-47 days) following the 3rd vaccination. The mean left ventricular ejection fraction was $61 \pm 7\%$ (range 53–71%), and regional wall motion abnormalities were present in one of the patients. Global T1 was increased in one of the patients, while focal T1 values were increased in 3 of the patients. Global T2 was increased in one of the patients, while focal T2 values were increased in all the patients. Global ECV was increased in 3 of the patients, while focal ECV was increased in all the patients. Median late gadolinium enhancement (LGE) was $4 \pm 3\%$ (range 1–9%), with the inferolateral segment as the most common location (3 of the 4 patients). All the patients met the Updated Lake Louise Criteria.

Conclusions: Patient characteristics and CMR imaging findings of myocarditis following the administration of the booster vaccine are relatively mild and consistent with those observed with the first two doses. Although larger-scale prospective studies are necessary, these initial findings are somewhat reassuring.

Keywords: myocarditis, BNT162b2 messenger RNA (mRNA) COVID-19 vaccination, third dose (booster), cardiac magnetic resonance imaging (CMR), COVID-19

INTRODUCTION

Myocarditis has been reported to be a possible rare adverse event following the first or second dose of Pfizer-BNT162b2 messenger RNA (mRNA) COVID-19 vaccination (1–4). Incidence of such post-vaccine myocarditis was reported to be highest among younger males, with most cases being mild or moderate with favorable clinical outcomes (1, 4). As reported by us (5) and others (6–8), cardiovascular magnetic resonance (CMR) imaging findings of these patients were consistently mild and in line with "classical myocarditis." Following the resurgence of COVID-19 morbidity, the Israeli Ministry of Health announced a campaign to administer the third dose (i.e., booster) of the BNT162b2 mRNA COVID-19 vaccine (Pfizer–BioNTech) to individuals who received the second dose > 5 months earlier, starting on July 13 (9). This third vaccine dose was reported to be effectively protected against severe COVID-19-related outcomes (9). Our aim in the current report was to describe the characteristics of patients referred for CMR with myocarditis following the administration of the BNT162b2 mRNA COVID-19 vaccine.

METHODS
Study Population
This study comprised consecutive patients who are members of Clalit Health Services (CHS), and who were referred for CMR at Mor Inside Ltd. (Kfar Saba, Israel), with a clinically suspected diagnosis of myocarditis within 21 days after receiving the third dose of the Pfizer-BNT162b2 mRNA COVID-19 vaccine between July 13, 2021, and November 11, 2021. Patient-specific data were available from referral letters and electronic medical records. Patients with prior history of myocarditis, with missing data of the third dose of the vaccine, or with an alternative competing diagnosis (i.e., COVID-19 infection) were excluded.

This study was approved by the CHS institutional review board and performed consistently with the Helsinki declaration. Exemption from informed consent was granted.

CMR Imaging
The patients underwent CMR imaging using a 1.5 T scanner (Ingenia; Philips Medical Systems). The CMR protocol included multiplanar cine imaging and late gadolinium enhancement (LGE) imaging. T1 mapping was performed using a balanced steady state free precession, single breath-hold modified inversion recovery Look-Locker (MOLLI). T2 mapping was performed using a navigator-gated black blood-prepared gradient spin-echo sequence. Native T1 and T2 mapping, and postcontrast T1 mapping were acquired in apical, mid-ventricular, and basal short-axis slices.

Data analysis was performed using a dedicated CMR workstation (Philips Intellispace Portal, version 11.0). Cardiac volume, function, and mass were measured using a semiautomated contour detection system, and extracellular volume (ECV) was calculated based on pre and postcontrast T1 images. Myocardial ROIs was placed accurately to minimize partial volume effects from adjacent blood pool or extra-myocardial tissues. Global T1 and T2 relaxation times and ECV were evaluated for the complete mid-ventricular slice using motion-corrected images as previously described (10). Consistent with Puntmann et al. (10), to avoid overestimation of T1 value due to partial volume effect, the apical slices were not analyzed. In addition, there are no differences in T1 value between basal and mid-ventricular slices (11), and in some cases, the basal slice may contain a part of the left ventricular outflow tract (11).

Regional T1, T2, and ECV were measured in LGE positive myocardium by manually drawing a region-of-interest (ROI) on the LGE image around the lesions and copying these ROIs to the corresponding T1 and T2 maps; respectively.

LGE was defined as an image intensity level ≥ 2 SDs above the mean of the remote myocardium. Abnormal native T1, T2, and ECV values were defined as >1,060 ms, >57 ms, and higher than 28%, respectively (12). The diameter of pericardial effusion was measured at the end-systolic frame, and pericardial LGE was considered present when enhancement involved parietal and visceral pericardial layers.

We evaluated the diagnosis of myocarditis by CMR using the Updated Lake Louise Criteria (13).

Statistical Analysis
A descriptive statistical methodology was used. Patient characteristics are presented as counts (%) for categorical variables and mean (±SD) or median (range) for continuous variables.

RESULTS

Overall, 4 patients met the inclusion criteria. A total of ¾ th (75%) were male, and the mean age was 27 ± 10 years (range: 18–44 years). Baseline characteristics are presented in **Table 1**. One of the patients had asthma, but the rest were otherwise healthy. The mean time from the third vaccine administration to the onset of symptoms was 5.7 5 ± 4.8 days (range 2–14). Of all the patients who experienced chest pain, ¾th (75%) had abnormal ECG mostly accounting for ST-segment elevations, and troponin levels were increased in all the patients, with peak values between 79 and 4,967 ng/L. Obstructive coronary artery disease was excluded in 3 (75%) of the patients, one had coronary angiography, and the other two had coronary computed tomography angiography.

The CMR imaging was performed after a median of 34 ± 15 days (range 8-47 days) following the 3rd vaccination. One of the patients underwent CMR during the acute phase, while the rest over a month following the acute episode. The CMR findings are presented in **Table 1**. CMR images of all the patients are presented in **Figure 1**.

The mean left ventricular ejection fraction was 61 ± 7% (range 53-71%), regional wall motion abnormalities were present in one of the patients only. Global T1 values were increased in one (25%) of the patients, while focal values were increased in 3 (75%) of the patients. Global T2 values were increased in one (25%) of the patients, while focal values were increased in all of the patients (100%). Global ECV was increased in 3 (75%) of the patients, while focal ECV was increased in all the patients (100%). LGE was present in all the patients; thus, all of the patients met the Updated Lake Louise Criteria. Mean LGE% was 4 ± 3% (range 1-9%), and the inferolateral segment was the most common location (3/4 patients). LGE patterns were as follows: epicardial 2 patients, mid-wall 1 patient, mid-wall and epicardial 1 patient. LGE in the pericardium was present in 2 of the 4 patients, and pericardial effusion was present in 2 of the 4 patients, circular in both. The diameter of pericardial effusion was 4 and 5 mm in the two latter patients.

TABLE 1 | Clinical characteristics and CMR findings of the study patients.

Age (years)	Sex	Past medical history	Symptoms	ECG	Peak Troponin (ng/L)	CAD ruled out	Time from 3rd vaccine and symptoms (days)	Time between 3rd vaccine and MRI (days)	LVEF %	Wall motion abnormality	LVEDV/BSA	LVESV/BSA	LV-mass/BSA	T1 global (ms)	T1 focal (ms)	T2 global (ms)	T2 focal (ms)	Global ECV (%)	Focal ECV (%)	LGE (%)	LGE localization	LGE pattern	LGE in pericard	Peri-cardial effusion	Diameter of effusion (mm)
21	M	None	Chest pain	Inferior STE	240	CA	4	8	53	Lateral wall	73.5	33.9	49.6	1,078 ±107	1,135 ±118	62 ± 8	69.2	30.1	36	9	Antero-lateral, infero-lateral (basal, mid) Lateral (apical)	Epicar-dial and mid-wall	Y	N	
44	F	None	Chest pain	Normal	80	CCT	2	40	63	N	70.6	25.8	31.7	1,039 ±70	1,077 ±66	52.4 ± 6	57.5	30.5	31.9	1	Apex, infero-septal (basal)	Mid-wall	Y	N	
26	M	Asthma	Chest pain	Diffuse STE	4,967	N	14	47	71	N	76.7	22.2	46.9	1,045 ±93	1,155 ±89	50 ± 6.7	58.1	34.2	44.9	3	Inferior and infero-lateral (basal)	Epicar-dial	N	Circular	5
18	M	None	Chest pain	Diffuse STE	79	CCT	3	42	59	N	74	31.4	45.8	1,008 ±70	1,041 ±80	49 ± 4.4	57.4	27.3	29.3	1	Inferior (basal)	Epicar-dial	N	Circular	4

M, male; Y, yes; N, no; LV, left ventricular; LVEDV, left ventricular end-diastolic volume; ECG, electrocardiogram; LVESV, left ventricular end-systolic volume; BSA, body surface are; LGE, late gadolinium enhancement; CAD, coronary artery disease; CA, coronary angiography; CCT, cardiac computed tomography; STE, ST-segment elevation.

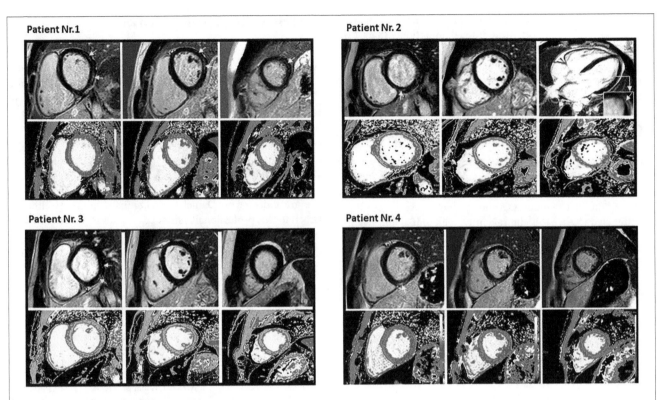

FIGURE 1 | Cardiac magnetic resonance imaging of the four patients who had myocarditis following the third dose of mRNA COVID-19 vaccination demonstrated late gadolinium enhancement (yellow arrows) and T1 mapping (lower row). Patient no. 1: Mid wall late gadolinium enhancement involving 9% of the myocardium with corresponding myocardial injury in native T1 mapping imaging in antero- and infero-lateral segments of basal and mid ventricular short-axis view, as well as in the lateral segment of apical short-axis view. Native T1 value was 1,135 ms, and T2 value was 69.2 ms. Peak troponin was 240 ng/L, and scan delay (from COVID-19 vaccine) was 8 days. Patient no. 2: Mid wall late gadolinium enhancement involving 1% of the myocardium with corresponding myocardial injury in native T1 mapping imaging in the lateral segment of apical and in the septal segment of the basal short-axis view. Native T1 value was 1,077 ms, and T2 value was 57.5 ms. Peak troponin was 80 ng/L, and scan delay (from COVID-19 vaccine) was 40 days. Patient no. 3: Epicardial late gadolinium enhancement involving 3% of the myocardium with corresponding myocardial injury in native T1 mapping imaging in the inferior and inferolateral segments of the basal short-axis view. Native T1 value was 1,155 ms, and T2 value was 58.1 ms. Peak troponin T was 4,967 ng/L, and scan delay (from COVID-19 vaccine) was 47 days. Patient no. 4: Mid wall late gadolinium enhancement involving 1% of the myocardium with corresponding myocardial injury in native T1 mapping imaging in inferior segments of the basal and mid-ventricular short axis view, as well as in the lateral segment of the apical short axis view. Native T1 value was 1,041 ms, and T2 value was 57.4 ms. Peak troponin T was 79 ng/L, and scan delay (from COVID-19 vaccine) was 42 days. Reference (normal) values: T1: 950–1,060 ms, T2: < 57 ms, and troponin T < 13 ng/L.

DISCUSSION

The present study consists, to our knowledge, of the first report describing CMR as well as clinical findings of patients with myocarditis following the administration of BNT162b2 mRNA COVID-19 booster (i.e., 3rd dose) vaccine. The baseline characteristics of the patients in this report are consistent with those of people who developed myocarditis following the first two doses, as previously reported (5–8); most were young men without a significant past medical history. However, it should be mentioned that one of the patients (25%) was a 44-year-old woman, which could imply less dominance of men with myocarditis following the 3rd vaccine, yet this is a small cohort thus such inferences are significantly limited. The CMR findings are overall mild, with two patients having ~1% LGE, and consistent with those previously reported following the first two doses of the vaccine (5–8). Although this could partially result from the delayed scan, it is probably consistent with the

favorable outcome of these patients. Findings are also similar to those reported on patients who recently recovered from COVID-19, suggesting potential etiological common pathways for myocardial involvement (10). The severity of the CMR findings (e.g., LGE percentage, T1 values, etc.) was greater in one patient, in whom CMR was performed during the acute phase compared with over a month delay in the other patients. Although this may imply the natural course of the inflammation, a selection bias with a more severe case scanned earlier cannot be ruled out. Nevertheless, and despite the delay in CMR in 3 of the patients, all the patients met the Updated Lake Louise Criteria (13).

LIMITATIONS

The causality between myocarditis and the vaccine cannot be unequivocally determined. However, temporal proximity between the two events and the very similar characteristics of the patients and previously reported CMR findings to support a probable causal association. An additional limitation is that CMR was performed over a month after the acute phase in 3 of the 4 patients, which might have attenuated some of the findings. We should also acknowledge the relatively small cohort, which limits the generalizability of the findings.

CONCLUSIONS

Patient characteristics and CMR findings of clinically suspected myocarditis following the administration of the booster vaccine are relatively mild and consistent with previous observations following the first two doses. Although more data are required to better characterize this clinical entity, these initial findings are somewhat reassuring with regard to the risk/benefit profile of the third dose of the vaccine.

REFERENCES

1. Witberg G, Barda N, Hoss S, Richer I, Wiessman M, Aviv Y, et al. Myocarditis after Covid-19 vaccination in a large Health Care Organization. *N Engl J Med.* (2021) 385:2132–9. doi: 10.1056/NEJMoa2110737
2. Montgomery J, Ryan M, Engler R, Hoffman D, McClenathan B, Collins L, et al. Myocarditis following immunization with mRNA COVID-19 vaccines in members of the US Military. *JAMA Cardiol.* (2021) 6:1202–6. doi: 10.1001/jamacardio.2021.2833
3. Shay DK, Shimabukuro TT, DeStefano F. Myocarditis occurring after immunization with mRNA-based COVID-19 vaccines. *JAMA Cardiol.* (2021) 6:1115–7. doi: 10.1001/jamacardio.2021.2821
4. Mevorach D, Anis E, Cedar N, Bromberg M, Haas E, Nadir E, et al. Myocarditis after BNT162b2 mRNA vaccine against Covid-19 in Israel. *N Engl J Med.* (2021) 385:2140–9. doi: 10.1056/NEJMoa2109730
5. Shiyovich A, Witberg G, Aviv Y, Eisen A, Orvin K, Wiessman M, et al. Myocarditis following COVID-19 vaccination: magnetic resonance imaging study. *Eur Heart J Cardiovasc Imag.* (2021) 2021:jeab230. doi: 10.1093/ehjci/jeab230
6. Shaw KE, Cavalcante JL, Han BK, Gössl M. Possible association between COVID-19 vaccine and myocarditis: clinical and CMR findings. *JACC Cardiovasc Imaging.* (2021) 14:1856–61. doi: 10.1016/j.jcmg.2021.06.002
7. Mansour J, Short RG, Bhalla S, Nathan CO. Acute myocarditis after a second dose of the mRNA COVID-19 vaccine: a report of two cases. *Clin Imaging.* (2021) 78:247–9. doi: 10.1016/j.clinimag.2021.06.019
8. Kim HW, Jenista ER, Wendell DC, Azevedo CF, Campbell MJ, Darty SN, et al. Patients with acute myocarditis following mRNA COVID-19 vaccination. *JAMA Cardiol.* (2021) 6:1196–201. doi: 10.1001/jamacardio.2021.2828
9. Barda N, Dagan N, Cohen C, Hernan MA, Lipsitch M, Kohane IS, et al. Effectiveness of a third dose of the BNT162b2 mRNA COVID-19 vaccine for preventing severe outcomes in Israel: an observational study. *Lancet.* (2021) 398:2093–100. doi: 10.1016/S0140-6736(21)02249-2
10. Puntmann VO, Carerj ML, Wieters I, Fahim M, Arendt C, Hoffmann J, et al. Outcomes of cardiovascular magnetic resonance imaging in patients recently recovered from coronavirus disease 2019 (COVID-19). *JAMA Cardiol.* (2020) 5:1265–73. doi: 10.1001/jamacardio.2020.3557
11. Puntmann VO, Valbuena S, Hinojar R, Petersen SE, Greenwood JP, Kramer CM, et al. Society for Cardiovascular Magnetic Resonance (SCMR) expert consensus for CMR imaging endpoints in clinical research: part I - analytical validation and clinical qualification. *J Cardiovasc Magnet Resonance.* (2018) 20:67. doi: 10.1186/s12968-018-0484-5
12. Bohnen S, Radunski UK, Lund GK, Ojeda F, Looft Y, Senel M, et al. Tissue characterization by T1 and T2 mapping cardiovascular magnetic resonance imaging to monitor myocardial inflammation in healing myocarditis. *Eur Heart J Cardiovasc Imaging.* (2017) 18:744–51. doi: 10.1093/ehjci/jex007
13. Ferreira VM, Schulz-Menger J, Holmvang G, Kramer CM, Carbone I, Sechtem U, et al. Cardiovascular magnetic resonance in nonischemic myocardial inflammation: expert recommendations. *J Am College Cardiol.* (2018) 72:3158–76. doi: 10.1016/j.jacc.2018.09.072

AUTHOR CONTRIBUTIONS

AS, AH, and RK conceived and planned the study. AS and AH reviewed the CMR tests, contributed to the interpretation of the results, and drafted the manuscript. AS, AH, YA, and GW obtained patient related clinical data and contributed to sample preparation. All authors provided critical feedback and helped shape the research, analysis, and manuscript. All authors contributed to the article and approved the submitted version.

ACKNOWLEDGMENTS

We are indebted to Daniel Outmezguine (Philips Healthcare, Israel) for his professional assistance.

27

COVID-19 Vaccination Associated Fulminant Myocarditis

Guanglin Cui[1,2], Rui Li[1,2], Chunxia Zhao[1,2] and Dao Wen Wang[1,2]*

[1] Division of Cardiology, Department of Internal Medicine, Tongji Hospital, Tongji Medical College, Huazhong University of Science and Technology, Wuhan, China, [2] Hubei Province Key Laboratory of Genetics and Molecular Mechanisms of Cardiological Disorders, Wuhan, China

Correspondence:
Dao Wen Wang
dwwang@tjh.tjmu.edu.cn

Herein, we describe a novel finding of fulminant myocarditis (FM) in two subjects the day after administration of the first dose of the currently available inactivated SARS-CoV-2 vaccine (Vero cell). Cardiac magnetic resonance imaging revealed extensive myocardial edema and necrosis. A pathologic evaluation of the endocardial biopsy tissues revealed inflammatory cell (lymphocytes) infiltration and interstitial edema, myocyte necrosis, and focal areas of fibrosis. A life-support-based comprehensive treatment regimen comprising mechanical circulatory support using intra-aortic balloon pulsation and immunomodulatory therapy—glucocorticoids and intravenous immunoglobulin—was used to treat the patients with FM; eventually, the patients recovered and were discharged. To our knowledge, these are the first two reported cases of FM, with no other identified cause or associated illness, after receiving the inactivated SARS-CoV-2 vaccine (Vero cell). These findings suggest a novel pathogenesis of myocarditis which mentions to pay more attention to this rare, but lethal complication of COVID-19 vaccination.

Keywords: myocarditis, COVID-19 vaccine, immunomodulatory therapy, myocyte necrosis, pathogenesis

BACKGROUND

Myocarditis refers to the inflammation of the heart muscle due to microbial infections, toxic substances, or autoimmune processes. Fulminant myocarditis, which is characterized by severe and sudden cardiac inflammation with cardiogenic shock and arrhythmias and a high mortality rate of approximately 40–70% (1, 2), is a less common, but not rare, clinical emergency; however, it is not specifically mentioned in the Dallas Criteria or in the report of the World Health Organization/International Society and Federation of Cardiology classification of cardiomyopathies (3). Since coronavirus disease (COVID-19) was first described in December 2019, COVID-19-related fulminant myocarditis has been reported several times (4–7). Current knowledge suggests that it is a combination of systemic inflammation due to cytokine storm, severe myocardial injury caused by the patient's immune response, and direct viral injury of the myocardium [since the identification of severe acute respiratory syndrome coronavirus 2 (SARS-CoV-2) particles in the reverse transcription polymerase chain reaction (RT-PCR) myocardial biopsy of rare patients], which suggests the eventual cardiotropism of the virus (8, 9). Currently, vaccines represent the most powerful approach in controlling the COVID-19 pandemic. However, several adverse events, especially vaccination-associated deaths, have been reported in the news and on social platforms (10, 11), and these adverse events often occur within 5–24 days of the vaccination. In this report, we describe a novel finding in two cases of fulminant myocarditis following the administration of the first dose of the currently available inactivated SARS-CoV-2 vaccine (Vero cell).

CASE PRESENTATION

Case 1

A 57-year-old woman presenting with chest distress, fatigue, fever, and chills for 4 days was hospitalized. Her highest recorded body temperature was 38.5°C. Her symptoms of chest tightness were aggravated, accompanied by palpitations. No discomfort, such as chest pain, nausea and vomiting, amaurosis and syncope, or acid regurgitation were observed. The woman had received the COVID-19 vaccine 4 days before. She had good health, apart from a history of hypertension.

Physical examination revealed a body temperature of 37.2°C, blood pressure of 102/58 mmHg, pulse of 99 bpm, and respiratory rate of 16 breaths/minute, and oxygen saturation of 99% while the patient was breathing ambient air. Physical examination of the heart revealed low and dull heart sounds.

Investigations

Biochemical analysis was performed when the patient was admitted (**Table 1**). Laboratory results reflected severe myocardial damage [troponin I > 50,000 pg/ml, creatine kinase (CK) 1,186 U/L, lactate dehydrogenase (LDH) 764 U/L], and elevated levels of white blood cell (WBC) (8.83×10^9/L) and neutrophils (92.6%) while decreased lymphocyte (0.44×10^9/L) levels. Additionally, high-sensitivity C-reactive protein, erythrocyte sedimentation rate, and inflammatory cytokines (ILβ, 8.9 pg/ml; TNFα, 11 pg/ml) were all elevated on the day of administration.

Given the patient's symptoms, two nucleic acid amplification tests for COVID-19 were performed, and the result was negative. Tests for influenza A and B, parainfluenza, respiratory syncytial virus, rhinovirus, adenovirus, and four common coronavirus strains known to cause illness in humans (HKU1, NL63, 229E, and OC43) as well as COVID-19 antibodies (IgG and IgM) were also negative.

The admission electrocardiogram showed a right bundle branch block (**Figure 1A**). Urgent coronary angiography excluded coronary artery disease (**Figures 2A–C**); therefore, transthoracic echocardiography (TTE) with strain analysis revealed diffuse left ventricular hypokinesia and increased thickness of the mid-ventricular septal wall (septal wall 13 mm; inferior wall 11 mm), and markedly reduced LV ejection fraction (LVEF 30%) (**Figures 3B,D**). Based on all these clinical and laboratory data, fulminant myocarditis was diagnosed, and treatments were immediately initiated with an intra-aortic balloon pump, which elevated the systolic blood pressure from 95 to 110 mm Hg and heart rate reduced from 100 to 85 bpm; intravenous drip of methylprednisolone (400 mg intravenous drip on the first day and then 200 mg per day for 4 more days) and intravenous immunoglobulin 20 g per day for 5 days. After these treatments, the patient's circulation stabilized and gradually recovered. On day 5, cardiac magnetic resonance (CMR) was performed, and the results revealed a corresponding extensive myocardial edema and necrosis with predominant subepicardial/mid-ventricular septal distribution highly suggestive of a myocarditis pattern

(**Figures 3G,H**). Additionally, late gadolinium enhancement imaging in different positions detected massive myocardial necrosis in the medial septum, thinning of the lateral wall of the myocardium, and fibrosis. Ventricular septal myoedema was observed on T1 mapping, and the value of myocardial T1 was significantly increased (1,364 ms, **Figure 3J**). Furthermore, endocardial biopsy was performed, and histological analysis showed mildly increased cardiomyocyte diameter with some perinuclear halos and dysmetric and dysmorphic nuclei, interstitial edema with lymphocytic aggregates, myocyte necrosis, and focal areas of fibrosis were observed (**Figure 3L**). All these results helped in establishing the final diagnosis of fulminant myocarditis, which is associated with the inactivated SARS-CoV-2 vaccination.

Case 2

A 63-year-old man had received a COVID-19 vaccine injection 4 days prior and was admitted for fever, fatigue of 3 days, and chest tightness for 1 day. The patient developed fever and fatigue 1 day after the vaccination, with the highest body temperature of 39°C, no palpitation, chest tightness, cough, dizziness, headache, abdominal pain, diarrhea, nausea, or vomiting. The patient visited the local clinic and took Tylenol orally, and his body temperature was within the normal range. One day before, the patient had sudden chest tightness, palpitation, dizziness, and loss of consciousness lasting for several seconds. An emergency electrocardiogram revealed a third-degree atrioventricular block (AVB) (**Figure 1B**). The patient was immediately transferred to Tongji Hospital directly through the chest pain center. His blood pressure was 90/60 mmHg, and his heart rate was 30 beats per minute with third AVB. Emergency coronary angiography revealed no obvious coronary stenosis. At this time, a diagnosis of fulminant myocarditis was suspected. After 20 mg intravenous dexamethasone, the patient was urgently implanted with a temporary pacemaker to maintain heart rate and was also implanted with an intra-aortic balloon pump to support his circulation; his blood pressure increased to 105/60 mm Hg. The patient was transferred to the cardiac intensive care unit.

Investigations

Physical examination revealed a body temperature of 36.2°C, blood pressure of 101/60 mmHg, pulse of 77 bpm (pacemaker heart rate, **Figure 1C**), respiratory rate of 18 bpm, and blood oxygen saturation of 99% while the patient was breathing ambient air. His heart sounds were low and dull. A biochemical analysis was also performed when the patient was admitted (**Table 1**). The results reflected severe myocardial damage (cTnI was 17,961.8 pg/ml, CK 586 U/L, LDH 401 U/L). The WBC was in a normal range (5.16×10^9/L) while elevated levels of neutrophils (90.1%) and decreased levels of lymphocyte (0.47×10^9/L). Immediate transthoracic echocardiography with strain analysis documented diffuse left ventricular hypokinesia and increased thickness in the mid-ventricular septal wall (13 mm), and LVEF severely reduced to 26% (**Figures 3A,C**). The patient was immediately treated as case one, including IVIG and methylprednisolone. After these treatments, including IABP

TABLE 1 | Clinical laboratory results.

Patient	Measure	Reference range	Illness Day 4, Hospital Day 1	Illness Day 6, Hospital Day 3	Illness Day 8, Hospital Day 5	Illness Day 10, Hospital Day 7
Case 1	White-cell count ($*10^9$/L)	3.5–9.5	8.83	14.66	11.76	7.94
	Red-cell count (10^{12}/L)	3.8–5.1	4.49	3.74	4.1	3.98
	Absolute neutrophil count ($*10^9$/L)	1.8–6.3	8.18	12.98	9.92	6.2
	Absolute lymphocyte count ($*10^9$/L)	1.1–3.2	0.44	1.02	1.22	1.23
	Platelet count ($*10^9$/L)	125.0–350.0	156	171	234	254
	Hemoglobin (g/L)	115.0–150.0	132	111	124	135
	Hematocrit (%)	35.0–45.0	39.3	34.3	36.9	40.2
	Sodium (mmol/L)	136.0–145.0	133.3	136.8	/	/
	Potassium (mmol/L)	3.5–5.1	3.47	4.41	3.69	4.17
	Chloride (mmol/L)	99.0–110.0	95.4	103.4	/	/
	Calcium (mmol/L)	2.20–2.55	2.19	2.14	/	/
	Bicarbonate radical (mmol/L)	22.0–29.0	20.7	22.7	26.6	22.2
	Glucose (mmol/L)	3.9–6.1	14.18	5.6	6.1	/
	Blood urea nitrogen (mmol/L)	2.6–7.5	6.26	10.10	7.93	11.75
	Creatinine (μmol/L)	45–84	79	63	59	69
	Total protein (g/L)	64.0–83.0	73.3	65.9	72	67.2
	Albumin (g/L)	35.0–52.0	36.3	30.4	28.9	31.5
	Total bilirubin (μmol/L)	≤21.0	18.6	4.4	3.4	5.7
	Procalcitonin (ng/ml)	0.02–0.05	0.6	/	/	0.33
	Alanine aminotransferase (U/L)	≤33	43	32	80	36
	Aspartate aminotransferase (U/L)	≤32	231	78	79	130
	Alkaline phosphatase (U/L)	35–105	106	85	98	86
	Fibrinogen (g/L)	2.0–4.0	5.93	3.22	/	/
	Lactate dehydrogenase (g/L)	135.0–214.0	764	688	629	550
	Prothrombin time (s)	11.5–14.5	13.4	13.4	/	/
	International normalized ratio	0.8–1.2	1.01	1.03	/	/
	Creatine kinase (U/L)	≤190	1186	846	647	274
	Venous lactate (mmol/L)	0.5–2.2	/	1.77	/	1.82
Case 2	White-cell count ($*10^9$/L)	3.5–9.5	5.16	9.36	7.81	4.87
	Red-cell count (10^{12}/L)	3.8–5.1	3.25	3.79	4.3	4.1
	Absolute neutrophil count ($*10^9$/L)	1.8–6.3	4.65	8.08	7.16	5.3
	Absolute lymphocyte count ($*10^9$/L)	1.1–3.2	0.47	0.64	0.38	0.98
	Platelet count ($*10^9$/L)	125.0–350.0	91	83	61	110
	Hemoglobin (g/L)	130.0–175.0	98	111	125	134
	Hematocrit (%)	40.0–50.0	29.7	34.2	38.6	42
	Sodium (mmol/L)	136.0–145.0	138.8	137.8	/	139.3
	Potassium (mmol/L)	3.5–5.1	3.86	3.97	4.08	4.18
	Chloride (mmol/L)	99.0–110.0	108.9	107.0	/	/
	Calcium (mmol/L)	2.20–2.55	2.08	1.95	/	/
	Bicarbonate radical (mmol/L)	22.0–29.0	17.9	22.8	26.6	25.7
	Glucose (mmol/L)	3.9–6.1	8.49	/	5.5	/
	Blood urea nitrogen (mmol/L)	3.6–9.5	8.14	7.7	5.68	5.9
	Creatinine (μmol/L)	59–104	83	76	72	77
	Total protein (g/L)	64.0–83.0	63.4	61.7	69.5	68.4
	Albumin (g/L)	35.0–52.0	34.4	30.1	31.2	33.8
	Total bilirubin (μmol/L)	≤26.0	5.8	4.9	4.3	6.9
	Procalcitonin (ng/ml)	0.02–0.05	0.03	/	/	/
	Alanine aminotransferase (U/L)	≤33	28	41	80	85
	Aspartate aminotransferase (U/L)	≤32	93	34	44	36
	Alkaline phosphatase (U/L)	40–130	45	42	52	51

(Continued)

TABLE 1 | Continued

Patient	Measure	Reference range	Illness Day 4, Hospital Day 1	Illness Day 6, Hospital Day 3	Illness Day 8, Hospital Day 5	Illness Day 10, Hospital Day 7
	Fibrinogen (g/L)	2.0–4.0	3.94	/	3.87	/
	Lactate dehydrogenase (g/L)	135.0–214.0	586	459	501	334
	Prothrombin time (s)	11.5–14.5	14.2	15.5	14.6	12
	International normalized ratio	0.8–1.2	1.09	/	/	/
	Creatine kinase (U/L)	≤190	586	687	423	211
	Venous lactate (mmol/L)	0.5–2.2	1.41	/	1.23	/

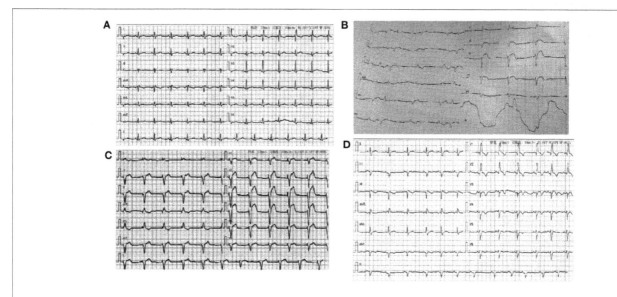

FIGURE 1 | (A) ECG for the woman patient when admitted to hospital: Sinus rhythm Right bundle branch block; **(B)** ECG of the man patient when admitted to hospital; V1–V3 lead ST-elevation and third-degree atrioventricular block; **(C)** ECG of the man patient when implanted with temporary pacing; **(D)** ECG of the man patient at discharge: Sinus rhythm, Right bundle branch block.

for circulatory support and immunomodulation therapy using sufficient doses of methylprednisolone and IVIG, the patients became stable soon. Five days later, his temporary pacemaker was withdrawn with regular sinus rhythm, and at this time, the CMR test revealed a corresponding extensive myocardial edema and necrosis with predominant subepicardial/mid-ventricular septal distribution highly suggestive of a myocarditis pattern (**Figures 3E,F**). Ventricular septal myoedema was observed on T1 mapping, and the value of myocardial T1 was significantly increased (1,380 ms in the male patient, **Figures 3I,J**).

Histological analysis of the endocardial biopsy confirmed the diagnosis of fulminant myocarditis with interstitial edema and lymphocytic lymphocyte infiltration (**Figure 3K**).

OUTCOME AND FOLLOW-UP

Case 1
After treatment for 10 days, her LVEF recovered to 52%, and she was discharged from the hospital with oral beta-blockers (47.5 mg/day), perindopril (4 mg/day), and prednisone 20 mg/day. At the first follow-up after 1 month, her LVEF was 60%, cTnI

level reduced from 12,000 pg/ml at discharge to 4,700 pg/ml and NT-proBNP reduced to close to normal levels (108 ng/L).

Case 2
After 9 days, the LVEF recovered to 59% with a normal sinus rhythm (**Figure 1D**) when he was discharged with oral beta-blockers (47.5 mg/day), perindopril (4 mg/day), and prednisone 20 mg/day. At the first follow-up after 1 month, her LVEF was 62%, cTnI level reduced from 17,961.8 pg/ml at discharge to 45 pg/ml and NT-proBNP reduced to normal levels (76 ng/L).

DISCUSSION

Previous studies reported only mild or moderate adverse events following the COVID-19 vaccine, including thrombosis and even pulmonary thrombosis (12). To the best of our knowledge, this is the first report of inactivated COVID-19 vaccine-associated fulminant myocarditis cases.

The two patients reported in this study had no previous history of myocarditis. They were in good health and had no

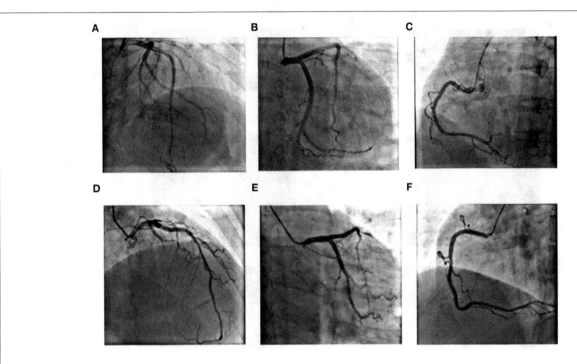

FIGURE 2 | Coronary angiography results for Case 1 **(A–C)**: **(A)** Left coronary artery: Cranial 30°; **(B)** Left coronary artery: Caudal 30°; **(C)** Right coronary artery: Left anterior oblique 45°; Coronary angiography results for Case 2 **(D–F)**: **(D)** Left anterior oblique 30° + Cranial 30°; **(E)** Left coronary artery: Caudal 30°; **(F)** Right coronary artery: Left anterior oblique 45°.

recent travel history. They were all at home in a community free of COVID-19 case. However, we found that they both had clinical symptoms that appeared the day after the COVID-19 vaccination. At present, we do not know whether the inactivated COVID-19 vaccine can directly cause myocarditis. However, based on the epidemiological analysis, these two cases of fulminant myocarditis may be possibly related to COVID-19 vaccination.

The term myocarditis refers to the inflammation of the heart muscle, which can be caused by infections, toxic substances, or autoimmune processes. A diagnosis of active myocarditis requires the presence of inflammatory infiltrates of non-ischemic origin in myocardial tissue associated with necrosis and/or degeneration of the adjacent cardiomyocytes. The diagnosis of myocarditis is a challenging diagnosis because of the heterogeneity of clinical presentations. Endomyocardial biopsy (EMB) is considered the reference standard for the diagnosis of myocarditis. In our report, both of our cases detected myocardial fibers, cardiomyocytes and myocardial interstitium all demonstrated edema of varying degrees with infiltration of chronic inflammatory (lymphocytic cells) cells, according to the Marburg criteria and Quantitative criteria (13, 14). Furthermore, myocyte necrosis and focal areas of fibrosis had also occurred in case 1. This phenomenon indicates the possibility of chronic transformation of acute myocarditis into inflammatory cardiomyopathy. The results of CMR imaging were also consistent with the typical findings of myocarditis. It is worth noting that the extent of LGE is a dynamic process in acute myocarditis, mainly related to tissue edema in the acute phase

that progressively disappears over time, whereas in the late phase, LGE mainly reflects postinflammatory replacement fibrosis. Moreover, immunohistochemistry is the current standard method used to evaluate infiltrating immune cells in tissues. However, the quantification and comparison of the different cell subsets are sometimes difficult. Immunohistochemistry-specific antibodies for leukocytes (CD45), macrophages (CD68), T cells (CD3) and their main subtypes, helper (CD4) and cytotoxic (CD8) cells, and B cells (CD19/CD20) can also increase the sensitivity of EMB. These measures will be helpful in the diagnosis and differential diagnosis of myocarditis.

At present, the underlying pathogenetic mechanisms of fulminant myocarditis are not known clearly, but may involve virus or other pathogen-induced initial myocardial injury and, more importantly, subsequent severe injury by aggravation of inflammatory cells and cytokine storm through pattern recognition receptors via both pathogen-associated molecular patterns and damage-associated molecular patterns (15–17). In these two patients, no evidence of other infections was detected. The possibility of COVID-19 vaccine-induced immune-related myocarditis was considered based on epidemiological history.

We do not know exactly how vaccine injection induces fulminant myocarditis. Under desired conditions, antigen vaccination is initially recognized by innate immune cells, such as dendritic cells and macrophages, engulfed by phagocytosis, and present pathogen-derived peptide antigens to naïve T cells, which then activate and instruct the development of antigen-specific adaptive immunity. However, inactivated COVID-19 virus contains RNAs and proteins and induces

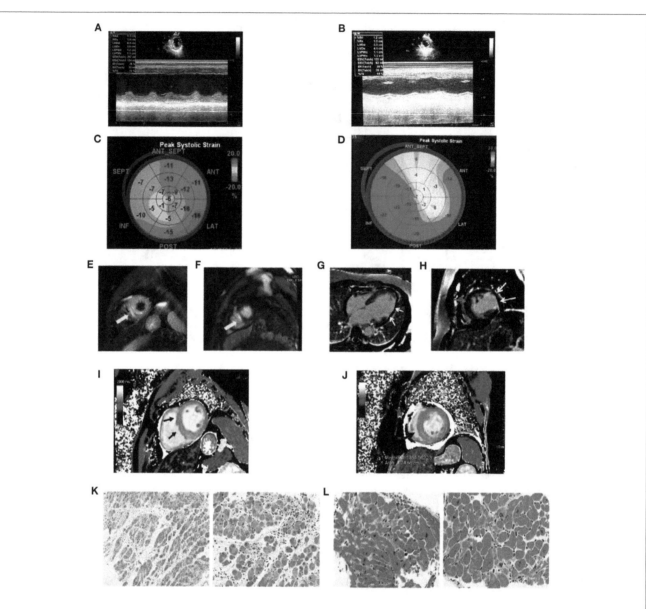

FIGURE 3 | The echocardiographic and cardiac magnetic resonance images recorded at admission and the findings of pathological specimens compatible with fulminant myocarditis. **(A)** LV ejection fraction was mildly reduced (EF value, 28%); **(B)** LV ejection fraction was mildly reduced (EF value = 30%); **(C)** Representative images of global longitudinal strains (GLS) presented as "bullseye" displays in case 1 (GLS = −12.1%); **(D)** Representative images of global longitudinal strains (GLS) presented as "bullseye" displays in case 2 (GLS = −9.8%); **(E)** Increased myocardial signal in the outer layer of the apical ventricular septum (edema) (arrow); **(F)** Late gadolinium enhancement imaging suggests myocardial enhancement in the outer layer of the apical ventricular septum (myocardial necrosis) (arrow); **(G)** Long-axis late gadolinium enhancement imaging suggests myocardial necrosis in the middle ventricular septum (red arrow), thinning, and enhancement of the lateral wall (yellow arrow); **(H)** Short axial late gadolinium enhancement imaging demonstrates myocardial necrosis in the middle ventricular septum (red arrow) with thinning of the lateral wall and formation of fibrosis (yellow arrow); **(I)** in T1 mapping, ventricular septal myocardial edema was observed, and the value of myocardial T1 was significantly increased, T1=1380 ms (normal value T1 = 1,180 ± 20 ms); **(J)** Myocardial edema in the lower interventricular septum was observed in T1 mapping, and the value of myocardial T1 was significantly increased, T1 = 1,364 ms (normal value T1 = 1,180 ± 20 ms); **(K)** Biopsy from myocardium showing myocardial fibers were slightly edematous and interstitial edema was accompanied by infiltration of inflammatory cells; **(L)** Biopsy from myocardium showing myocardial atrophy, hypertrophy of some cardiomyocytes, myocardial interstitial edema, local fibrosis, scattered focal necrosis of cardiomyocytes accompanied by infiltration of inflammatory cells.

a non-adaptive response, resulting in an overactivated inflammatory response, such as myocarditis or lethal fulminant myocarditis (15–18).

The mainstay of treatment for fulminant myocarditis is immunoregulatory therapy and an optimal heart failure medical regimen. Moreover, EMB is the basis for safe (infection-negative) immunosuppression or antiviral treatment. Our center has accumulated a lot of practical experience in the treatment of fulminant myocarditis, including COVID-19 related myocarditis (2, 6, 19, 20). In our report, a life-support-based comprehensive treatment regimen was preferentially used to treat the patients according to expert consensus recommendations (21). In this treatment regimen, mechanical circulatory support is based and simultaneously, immunomodulatory therapy using sufficient doses of glucocorticoids and intravenous immunoglobulin plays an important role in the treatment of myocardial injury and the regulation of inflammatory response. In a previous study, we demonstrated that early application of IABP is sufficient to stabilize circulation in most patients with fulminant myocarditis (2). A combination of glucocorticoid and IVIG can modulate the overactivated immune response and inhibit severe cardiac inflammation (22–25); therefore, it was successfully used in these two cases.

SUMMARY

Both the clinical and endomyocardial biopsy analyses of these two cases related to the SARS-CoV-2 vaccines confirmed the diagnosis of fulminant myocarditis; hence, based on the frequency and social importance of vaccination, vaccine-related adverse reactions should be further investigated and pay close attention in a larger population and in different ethnic groups because fulminant myocarditis is lethal.

Limitations and Strengths

Strengths: This case serves as a reminder of the importance of the possibility of COVID-19 vaccine-induced immune-related myocarditis and its management. Weaknesses: Several mRNA COVID-19 vaccine-related myocarditis have been reported before. In this case, thorough etiologic tests for myocarditis did not reveal any specific cause for viral myocarditis. The mechanism is uncertain and there is no specific diagnostic method for this etiology. It is also unclear why patients do not have COVID abs after receiving vaccinations. The etiologic diagnosis of the inactivated COVID-19 vaccine-related myocarditis would be dependent on the manner of exclusion in a case with a temporal relationship. We need to wait for further cases to confirm this epidemiological relationship.

AUTHOR CONTRIBUTIONS

GC participated in the research design, carried out the epidemiological investigation, performed statistical analyses, and drafted the manuscript. RL and CZ collected samples, participated in the epidemiological investigation, and collected samples for this study. DW participated in the research design, carried out the epidemiological investigation. All authors have read and approved the final manuscript.

ACKNOWLEDGMENTS

We thank Dr. Haojie Li, for the clinical contribution. We also thank the patients, the nurses and clinical staff who are providing care for the patient.

REFERENCES

1. Cooper Jr LT. Myocarditis. *N Engl J Med.* (2009) 360:1526–38. doi: 10.1056/NEJMra0800028
2. Li S, Xu S, Li C, Ran X, Cui G, He M, et al. A life support-based comprehensive treatment regimen dramatically lowers the in-hospital mortality of patients with fulminant myocarditis: a multiple center study. *Sci China Life Sci.* (2019) 62:369–80. doi: 10.1007/s11427-018-9501-9
3. Aretz HT, Billingham ME, Edwards WD, Factor SM, Fallon JT, Fenoglio JJ. Jr., et al. Myocarditis A histopathologic definition and classification. *Am J Cardiovasc Pathol.* (1987) 1:3–14.
4. Kallel O, Bourouis I, Bougrine R, Housni B, El Ouafi N, Ismaili N. Acute myocarditis related to Covid-19 infection: 2 cases report. *Ann Med Surg.* (2021) 66:102431. doi: 10.1016/j.amsu.2021.102431
5. Zeng JH, Liu YX, Yuan J, Wang FX, Wu WB Li JX, et al. First case of COVID-19 complicated with fulminant myocarditis: a case report and insights. *Infection.* (2020) 48:773–7. doi: 10.1007/s15010-020-01424-5
6. Chen C, Zhou Y, Wang DW. SARS-CoV-2: a potential novel etiology of fulminant myocarditis. *Herz.* (2020) 45:230–2. doi: 10.1007/s00059-020-04909-z
7. Guzik TJ, Mohiddin SA, Dimarco A, Patel V, Savvatis K, Marelli-Berg FM, et al. COVID-19 and the cardiovascular system: implications for risk assessment, diagnosis, and treatment options. *Cardiovasc Res.* (2020) 116:1666–87. doi: 10.1093/cvr/cvaa106
8. Magadum A, Kishore R. Cardiovascular manifestations of COVID-19 infection. *Cells.* (2020) 9:9112508. doi: 10.3390/cells9112508
9. Valverde I, Singh Y. Sanchez-de-Toledo J, Theocharis P, Chikermane A, Di Filippo S, et al. Acute cardiovascular manifestations in 286 children with multisystem inflammatory syndrome associated with COVID-19 infection in Europe. *Circulation.* (2021) 143:21–32. doi: 10.1161/CIRCULATIONAHA.120.050065
10. Kaur RJ, Dutta S, Bhardwaj P, Charan J, Dhingra S, Mitra P, et al. Adverse events reported from COVID-19 vaccine trials: a systematic review. *Indian J Clin Biochem.* 2021:1–13. doi: 10.1007/s12291-021-00968-z
11. Witberg G, Barda N, Hoss S, Richter I, Wiessman M, Aviv Y, et al. Myocarditis after Covid-19 vaccination in a large health care organization. *N Engl J Med.* (2021) 385:2132–9. doi: 10.1056/NEJMoa2110737
12. Hippisley-Cox J, Patone M, Mei XW, Saatci D, Dixon S, Khunti K, et al. Risk of thrombocytopenia and thromboembolism after covid-19 vaccination and SARS-CoV-2 positive testing: self-controlled case series study. *BMJ.* (2021) 374:n1931. doi: 10.1136/bmj.n1931
13. Maisch B, Portig I, Ristic A, Hufnagel G, Pankuweit S. Definition of inflammatory cardiomyopathy (myocarditis): on the way to consensus. A status report. *Herz.* (2000) 25:200–9. doi: 10.1007/s000590050007
14. Caforio AL, Pankuweit S, Arbustini E, Basso C, Gimeno-Blanes J, Felix SB, et al. Current state of knowledge on aetiology, diagnosis, management, and therapy of myocarditis: a position statement of the European Society of Cardiology Working Group on Myocardial and Pericardial Diseases. *Eur Heart J.* (2013) 34:2636-48, 48a–48d. doi: 10.1093/eurheartj/eht210
15. Gong T, Liu L, Jiang W, Zhou R. DAMP-sensing receptors in sterile inflammation and inflammatory diseases. *Nat Rev Immunol.* (2020) 20:95–112. doi: 10.1038/s41577-019-0215-7
16. Takeda K, Akira S. Toll-like receptors in innate immunity. *Int Immunol.* (2005) 17:1–14. doi: 10.1093/intimm/dxh186
17. Boyd JH, Mathur S, Wang Y, Bateman RM, Walley KR. Toll-like receptor stimulation in cardiomyocytes decreases contractility and initiates an NF-kappaB dependent inflammatory response. *Cardiovasc Res.* (2006) 72:384–93. doi: 10.1016/j.cardiores.2006.09.011
18. Quagliariello V, Bonelli A, Caronna A, Lombari MC, Conforti G, Libutti M, et al. SARS-CoV-2 infection: NLRP3 inflammasome as plausible target

to prevent cardiopulmonary complications? *Eur Rev Med Pharmacol Sci.* (2020) 24:9169–71.

19. Chen C, Li H, Hang W, Wang DW. Cardiac injuries in coronavirus disease 2019 (COVID-19). *J Mol Cell Cardiol.* (2020) 145:25–9. doi: 10.1016/j.yjmcc.2020.06.002

20. Ammirati E, Wang DW. SARS-CoV-2 inflames the heart. The importance of awareness of myocardial injury in COVID-19 patients. *Int J Cardiol.* (2020) 311:122–3. doi: 10.1016/j.ijcard.2020.03.086

21. Wang D, Li S, Jiang J, Yan J, Zhao C, Wang Y, et al. Chinese society of cardiology expert consensus statement on the diagnosis and treatment of adult fulminant myocarditis. *Sci China Life Sci.* (2019) 62:187–202. doi: 10.1007/s11427-018-9385-3

22. Hang W, Chen C, Seubert JM, Wang DW. Fulminant myocarditis: a comprehensive review from etiology to treatments and outcomes. *Signal Transduct Target Ther.* (2020) 5:287. doi: 10.1038/s41392-020-00360-y

23. Guilliams M, Bruhns P, Saeys Y, Hammad H, Lambrecht BN. The function of Fcgamma receptors in dendritic cells and macrophages. *Nat Rev Immunol.* (2014) 14:94–108. doi: 10.1038/nri3582

24. Pincetic A, Bournazos S, DiLillo DJ, Maamary J, Wang TT, Dahan R, et al. Type I and type II Fc receptors regulate innate and adaptive immunity. *Nat Immunol.* (2014) 15:707–16. doi: 10.1038/ni.2939

25. Anthony RM, Nimmerjahn F, Ashline DJ, Reinhold VN, Paulson JC, Ravetch JV. Recapitulation of IVIG anti-inflammatory activity with a recombinant IgG Fc. *Science.* (2008) 320:373–6. doi: 10.1126/science.1154315

28

Post-ST-Segment Elevation Myocardial Infarction Follow-Up Care during the COVID-19 Pandemic and the Possible Benefit of Telemedicine

Audrey A. Y. Zhang [1†], Nicholas W. S. Chew [1*†], Cheng Han Ng [2], Kailun Phua [3],
Yin Nwe Aye [1], Aaron Mai [2], Gwyneth Kong [2], Kalyar Saw [1], Raymond C. C. Wong [1,2],
William K. F. Kong [1,2], Kian-Keong Poh [1,2], Koo-Hui Chan [1,2], Adrian Fatt-Hoe Low [1,2],
Chi-Hang Lee [1,2], Mark Yan-Yee Chan [1,2], Ping Chai [1,2], James Yip [1,2], Tiong-Cheng Yeo [1,2],
Huay-Cheem Tan [1,2] and Poay-Huan Loh [1,2]

[1] Department of Cardiology, National University Heart Centre, National University Health System, Singapore, Singapore,
[2] Yong Loo Lin School of Medicine, National University of Singapore, Singapore, Singapore, [3] Department of Medicine,
National University Hospital, Singapore

*Correspondence:
Nicholas W. S. Chew
nicholas_ws_chew@nuhs.edu.sg

† These authors have contributed
equally to this work

Background: Infectious control measures during the COVID-19 pandemic have led to the propensity toward telemedicine. This study examined the impact of telemedicine during the pandemic on the long-term outcomes of ST-segment elevation myocardial infarction (STEMI) patients.

Methods: This study included 288 patients admitted 1 year before the pandemic (October 2018–December 2018) and during the pandemic (January 2020–March 2020) eras, and survived their index STEMI admission. The follow-up period was 1 year. One-year primary safety endpoint was all-cause mortality. Secondary safety endpoints were cardiac readmissions for unplanned revascularisation, non-fatal myocardial infarction, heart failure, arrythmia, unstable angina. Major adverse cardiovascular events (MACE) was defined as the composite outcome of each individual safety endpoint.

Results: Despite unfavorable in-hospital outcomes among patients admitted during the pandemic compared to pre-pandemic era, both groups had similar 1-year all-cause mortality (11.2 vs. 8.5%, respectively, $p = 0.454$) but higher cardiac-related (14.1 vs. 5.1%, $p < 0.001$) and heart failure readmissions in the pandemic vs. pre-pandemic groups (7.1 vs. 1.7%, $p = 0.037$). Follow-up was more frequently conducted via teleconsultations (1.2 vs. 0.2 per patient/year, $p = 0.001$), with reduction in physical consultations (2.1 vs. 2.6 per patient/year, $p = 0.043$), during the pandemic vs. pre-pandemic era. Majority achieved guideline-directed medical therapy (GDMT) during pandemic vs. pre-pandemic era (75.9 vs. 61.6%, $p = 0.010$). Multivariable Cox regression demonstrated achieving medication target doses (HR 0.387, 95% CI 0.164–0.915, $p = 0.031$) and GDMT (HR 0.271, 95% CI 0.134–0.548, $p < 0.001$) were independent predictors of lower 1-year MACE after adjustment.

Conclusion: The pandemic has led to the wider application of teleconsultation, with increased adherence to GDMT, enhanced medication target dosing. Achieving GDMT was associated with favorable long-term prognosis.

Keywords: COVID-19, telemedicine, telehealth, ST-segment elevation myocardial infarction, pandemic

INTRODUCTION

The coronavirus-2019 (COVID-19) pandemic has demanded the rapid adaptation of healthcare operations in implementing measures to reduce the infectious rate but to also maintain the standard of patient care. Patients with cardiovascular disease are at increased risk of contracting the COVID-19 infection with a poorer outcome (1). The universally adopted strategy of social distancing as a measure to "flatten the curve" have resulted in a decrease in traditional physical consultations and the wider adaptation of teleconsultations. Teleconsultations, or telemedicine in general, offers virtual clinic consultations and monitoring which has gained traction as appropriate viable alternative for safe and efficient medical care. Its role has gained attention given the benefits of removing the risk of hospital exposure for these vulnerable patients during the pandemic. As the application of telemedicine expands, it becomes increasingly important to understand its impact on patient care and clinical outcomes.

During the pandemic, there has been a substantial reduction in patients presenting with ST-segment elevation myocardial infarction (STEMI) requiring primary percutaneous coronary intervention (PPCI) compared to the pre-pandemic era (2). Despite the decrease in PPCI case volume, the opposite effect of worse overall in-hospital STEMI performance metrics and short-term clinical outcomes were observed during the pandemic (3, 4). At present, little is known about the follow-up care of these STEMI patients during the pandemic and the potential role of telemedicine in the management of such patients following hospital discharge. This study is the first to examine the trend in teleconsultations for post-STEMI patients during the pandemic, and its association with optimal medical therapy, target medication doses, cardiovascular risk factor control and long-term clinical outcomes.

METHODS

Setting and Design

This is a retrospective single-center study of patients with STEMI who presented to a major PCI-capable hospital in Singapore, and survived the index STEMI admission. Consecutive patients were enrolled into two study groups according to the date of their index admission: (1) Pre-pandemic, from 1 October 2018 to 31 December 2018, and (2) pandemic, from 1 January 2020 to 31 March 2020. Those who did not survive the index admission were excluded from the study. There were no patients who were admitted during both study periods. The follow-up was 1 year following the index STEMI admission. For at least 1 year post-STEMI, the cardiologists of the center visit would traditionally follow up with these patients closely whilst on dual-antiplatelet therapy. It was highly unlikely for these patients to be followed up by other cardiologists outside of the center visit, although these patients might be followed up by doctors from other sub-specialties based on their comorbidities. The time period for the pre-pandemic group was carefully chosen to allow a control with the closest temporal proximity to the COVID-19 pandemic period, without its 1-year post-STEMI follow-up being affected by the pandemic.

During the pandemic, particularly when the Disease Outbreak Response was heightened to its second highest level on 7 February 2020, the standard post-STEMI care after hospital discharge had to be rapidly revamped with increased adaptation of telemedicine. This involved virtual consultations that were conducted via a secure audio-visual telecommunication system between the patients and healthcare providers. Patients were encouraged to subscribe to the hospital telemedicine service and were either provided with or used their own equipment to measure blood pressure, pulse rate and body weight. Patients were also offered remote vital signs monitoring conducted daily for 1 month post-STEMI. Prescriptions were optimized based on the virtual assessment and delivered to the patient's homes. The main goal of teleconsultation during the COVID-19 pandemic was not to provide superior care to the standard face-to-face consultations, but to provide these patients with "health maintenance strategy" individualized to their needs and risk factor control targets (5, 6). The teleconsultation integrated virtual consultations, symptomology assessment, evaluation of home monitoring vitals such as blood pressure, patient education, drug tolerance and adherence, quality of life, and anticoagulation tolerance (7). Physical face-to-face consultations were still conducted, albeit less frequently, during the pandemic and these consultations involved serum testing for cardiovascular risk factor control. Serum measurements of glycated A1c (HbA1c), low-density lipoprotein (LDL) cholesterol, creatinine, estimated glomerular filtration rates (eGFR) and international normalized ratio (INR) (as appropriate) were taken during the physical consultations. Hence, these study periods were carefully chosen to compare the effectiveness of telemedicine on post-STEMI care during the pandemic, vs. the standard post-STEMI care during the pre-pandemic era. Patients with recurrent STEMI presentations during subsequent study periods were excluded to avoid duplication. During the pandemic, the hospital was actively involved in the care for COVID-19 patients.

None of the patients in the study were diagnosed with COVID-19. In our institution, the COVID-19 patients would be co-managed by the pandemic and the Cardiology inpatient teams. Once the COVID-19 patients have been de-isolated with negative COVID-19 polymerase chain reaction tests, they will be transferred under the Cardiology team's care. All patients, regardless of the COVID-19 status, will be reviewed outpatient in the Cardiology clinics. The COVID-19 status of the patients do not have any implications on their post-STEMI management.

Data Collection

Data on demographic and clinical characteristics were retrospectively collected from the hospital STEMI registry. This included past medical history, cardiovascular risk factors, presentation type, presentation route, complications during index admission, and medications on discharge. Angiographic data were also collected from the electronic medical records. Follow-up outpatient data on the number of outpatient consultations (including physical consultations, teleconsultations and cardiac rehabilitation), remote vital signs monitoring uptake, reported symptoms in clinic, and post-discharge medications were obtained. Serial measurements of Hba1c, LDL, and systolic blood pressure during the follow-up period were collected.

Guideline-directed medical therapy for STEMI was defined as being on dual antiplatelet therapy (aspirin and P2Y12 inhibitor), statin, β-blocker, with the option of angiotensin-converting enzyme inhibitor or angiotensin receptor blocker (ACEI/ARB) if the post-STEMI left ventricular ejection fraction (LVEF) was ≤40% or the patient had diabetes mellitus (8, 9), unless these medications were clinically contraindicated in the individual. Patients who were on oral anticoagulation had to complete a month of triple antithrombotic therapy followed by concomitant oral anticoagulation and single antiplatelet, to be considered as being on guideline-directed medical therapy. β-blocker and angiotensin-converting enzyme inhibitors (ACEI) or angiotensin II receptor blocker (ARB) doses were recorded on discharge and at follow-up clinic. Achieving target dose intensity of β-blocker and ACEI/ARB was based on the type and dose of the medication in accordance to a standardized algorithm as defined by our previous study (10). Guideline-directed medical therapy at follow-up was recorded in any of the outpatient clinic visits during the first year post-STEMI. The presence of guideline-directed medical therapy during the outpatient follow-up was used for the multivariable analyses. Our institution adopted the protocol for dual antiplatelet therapy in accordance to the European Society of Cardiology (11) and American College of Cardiology/American Heart Association (12) guidelines in administering a potent P2Y$_{12}$ inhibitor (prasugrel or ticagrelor), or clopidogrel if these are unavailable or contraindicated, and is usually prescribed before percutaneous coronary intervention is performed. Dual antiplatelet therapy was maintained over 12 months unless contraindicated.

Study Outcomes

All study outcomes were measured during the 1-year follow-up from the discharge date of the index admission. The primary safety endpoint was all-cause mortality. Secondary safety endpoints were cardiac readmissions for unplanned revascularisation, non-fatal MI, heart failure, arrhythmia, unstable angina, and major adverse cardiovascular events (MACE). MACE was defined as the composite outcome of each individual safety endpoints.

Secondary efficacy outcomes measured were (1) prescription of guideline-directed medical therapy, (2) achieving target dose intensities of β-blocker and ACEI/ARB (10), and (3) cardiovascular risk factor control (systolic blood pressure, LDL, and HbA1c).

Statistical Analyses

Categorical variables were described as percentages and continuous variables as mean with standard deviation (SD). Continuous variables were assessed with one-way analysis of variance (ANOVA). Categorical variables were evaluated with Pearson's chi-square test (or Fisher's Exact Test where appropriate). The multivariable Cox regression model was constructed to evaluate the association of telemedicine and 1-year MACE, as well as telemedicine and all-cause mortality, which included variables such as achieving medication target doses, guideline-directed medical therapy, remote vital signs monitoring, age, diabetes mellitus, chronic kidney disease, LVEF, smoking status, admission in the pandemic era, and presented with out-of-hospital cardiac arrest and/or cardiogenic shock. These co-variates were carefully chosen as they are traditional prognostic factors in STEMI patients.

Furthermore, *post-hoc* logistic regression was performed to evaluate the association of telemedicine and achieving guideline-directed medical therapy or medication target doses, which included co-variates such as age, smoking status, admission in the pandemic era, out-of-hospital cardiac arrest and cardiogenic shock, LVEF, gender, ethnicity, and presence of symptoms post-discharge. A p-value of < 0.05 was considered statistically significant. All statistical analyses were performed using IBM SPSS Statistics for Windows, Version 25.0. Armonk, NY. This study was conducted in accordance to the revised Declaration of Helsinki and approved by the institutional and local ethics committee (NHG DSRB No. 2013/00442). As the study involved retrospective analysis of clinically acquired data, the institutional review board waived the need for written patient consent.

RESULTS

Baseline Characteristics

Table 1 displays the baseline characteristics of the study population. A total of 320 patients with STEMI who underwent primary PCI were reviewed retrospectively from the local STEMI registry. A total of 17 patients were lost to follow-up, with 6 patients from the pre-pandemic era and 11 from the pandemic era. All patients included in the analysis completed 1-year of follow-up. There were 15 inpatient deaths, 9 and 6 of whom were from the pandemic and pre-pandemic eras, respectively. After excluding inpatient deaths in the index hospitalization, 288 patients who survived their index admission were recruited in the study analysis. There were 170 (59.0%) STEMI patients in the pandemic group, and 118 (41.0%) in the pre-pandemic group. Baseline demographic characteristics and past medical history were similar between both groups. There were more evolved MI

TABLE 1 | Baseline characteristics of study participants with ST-segment elevation myocardial infarction during index admission according to pre-pandemic or pandemic era.

	Total (n = 288)	Pandemic (n = 170)	Pre-pandemic (n = 118)	P-value
Demographic				
Age, years	59 (13)	59 (13)	58 (12)	0.626
Sex, female	46 (16.0)	29 (17.1)	17 (14.4)	0.546
Ethnicity				0.448
Chinese	142 (49.3)	88 (51.8)	54 (45.8)	
Malay	58 (20.1)	29 (17.1)	29 (24.6)	
Indian	66 (22.9)	39 (22.9)	27 (22.9)	
Other	22 (7.6)	14 (8.2)	8 (6.8)	
Medical history				
Smoking status				0.952
Non-smoker	130 (45.1)	78 (45.9)	52 (44.1)	
Active smoker	124 (43.1)	72 (42.4)	52 (44.1)	
Ex-smoker	34 (11.8)	20 (11.8)	14 (11.9)	
Hypertension	169 (58.7)	98 (57.6)	71 (60.2)	0.669
Diabetes	113 (39.2)	70 (41.2)	43 (36.4)	0.418
Hyperlipidaemia	179 (62.2)	100 (58.8)	79 (66.9)	0.162
Previous myocardial infarction	38 (13.2)	20 (11.8)	18 (15.3)	0.389
Previous PCI	45 (15.6)	21 (12.4)	24 (20.3)	0.066
Previous CABG	5 (1.7)	1 (0.6)	4 (3.4)	0.073
Stroke	14 (4.9)	8 (4.7)	6 (5.1)	0.883
Chronic kidney disease	23 (8.0)	15 (8.8)	8 (6.8)	0.529
Atrial fibrillation	8 (2.8)	4 (2.4)	4 (3.4)	0.598
Previous heart failure	9 (3.1)	6 (3.5)	3 (2.5)	0.636
Family history of premature CAD	37 (12.8)	28 (16.5)	9 (7.6)	**0.027**
Index admission				
Presentation type				**<0.001**
STEMI	248 (86.1)	136 (80.0)	112 (94.9)	
Evolved MI	23 (8.0)	23 (13.5)	0	
Out-of-hospital cardiac arrest	17 (5.9)	11 (6.5)	6 (5.1)	
Presentation route				0.156
Direct visit	199 (69.1)	112 (65.9)	87 (73.7)	
Interhospital transfers	89 (30.9)	58 (34.1)	31 (26.3)	
Complications				
Heart failure (Killip class 3)	34 (11.8)	26 (15.3)	8 (6.8)	**0.028**
Sepsis	23 (8.0)	18 (10.7)	5 (4.2)	**0.049**
New onset atrial fibrillation	16 (5.6)	14 (8.2)	2 (1.7)	**0.017**
Major bleed	27 (9.4)	18 (10.6)	9 (7.6)	0.397
Cardiogenic shock	21 (7.3)	13 (7.6)	8 (6.8)	0.781
Stroke	3 (1.0)	3 (1.8)	0	0.147
Acute kidney injury	53 (18.4)	27 (15.9)	26 (22.0)	0.185
Inotrope requirement	34 (11.8)	22 (12.9)	12 (10.2)	0.473
Requiring intubation	36 (12.5)	25 (14.7)	11 (9.3)	0.174
Requiring CABG	7 (2.5)	5 (3.2)	2 (1.7)	0.442
Length of stay, days	6 (7)	6 (8)	5 (5)	0.226
LVEF on discharge, %	46 (12)	44 (13)	49 (10)	**0.002**
Angiographic characteristics				
Radial access	210 (73.0)	128 (75.3)	82 (70.1)	0.451
Multivessel disease	140 (48.6)	85 (50.0)	55 (46.6)	0.571
Number of stents				0.616
0	36 (19.3)	30 (19.7)	6 (17.1)	

(Continued)

TABLE 1 | Continued

	Total (*n* = 288)	Pandemic (*n* = 170)	Pre-pandemic (*n* = 118)	*P*-value
1	120 (64.2)	95 (62.5)	25 (71.4)	
2	26 (13.9)	22 (14.5)	4 (11.4)	
3	5 (2.7)	5 (3.3)	0	
Door-to-balloon time, minutes	88 (145)	96 (172)	80 (103)	0.390
Discharge medications	269 (93.4)	160 (94.1)	109 (92.4)	0.557
Aspirin				
P2Y12 inhibitor	281 (97.6)	170 (100)	111 (94.1)	**0.001**
Oral anticoagulation	13 (4.5)	8 (4.7)	5 (4.2)	0.851
Betablocker	231 (82.5)	136 (84.0)	95 (80.5)	0.454
ACEI/ARB	191 (68.2)	113 (69.8)	78 (66.1)	0.517
Statin	269 (93.7)	157 (92.9)	112 (94.9)	0.488
Guideline-directed medical therapy	220 (76.4)	131 (77.1)	83 (75.4)	0.748

Categorical data presented as n (%). Continuous data presented as mean values (standard deviation).
ACEI, angiotensin converting enzyme inhibitor; ARB, angiotensin receptor blocker; CABG, coronary artery bypass graft; CAD, Coronary artery disease; LVEF, left ventricular ejection fraction; MI, myocardial infarction; PCI, percutaneous coronary intervention; STEMI, ST segment elevation myocardial infarction.
Statistically significant P values are highlighted in bold.

TABLE 2 | Characteristics of study participants with ST-segment elevation myocardial infarction during 1-year follow-up based on pre-pandemic or pandemic era.

	Total (*n* = 288)	Pandemic (*n* = 170)	Pre-pandemic (*n* = 118)	*P*-value
Outpatient consultations				
Total consultations	3.6 (3.1)	4.1 (3.5)	2.7 (2.2)	**<0.001**
Physical consultations	2.4 (1.7)	2.1 (1.6)	2.6 (1.7)	**0.043**
Teleconsultations	0.8 (1.7)	1.2 (1.9)	0.2 (1.1)	**0.001**
Cardiac rehabilitation	0.17 (0.74)	0.1 (0.7)	0.3 (0.7)	**<0.001**
Remote vital signs monitoring	97 (33.7)	59 (34.7)	38 (32.2)	0.659
Reported symptoms				
Typical chest pain	3 (1.2)	1 (0.7)	2 (1.9)	0.386
Atypical chest pain	22 (8.7)	12 (8.2)	10 (9.3)	0.741
Dyspnoea	21 (8.3)	10 (6.8)	11 (10.3)	0.320
Palpitations	3 (1.2)	3 (2.0)	0	0.137
Orthopnoea/PND/lower limb oedema	30 (11.8)	20 (13.6)	10 (9.3)	0.299
Post-discharge medications				
Aspirin	269 (93.4)	160 (94.1)	109 (92.4)	0.557
P2Y12 inhibitor	251 (87.8)	154 (90.6)	97 (83.6)	0.077
Oral anticoagulation	22 (7.6)	12 (7.1)	10 (8.5)	0.656
Beta-blocker	220 (76.9)	136 (80.0)	84 (72.4)	0.135
ACEI/ARB	202 (70.6)	126 (74.1)	76 (65.6)	0.117
Statin	263 (92.0)	158 (92.9)	105 (90.5)	0.459

Categorical data presented as n (%). Continuous data presented as mean values (standard deviation).
ACEI, angiotensin converting enzyme inhibitor; ARB, angiotensin receptor blocker; PND, paroxysmal nocturnal dyspnea.
Total consultations include physical and teleconsultations.
Statistically significant P values are highlighted in bold.

(13.5% vs. none, $p < 0.001$) and out-of-hospital cardiac arrest (6.5 vs. 5.1%, $p < 0.001$) in the pandemic group compared to the pre-pandemic group. Those who were admitted during the pandemic had higher incidence of unfavorable inpatient clinical progress compared to those admitted during the pre-pandemic era, such as Killip class 3 heart failure (15.3 vs. 6.8%, $p = 0.028$), sepsis (10.7 vs. 4.2%, $p = 0.049$), new onset atrial fibrillation (8.2 vs. 1.7%, $p = 0.017$) and lower LVEF (44 vs. 49%, $p = 0.002$). Importantly, there was no difference in discharge medications between the pandemic and pre-pandemic groups, apart from P2Y12 inhibitor use (100 vs. 94.1%, $p = 0.001$, respectively). Of the 7 patients discharged without P2Y12 inhibitor, only 1 was on concomitant oral anticoagulation with aspirin. The prescription of guideline-directed medical therapy on discharge between both groups was similar ($p = 0.748$).

Telemedicine, Guideline-Directed Medical Therapy, Target Drug Dose Intensity, and Cardiovascular Risk Factor Control

The characteristics of study participants during follow-up are described in **Table 2**. The average number of physical consultations per patient over a 1-year period during the pandemic was lower than that in the pre-pandemic era (2.1 vs. 2.6 visits per patient per year, respectively, $p = 0.043$). Conversely, there was higher average number of teleconsultations per patient during the pandemic compared to the pre-pandemic era over the 1-year follow-up (1.2 vs. 0.2 teleconsultations per patient per year, respectively, $p = 0.001$). Cardiac rehabilitation visits were fewer during the pandemic compared to pre-pandemic era (mean of 0.1 vs. 0.3 per patient per year, respectively, $p < 0.001$).

During follow-up, all first visit post-myocardial infarction clinic consultations were physical consultations. The mean duration from discharge to first physical consultation was longer during the pandemic compared to pre-pandemic era (50 ± 39 vs. 39 ± 31 days, respectively, $p = 0.005$), with also longer mean duration between the first physical consultation to second physical consultation during the pandemic compared to pre-pandemic era (128 ± 84 vs. 98 ± 67 days, respectively,

$p = 0.008$). There was no statistical difference in the uptake of remote vital signs monitoring between both study groups.

The pandemic era observed a significantly greater proportion of patients being on guideline-directed medical therapy (75.9%) compared to the pre-pandemic era (61.6%, $p = 0.010$) on follow-up. There was a trend towards achieving medication target doses in both β-blocker (19.4 vs. 15.3%, respectively, $p = 0.363$) and ACEI/ARB (9.5 vs. 5.9%, respectively, $p = 0.278$) during the pandemic compared to the pre-pandemic era.

We observed some differences in cardiovascular risk factor control and laboratory measurements from admission to outpatient surveillance between the pandemic and pre-pandemic periods. Firstly, LDL during index admission was similar in both pandemic and pre-pandemic groups (3.09 vs. 3.14 mmol/L, respectively, $p = 0.588$). Throughout the 1-year follow-up, similar improvement in LDL was achieved in the pandemic and pre-pandemic groups on the first clinic visit (1.81 vs. 1.52 mmol/L, respectively, $p = 0.124$), second visit (1.73 vs. 1.69 mmol/L, respectively, $p = 0.788$) and third visit (1.95 vs. 1.24 mmol/L, respectively, $p = 0.179$). Secondly, the percentage of patients with Hba1c ≥7% was similar between the pandemic and pre-pandemic eras during admission (30.7 vs. 29.0%, respectively, $p = 0.536$) and first clinic visit (29.4 vs. 32.6%,

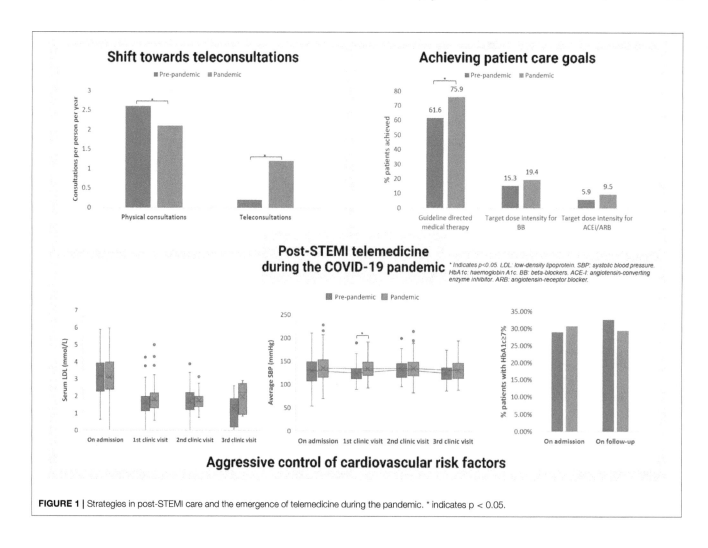

FIGURE 1 | Strategies in post-STEMI care and the emergence of telemedicine during the pandemic. * indicates p < 0.05.

respectively, $p = 0.734$). Thirdly, the average systolic blood pressure measured on discharge (134 vs. 128 mmHg, $p = 0.09$) and first clinic visit (133 vs. 123 mmHg, $p < 0.001$) was higher during the pandemic vs. the pre-pandemic eras; however such difference was no longer observed subsequently during the second (132 vs. 131 mmHg, $p = 0.235$) and third visit (130 vs. 123 mmHg, $p = 0.174$). These findings are summarized in **Figure 1**.

Study Safety End-Point

The 1-year all-cause mortality rates were similar between both groups ($p = 0.454$). However, there was an overall increased cardiac readmissions in the pandemic vs. the pre-pandemic era (14.1 vs. 5.1%, $p < 0.001$). There were increased heart failure readmissions in the pandemic (7.1%) compared to pre-pandemic era (1.7%, $p = 0.037$). No differences in unplanned revascularisation ($p = 0.787$), non-fatal MI ($p = 0.336$), arrhythmia ($p = 0.239$), unstable angina ($p = 0.701$) and MACE ($p = 0.112$) were observed between the two groups (**Table 3**).

On the multivariable Cox regression analysis, there was no significant association between teleconsultation and 1-year MACE [adjusted hazards ratio [aHR] 1.938, 95% confidence interval [CI] 0.896–4.190, $p = 0.093$]. Patients who achieved medication target doses (aHR 0.387, 95% CI 0.164–0.915, $p = 0.031$) and guideline-directed medical therapy (aHR 0.271, 95% CI 0.134–0.548, $p < 0.001$) were significantly associated with decreased rates of MACE after adjusting for important confounders (**Table 4**). There was also no significant association between teleconsultation and 1-year all-cause mortality (aHR 0.867, 95% CI 0.203–3.706, $p = 0.847$) after adjusting for important confounders (**Supplementary Material 1**)

In addition, the association between telemedicine and guideline-directed medical therapy or medication target doses was explored. *Post-hoc* multivariable logistic regression demonstrated that having teleconsultations was significantly associated with achieving guideline-directed medical

therapy [odds ratio [OR] 3.472, 95% CI 1.537–7.843, $p = 0.003$] but not achieving medication target doses (OR 1.272, 95% CI 0.636–2.542, $p = 0.496$), after adjusting for important confounders.

DISCUSSION

The conventional post-STEMI care has been drastically affected by the COVID-19 pandemic, and healthcare institutions have been required to adapt quickly to the stringent infectious control measures without compromising STEMI care. To our knowledge, this study is the first to systematically examine real-world data of the impact of COVID-19 pandemic on the standard of follow-up care and outcomes of STEMI patients over the ensuing year following hospital discharge. Our study has revealed several important findings. Firstly, despite exclusion of those who died while inpatient, patients admitted with STEMI during the pandemic had worse in-hospital outcomes such as increased rates of sepsis, new onset atrial fibrillation, heart failure and reduced left ventricular ejection fraction, compared to the pre-pandemic counterparts. Yet, during the 1-year follow-up, both these groups of patients had similar rates of all-cause mortality, but there were more frequent overall cardiac readmissions and heart failure readmission among those admitted during the pandemic era. This was in conjunction with the wider adaptation of teleconsultations, albeit a reduction of physical consultations, during the pandemic. Secondly, there were significantly more patients achieving guideline-directed medical therapy during the pandemic compared to the pre-pandemic era. Thirdly, there was also a trend toward increased rate of achieving medication target doses of β-blocker and ACEI/ARB therapy during the pandemic vs. the pre-pandemic era. Despite this, patients in the pandemic era had substantially higher mean LDL levels

TABLE 3 | Safety and efficacy end-points of the study population during 1-year follow-up post-index ST-segment elevation myocardial infarction admission.

	Total (n = 288)	Pandemic (n = 170)	Pre-pandemic (n = 118)	P-value
Safety end-point				
All-cause mortality	29 (10.1)	19 (11.2)	10 (8.5)	0.454
Cardiac readmission				
Unplanned revascularisation	3 (1.0)	2 (1.2)	1 (0.8)	0.787
Non-fatal MI	5 (1.7)	4 (2.4)	1 (0.8)	0.336
Heart failure	14 (4.9)	12 (7.1)	2 (1.7)	**0.037**
Arrythmia	2 (0.7)	2 (1.2)	0	0.239
Unstable angina	6 (2.1)	4 (2.4)	2 (1.7)	0.701
Major adverse cardiac events	59 (20.4)	43 (25.2)	16 (13.6)	0.112
Efficacy end-point				
Guideline-directed medical therapy	202 (70.2)	129 (75.9)	72 (61.6)	**0.010**
Achieving target dose intensity				
ACEI/ARB	23 (8.0)	16 (9.5)	7 (5.9)	0.278
Beta-blocker	51 (17.7)	33 (19.4)	18 (15.3)	0.363

Categorical data presented as n (%).
ACEI, angiotensin converting enzyme inhibitor; ARB, angiotensin receptor blocker; MI, myocardial infarction.
Statistically significant P values are highlighted in bold.

TABLE 4 | Cox regression for 1-year MACE in patients who survived index admission of STEMI.

Variables	Adjusted hazards ratio (95% confidence ratio)	p-value
Teleconsultation	1.938 (0.896–4.190)	0.093
Achieving medication target doses	0.387 (0.164–0.915)	**0.031**
Post-discharge guideline-directed medical therapy	0.271 (0.134–0.548)	**<0.001**
Remote vital signs monitoring	0.512 (0.216–1.213)	0.128
Age	1.024 (1.000–1.050)	0.055
Diabetes mellitus	1.369 (0.706–2.655)	0.353
Chronic kidney disease	3.057 (1.291–7.238)	**0.011**
Left ventricular ejection fraction	0.944 (0.921–0.969)	**<0.001**
Smoker/Ex-smoker	0.609 (0.297–1.246)	0.174
Out-of-hospital cardiac arrest/cardiogenic shock	0.842 (0.348–2.037)	0.702
Admission in pandemic era	1.905 (0.827–4.390)	0.130

Statistically significant P values are highlighted in bold.

on follow-up, albeit statistically non-significant, than those in the pre-pandemic era. Fourthly, for patients who survived the index STEMI admission, achieving medication target doses and guideline-directed medical therapy during the follow-up were independently associated with a lower 1-year MACE. Even though teleconsultation was not an independent predictor of MACE, our findings highlight that teleconsultation had a significant association with achieving guideline-directed medical therapy during follow-up.

As demonstrated by a recent meta-analysis on the global impact of the COVID-19 pandemic on STEMI care (3), short-term STEMI outcomes have been shown to be unfavorable with delayed symptom onset-to-door time, door-to-balloon time, lower LVEF on discharge, suboptimal reperfusion following PCI, increased duration of intensive care unit stay and increased in-hospital mortality during the pandemic era compared to the pre-pandemic era. Similarly, our study has shown worse STEMI metrics during the index admission even after excluding those who did not survive. There were higher overall cardiac related readmissions, particularly heart failure readmissions, in the pandemic compared to pre-pandemic eras. The study sample size, however, might be too small to detect small significant differences in readmission rates in the other subgroups. Despite this, our findings revealed similar 1-year follow-up mortality between both groups. Moreover, achieving medication target doses and guideline-directed medical therapy during follow-up are independent predictors of reducing the risk of MACE. Whether teleconsultation affects the overall outcome of patients with STEMI remains to be investigated. However, it allows for safer and regular follow-up during the pandemic, with drug optimisation for patients in the early post-STEMI period. Importantly, as demonstrated by the present study that patients admitting during the pandemic had worse clinical outcomes during the index admission, this could have increased the demand for closer outpatient surveillance with increased teleconsultations particularly for patients with worse severity of cardiac disease. This might be reflected by the large standard deviation of the average number of teleconsultations in this study. Telemedicine indeed offers a synergistic avenue, in conjunction with physical consultations, in enhancing more frequent

surveillance which is particularly important during the pandemic whilst maintaining the stringent infection control measures. Beyond the pandemic, teleconsultation has been shown to be cost-effective particularly for patients with myocardial infarction, as this important window of follow-up helps ameliorate adverse post-STEMI remodeling, and reduces the potential for the detrimental consequences of chronic heart failure (13).

Our recent published data displayed an increase in STEMI cases during the pandemic compared to the pre-pandemic era, which was partly due to the our regional STEMI network strategy in centralizing primary PCI service at our hospital, taking advantage of the geographical proximity of healthcare hospitals within the West of Singapore allowing timely inter-hospital transfers (14). Our previous study (4) also demonstrated that no significant door-to-balloon delay in inter-hospital transfers between the pandemic and pre-pandemic periods. This allowed the other hospitals to divert resources in providing care for the COVID-19 cases. Moreover, patients admitted during the pandemic had higher incidence of heart failure, sepsis, atrial fibrillation and lower LVEF, compared to those in the pre-pandemic period, which might play a role on the follow-up requirements during the pandemic.

Although telemedicine is a viable alternative, it is not a complete replacement for physical face-to-face consultations. In our study, there was increased overall cardiac related and heart failure readmissions during the pandemic compared to the pre-pandemic era. This could partly be due to the increased in-hospital complications during the pandemic era, such as increased prevalence of Killip class 3 heart failure at presentation and lower LVEF, compared to the pre-pandemic era. However, one might speculate that this observation suggests the limitation of teleconsultation follow-up when it comes to patients at risk of heart failure especially during the early stage following STEMI since it is limited by the absence of face-to-face clinical examination of fluid status and the lack of traditional parameter measurements in clinics such as body weight (15, 16). Nevertheless, the increasing evidence for telemedicine in heart failure management appears promising with several reviews demonstrating significant reduction in heart failure-related hospital admission compared to the conventional care

(17–21). Various trials including Telemedical Interventional Monitoring in Heart Failure (TIM-HF I and TIM-HF II) have shown improved patient education, medication adherence rates, lower mortality, overall hospital admissions and heart failure admissions, with improved quality of life for patients and reduced healthcare costs with the use of telemedicine (22, 23). Hence, patients might require closer monitoring during early stage following STEMI especially those with unfavorable risk factors such as lower LVEF (10).

Teleconsultations allow rapid titration of guideline-directed medical therapy and the increased likelihood of achieving medication target doses. Despite the restrictions during the pandemic, patients were more likely to be on guideline-directed medical therapy with similar medication target dose intensities, compared to their pre-pandemic counterparts. Our study echoes previous landmark trials such that patients achieving guideline-directed medical therapy and target doses have significantly lower rate of MACE (24, 25), especially in the setting of reduced LVEF. Several reviews demonstrated significant benefits in telemedicine for HbA1c (26, 27) and LDL reductions (28, 29), although the evidence for telemedical interventions on lowering blood pressure and body mass index remains mixed (30–32). However, our study highlights the concerns regarding aggressive cardiovascular risk factor control during the pandemic. Even though we demonstrated non-significant differences between pandemic and pre-pandemic groups in terms of LDL control over the 1-year follow-up period, the absolute differences between the serial LDL levels are clinically significant. Clinicians need to be aware of the potentiality of inadequate cardiovascular risk factor control particularly in the pandemic when lifestyle and diet might be changed during the lockdown. Teleconsultation remains the cornerstone of post-STEMI care during the pandemic with timely consultations, prompt initiation and titration of optimal medical therapy, whilst ensuring social distancing and reducing the patient's exposure to the hospital. As it will take time for the telemedicine program to adapt and evolve with the dynamic demands of the pandemic, it is a possibility that there might be variations in follow-up efficacy and efficiency within each of the study groups. However, given the small study sample size, the correlation of monthly variations with clinical outcomes is likely to be underpowered to draw any conclusions. Nevertheless, these are invaluable lessons that we should take beyond the pandemic in reducing waiting and traveling time, and clinic delays, whilst maintaining the standard of post-STEMI care (33–35). The institution is constantly evolving its telemedicine programmes in conjunction with regular physical consultations, and also integrating allied health care practitioner-led remote intensive management in addition to the cardiologist-led standard care (10).

Further studies are needed to evaluate patient's perspective and potential hurdles of telemedicine. Potential hurdles to implementation of telemedicine include patient-related factors associated with older age, low health literacy, cognitive dysfunction, privacy and security concerns (6, 36, 37). In the face of constant evolution of modalities to deliver digital healthcare, the European Society of Cardiology recommends the development of specific training programs for patients, caregivers and medical staff to assist them in understanding the capabilities and limitations of telemedicine (36).

CLINICAL IMPLICATIONS

With enhanced pandemic control measures, there is a pressing need to reduce physical consultations. Telemedicine plays an important role during the pandemic to bridge this gap in providing adequate follow-up to ensure optimisation of medical therapy post-STEMI and maintaining intensive cardiovascular risk factor control (21). It has, at least in part, contributed to the comparable 1-year post-STEMI outcomes between the pandemic and pre-pandemic eras among our patients, despite the adverse in-hospital STEMI metrics observed during the pandemic. These lessons from the pandemic serve a vital and broader role for the future with the emergence of telemedicine in post-STEMI care.

LIMITATIONS

Although this study is the first to examine the feasibility, efficacy, and safety of telemedicine in post-STEMI care during the pandemic, our study has several limitations that merit consideration. Firstly, this is a single-center retrospective observational study with a small sample size, and hence it is not possible to infer causality between telemedicine and the observed clinical outcomes. Nevertheless, our study offers real-world data based on consecutive patients enrolled in our STEMI database, and it reflects the actual follow-up processes that transitioned from physical consultations to teleconsultations during the pandemic. Secondly, the care provided to our control group (pre-pandemic group) might not be representative of care standard that was in line with the current recommendations. Nevertheless, it was chosen as it was the most recent period possible during which the 1-year follow-up care was not affected by the pandemic. Thirdly, teleconsultation was not standardized across all attending physicians and follow-up intervals varied among the patients given the nature of the study and resource constraints during the pandemic. Fourthly, the general attitudes to health and the stresses faced by patients and healthcare providers may also differ during pre-pandemic and pandemic era. For example, the pandemic might motivate the adoption of healthier lifestyle and healthier choices; on the other hand, the social distancing and compulsory home isolation may compel a more sedentary lifestyle (38). New challenges for healthcare providers during the pandemic include the need to comply to social distancing while ensuring the rapport with patients and quality of care are not compromised, and also identifying patients at higher risk of complications in a remote setting (39). However, this study was not designed to evaluate these additional factors which might have an impact on clinical outcomes and cardiovascular risk factor control.

However, our study findings represent actual clinical practice based on the physician's clinical judgment and discretion. Moreover, telemedicine consists of both virtual telehealth clinics and the utility of digital healthcare technologies. However, our study was not designed to evaluate the deliverance of digital healthcare. Overall, the results of the study need to be interpreted with caution, as the study observations might be related to the complex interplay between the COVID-19 pandemic, telemedicine and other non-measurable factors. This retrospective cohort provides, for the first time, real-world data of the dynamic change in hospital follow-up processes in STEMI follow-up with drastic decrease in physical consultations due to social distancing policies and the rapid emergence of telemedicine. With the inherent limitations of a real-world cohort study in this ever-changing landscape during a pandemic, the preliminary findings shed light on the invaluable lessons of teleconsultation adaptation, but controlling for external influences of the pandemic is evidently not possible. Furthermore, we were not able to evaluate if the number of total consultations correlated with improvement in outcomes as the number of consultations was determined by both the routine follow-up as well as the patient's individual need for closer surveillance.

CONCLUSION

Despite the unfavorable in-hospital STEMI metrics of patients admitted during the pandemic, their 1-year mortality rate was similar to those admitted during the pre-pandemic era.

The pandemic led to wider adaptation of teleconsultation which might partly contribute to increased use of guideline-directed medical therapy and meeting medication target dosing. Guideline-directed medical therapy was associated with better outcomes regardless of telemedicine or the pandemic. Telemedicine, at its core, should not be considered a replacement of the traditional face-to-face doctor-patient interactions, but a synergistic extension of post-STEMI care. The invaluable lessons of telemedicine during the pandemic should be extended for future post-STEMI care.

IRB INFORMATION

This study was approved by the local institution review board (NHG DSRB No. 2013/00442).

AUTHOR CONTRIBUTIONS

All authors listed have made a substantial, direct and intellectual contribution to the work, and approved it for publication.

REFERENCES

1. Ganatra S, Hammond SP, Nohria A. The novel coronavirus disease (COVID-19) threat for patients with cardiovascular disease and cancer. *JACC CardioOncol.* (2020) 2:350–55. doi: 10.1016/j.jaccao.2020.03.001
2. De Luca G, Verdoia M, Cercek M, Jenson LO, Vavlukis M, Calmac L, et al. Impact of COVID-19 pandemic on mechanical reperfusion for patients with STEMI. *J Am Coll Cardiol.* (2020) 76:2321–30. doi: 10.1016/j.jacc.2020.09.546
3. Chew NW, Ow ZGW, Teo VXY, Heng RRY, Ng CH, Lee CH, et al. The global impact of the COVID-19 pandemic on STEMI care: a systematic review and meta-analysis. *Can J Cardiol.* (2021) 37:1450–9. doi: 10.1016/j.cjca.2021.04.003
4. Chew NW, Sia CH, Wee HL, Loh JDB, Rastogi S, Kojodjojo P, et al. Impact of the COVID-19 pandemic on door-to-balloon time for primary percutaneous coronary intervention - results from the Singapore Western STEMI Network. *Circ J.* (2021) 85:139–49. doi: 10.1253/circj.CJ-20-0800
5. Cleland JGF, Clark RA, Pellicori P, Inglis SC. Caring for people with heart failure and many other medical problems through and beyond the COVID-19 pandemic: the advantages of universal access to home telemonitoring. *Eur J Heart Fail.* (2020) 22:995–8. doi: 10.1002/ejhf.1864
6. Tersalvi G, Winterton D, Cioffi GM, Ghidini S, Roberto M, Biasco L, et al. Telemedicine in heart failure during COVID-19: a step into the future. *Front Cardiovasc Med.* (2020) 7:612818. doi: 10.3389/fcvm.2020.612818
7. Nan J, Jia R, Meng S, Jin Y, Chen W, Hu H. The impact of the COVID-19 pandemic and the importance of telemedicine in managing acute st segment elevation myocardial infarction patients: preliminary experience and literature review. *J Med Syst.* (2021) 45:9. doi: 10.1007/s10916-020-01703-6
8. O'Gara PT, Kushner FG, Ascheim DD, Casey DE Jr, Chung MK, de Lemos JA, et al. 2013 ACCF/AHA guideline for the management of ST-elevation myocardial infarction: a report of the American College of Cardiology

Foundation/American Heart Association Task Force on Practice Guidelines. *Circulation.* (2013) 127:e362–425. doi: 10.1161/CIR.0b013e3182742c84
9. Ibanez B, James S, Agewall S, Antunes MJ, Bucciarelli-Ducci C, Bueno H, et al. 2017 ESC Guidelines for the management of acute myocardial infarction in patients presenting with ST-segment elevation: the Task Force for the management of acute myocardial infarction in patients presenting with ST-segment elevation of the European Society of Cardiology (ESC). *Eur Heart J.* (2018) 39:119–77. doi: 10.1093/eurheartj/ehx393
10. Chan MY, Koh KWL, Poh SC, Marchesseau S, Singh D, Han Y, et al. Remote postdischarge treatment of patients with acute myocardial infarction by allied health care practitioners vs standard care: the IMMACULATE randomized clinical trial. *JAMA Cardiol.* (2020) 6:830–5. doi: 10.1001/jamacardio.2020.6721
11. Valgimigli M, Bueno H, Byrne RA, Collet JP, Costa F, Jeppsson A, et al. 2017 ESC focused update on dual antiplatelet therapy in coronary artery disease developed in collaboration with EACTS: the Task Force for dual antiplatelet therapy in coronary artery disease of the European Society of Cardiology (ESC) and of the European Association for Cardio-Thoracic Surgery (EACTS). *Eur Heart J.* (2018) 39:213–60. doi: 10.1093/eurheartj/ehx419
12. Levine GN, Bates ER, Bittl JA, Brindis RG, Fihn SD, Fleisher LA, et al. 2016 ACC/AHA guideline focused update on duration of dual antiplatelet therapy in patients with coronary artery disease. *Circulation.* (2016) 134:e123–55. doi: 10.1161/CIR.0000000000000404
13. Roth GA, Johnson C, Abajobir A, Abd-Allah F, Abera SF, Abyu G, et al. Global, regional, and national burden of cardiovascular diseases for 10 causes, 1990 to 2015. *J Am Coll Cardiol.* (2017) 70:1–25. doi: 10.1016/j.jacc.2017.04.052
14. Phua K, Chew NWS, Sim V, Zhang AA, Rastogi S, Kojodjojo P, et al. One-year outcomes of patients with ST-segment elevation myocardial infarction during the COVID-19 pandemic. *J Thromb Thrombolysis.* (2021) 1–11 doi: 10.1007/s11239-021-02557-6
15. Tse G, Chan C, Gong M, Meng L, Zhang J, Su XL, et al. Telemonitoring and hemodynamic monitoring to reduce hospitalization rates in heart

failure: a systematic review and meta-analysis of randomized controlled trials and real-world studies. *J Geriatr Cardiol.* (2018) 15:298–309. doi: 10.11909/j.issn.1671-5411.2018.04.008

16. Emani S. Remote monitoring to reduce heart failure readmissions. *Curr Heart Fail Rep.* (2017) 14:40–7. doi: 10.1007/s11897-017-0315-2

17. Conway A, Inglis SC, Clark RA. Effective technologies for noninvasive remote monitoring in heart failure. *Telemed J E Health.* (2014) 20:531–8. doi: 10.1089/tmj.2013.0267

18. Kotb A, Cameron C, Hsieh S, Wells G. Comparative effectiveness of different forms of telemedicine for individuals with heart failure (HF): a systematic review and network meta-analysis. *PLoS ONE.* (2015) 10:e0118681. doi: 10.1371/journal.pone.0118681

19. Piotrowicz E. The management of patients with chronic heart failure: the growing role of e-Health. *Expert Rev Med Devices.* (2017) 14:271–277. doi: 10.1080/17434440.2017.1314181

20. Yun JE, Park JE, Park HY, Lee HY, Park DA. Comparative effectiveness of telemonitoring versus usual care for heart failure: a systematic review and meta-analysis. *J Card Fail.* (2018) 24:19–28. doi: 10.1016/j.cardfail.2017.09.006

21. Carbo A, Gupta M, Tamariz L, Palacio A, Levis S, Nemeth Z, et al. Mobile technologies for managing heart failure: a systematic review and meta-analysis. *Telemed J E Health.* (2018). doi: 10.1089/tmj.2017.0269

22. Koehler F, Winkler S, Schieber M, Sechtem U, Stangl K, Böhm M, et al. Telemedical Interventional Monitoring in Heart Failure (TIM-HF), a randomized, controlled intervention trial investigating the impact of telemedicine on mortality in ambulatory patients with heart failure: study design. *Eur J Heart Fail.* (2010) 12:1354–62. doi: 10.1093/eurjhf/hfq199

23. Koehler F, Koehler K, Prescher S, Sechtem U, Stangl K, Böhm M, et al. Mortality and morbidity 1 year after stopping a remote patient management intervention: extended follow-up results from the telemedical interventional management in patients with heart failure II (TIM-HF2) randomised trial. *Lancet Digit Health.* (2020) 2:e16–24. doi: 10.1016/S2589-7500(19)30195-5

24. Dargie HJ. Effect of carvedilol on outcome after myocardial infarction in patients with left-ventricular dysfunction: the CAPRICORN randomised trial. *Lancet.* (2001) 357:1385–90. doi: 10.1016/S0140-6736(00)04560-8

25. Effect of ramipril on mortality and morbidity of survivors of acute myocardial infarction with clinical evidence of heart failure. The Acute Infarction Ramipril Efficacy (AIRE) Study Investigators. *Lancet.* (1993) 342:821–8.

26. Eberle C, Stichling S. Clinical improvements by telemedicine interventions managing type 1 and type 2 diabetes: systematic meta-review. *J Med Internet Res.* (2021) 23:e23244. doi: 10.2196/23244

27. Eberle C, Stichling S. Effect of Telemetric interventions on glycated hemoglobin A1c and management of type 2 diabetes mellitus: systematic meta-review. *J Med Internet Res.* (2021) 23:e23252. doi: 10.2196/23252

28. Akbari M, Lankarani KB, Naghibzadeh-Tahami A, Tabrizi R, Honarvar B, Kolahdooz F, et al. The effects of mobile health interventions on lipid profiles among patients with metabolic syndrome and related disorders: a systematic review and meta-analysis of randomized controlled trials. *Diabetes Metab Syndr.* (2019) 13:1949–55. doi: 10.1016/j.dsx.2019.04.011

29. Lau D, McAlister FA. Implications of the COVID-19 pandemic for cardiovascular disease and risk-factor management. *Can J Cardiol.* (2021) 37:722–32. doi: 10.1016/j.cjca.2020.11.001

30. Parati G, Pellegrini D, Torlasco C. How digital health can be applied for preventing and managing hypertension. *Curr Hypertens Rep.* (2019) 21:40. doi: 10.1007/s11906-019-0940-0

31. Timpel P, Oswald S, Schwarz PEH, Harst L. Mapping the evidence on the effectiveness of telemedicine interventions in diabetes, dyslipidemia, and hypertension: an umbrella review of systematic reviews and meta-analyses. *J Med Internet Res.* (2020) 22:e16791. doi: 10.2196/16791

32. Huang JW, Lin YY, Wu NY. The effectiveness of telemedicine on body mass index: a systematic review and meta-analysis. *J Telemed Telecare.* (2019) 25:389–401. doi: 10.1177/1357633X18775564

33. Kronenfeld JP, Penedo FJ. Novel Coronavirus (COVID-19): telemedicine and remote care delivery in a time of medical crisis, implementation, and challenges. *Transl Behav Med.* (2021) 11:659–63. doi: 10.1093/tbm/ibaa105

34. Orlando JF, Beard M, Kumar S. Systematic review of patient and caregivers' satisfaction with telehealth videoconferencing as a mode of service delivery in managing patients' health. *PLoS ONE.* (2019) 14:e0221848. doi: 10.1371/journal.pone.0221848

35. Knox L, Rahman RJ, Beedie C. Quality of life in patients receiving telemedicine enhanced chronic heart failure disease management: a meta-analysis. *J Telemed Telecare.* (2017) 23:639–49. doi: 10.1177/1357633X16660418

36. Frederix I, Caiani EG, Dendale P, Anker S, Bax J, Böhm A, et al. ESC e-cardiology working group position paper: overcoming challenges in digital health implementation in cardiovascular medicine. *Eur J Prev Cardiol.* (2019) 26:1166–77. doi: 10.1177/2047487319832394

37. Walker RC, Tong A, Howard K, Palmer SC. Patient expectations and experiences of remote monitoring for chronic diseases: Systematic review and thematic synthesis of qualitative studies. *Int J Med Inform.* (2019) 124:78–85. doi: 10.1016/j.ijmedinf.2019.01.013

38. Esther T. Van der Werf, Martine Busch, Meik C. Jong, Hoenders HJR. Lifestyle changes during the first wave of the COVID-19 pandemic: a cross-sectional survey in the Netherlands. *BMC Public Health.* (2021) 21:1226. doi: 10.1186/s12889-021-11264-z

39. Verhoeven V, Tsakitzidis G, Philips H, Royen PV. Impact of the COVID-19 pandemic on the core functions of primary care: will the cure be worse than the disease? A qualitative interview study in Flemish GPs. *BMJ Open.* (2020) 10:e039674. doi: 10.1136/bmjopen-2020-039674

29

Impact of Angiotensin-Converting Enzyme Inhibitors and Angiotensin Receptor Blockers on the Inflammatory Response and Viral Clearance in COVID-19 Patients

Linna Huang [1,2,3†], Ziying Chen [1,2,3,4†], Lan Ni [5], Lei Chen [6], Changzhi Zhou [7], Chang Gao [8], Xiaojing Wu [1,2,3], Lin Hua [9], Xu Huang [1,2,3], Xiaoyang Cui [1,2,3], Ye Tian [1,2,3], Zeyu Zhang [1,2,3] and Qingyuan Zhan [1,2,3*]

[1] Center for Respiratory Diseases, China-Japan Friendship Hospital, Beijing, China, [2] Department of Pulmonary and Critical Care Medicine, China-Japan Friendship Hospital, Beijing, China, [3] National Clinical Research Center for Respiratory Diseases, Beijing, China, [4] Peking University Health Science Center, Beijing, China, [5] Department of Pulmonary and Critical Care Medicine, Zhongnan Hospital of Wuhan University, Wuhan, China, [6] Department of Pulmonary and Critical Care Medicine, Tongji Hospital, Tongji Medical College, Huazhong University of Science and Technology, Wuhan, China, [7] Department of Pulmonary and Critical Care Medicine, The Central Hospital of Wuhan, Wuhan, China, [8] Department of Critical Care Medicine, The First Affiliated Hospital of Soochow University, Suzhou, China, [9] School of Biomedical Engineering, Capital Medical University, Beijing, China

*Correspondence:
Qingyuan Zhan
drzhanqy@163.com

[†] These authors have contributed
equally to this work

Objectives: To evaluate the impact of angiotensin-converting enzyme inhibitors (ACEIs) or angiotensin receptor blockers (ARBs) on the inflammatory response and viral clearance in coronavirus disease 2019 (COVID-19) patients.

Methods: We included 229 patients with confirmed COVID-19 in a multicenter, retrospective cohort study. Propensity score matching at a ratio of 1:3 was introduced to eliminate potential confounders. Patients were assigned to the ACEI/ARB group ($n = 38$) or control group ($n = 114$) according to whether they were current users of medication.

Results: Compared to the control group, patients in the ACEI/ARB group had lower levels of plasma IL-1β [(6.20 ± 0.38) vs. (9.30 ± 0.31) pg/ml, $P = 0.020$], IL-6 [(31.86 ± 4.07) vs. (48.47 ± 3.11) pg/ml, $P = 0.041$], IL-8 [(34.66 ± 1.90) vs. (47.93 ± 1.21) pg/ml, $P = 0.027$], and TNF-α [(6.11 ± 0.88) vs. (12.73 ± 0.26) pg/ml, $P < 0.01$]. Current users of ACEIs/ARBs seemed to have a higher rate of vasoconstrictive agents (20 vs. 6%, $P < 0.01$) than the control group. Decreased lymphocyte counts [(0.76 ± 0.31) vs. (1.01 ± 0.45)*10^9/L, $P = 0.027$] and elevated plasma levels of IL-10 [(9.91 ± 0.42) vs. (5.26 ± 0.21) pg/ml, $P = 0.012$] were also important discoveries in the ACEI/ARB group. Patients in the ACEI/ARB group had a prolonged duration of viral shedding [(24 ± 5) vs. (18 ± 5) days, $P = 0.034$] and increased length of hospitalization [(24 ± 11) vs. (15 ± 7) days, $P < 0.01$]. These trends were similar in patients with hypertension.

Conclusions: Our findings did not provide evidence for a significant association between ACEI/ARB treatment and COVID-19 mortality. ACEIs/ARBs might decrease proinflammatory cytokines, but antiviral treatment should be enforced, and hemodynamics should be monitored closely. Since the limited influence on the ACEI/ARB treatment, they should not be withdrawn if there was no formal contraindication.

Keywords: ACE inhibitor, ARB, inflammatory response, viral clearance, COVID-19

INTRODUCTION

Up to March 31, 2020, the total number of patients with coronavirus disease 2019 has risen sharply to nearly 700,000 globally, with a mortality rate of nearly 5%. Meanwhile, this epidemic seems to be spreading at an exponential rate and has become an urgent public health emergency of international concern.

Several large retrospective studies have revealed that pre-existing cardiovascular disease and diabetes were the most frequent comorbidities of coronavirus disease 2019 (COVID-19) patients (1–3); these patients even had a higher risk of mortality (4, 5) than those with underlying respiratory disease. Angiotensin-converting enzyme inhibitors (ACEIs) and angiotensin receptor blockers (ARBs) are widely prescribed for these patients. ACEIs/ARBs have an impact on the renin-angiotensin system (RAS) and are postulated to attenuate pulmonary and systemic inflammatory responses, reducing the severity and mortality of viral pneumonia-related acute respiratory distress syndrome (6–8), ultimately by angiotensin-converting enzyme 2 (ACE2) upregulation through the ACE2-Ang-(1-7)-Mas axis (9).

The molecular biology of severe acute respiratory syndrome coronavirus 2 (SARS-CoV-2) is well-established, as it appears to bind to its target cells through ACE2, which is expressed by epithelial cells of the lung, to enable it to infect host cells (10, 11). The expression of ACE2 is substantially increased in patients who are treated with ACE inhibitors and ARBs (12), which promotes SARS-CoV-2 entry into the body, increasing the risk of developing COVID-19 (13, 14).

The controversial pathogenesis as well as the mixed results of several clinical studies (15, 16) of pneumonia with other pathogens made it difficult for physicians to determine whether the use of ACE inhibitors or ARBs should be terminated in patients with COVID-19.

To date, the actual impact of ACE inhibitor and ARB prescriptions on COVID-19 patients has not been assessed in current studies. Therefore, we aimed to evaluate the clinical manifestations and outcomes, especially inflammatory responses and viral clearance, by a multicenter, retrospective cohort study.

MATERIALS AND METHODS

Study Design and Population

We retrospectively included patients with microbiologically confirmed cases of COVID-19 according to the World Health Organization (WHO) (17) and official Chinese guidelines (18) in a multicenter retrospective cohort study performed at three tertiary hospitals in Wuhan, Hubei Province, China (Tongji Hospital, Tongji Medical College, Huazhong University of Science and Technology; Zhongnan Hospital of Wuhan University; and the Central Hospital of Wuhan) from February 15, 2020 to March 25, 2020. Patients included in our study were all assessed for eligibility on the basis of positive SARS-CoV-2 nucleic acid testing results by reverse transcription-polymerase chain reaction (RT-PCR) with nasopharyngeal swab samples. However, it was not possible to determine whether the patients had pneumonia, as not all were available for CT scans.

Exclusion Criteria

(1) Patients younger than 18 years old.

(2) Patients still hospitalized at the end of the study.

All patients were treated according to the standard protocols for antiviral, antibiotic, glucocorticoid, and Chinese medicine treatments.

The ethics committee of China-Japan Friendship Hospital approved this study (2020-21-K16). Written informed consent was waived due to the rapid emergence of this infectious disease.

Group Division

We divided the patients into two groups. The ACEI/ARB group included patients who were current users of ACE inhibitors or ARB medication, while non-current users were included as the control group. Patients in the ACEI/ARB group were further divided into subgroups of a continued medication group and a terminated medication group according to the application of ACE inhibitors or ARBs during hospitalization.

Data Collection and Analysis

We collected data on the following parameters from the hospital electronic medical record systems, nursing records, laboratory examination systems, and radiological examinations and obtained standardized data collection forms: demographic characteristics, comorbidities, medication history within 1 month, symptoms at admission, laboratory finding changes from day 1 to day 14, radiological manifestations, treatment during hospitalization and outcome data that contained the rate of in-hospital death and progression, the duration of viral shedding, the length of hospital stay and the time from onset to death or discharge. The primary outcome was mortality at discharge, while the secondary outcomes we observed included the duration of hospital stay, the duration of viral shedding and the differences in inflammatory cytokines.

Patients with cardiovascular disease and diabetes are often taking a combination of medications with statins (19) and oral hypoglycemic agents, especially thiazolidinediones, which have been reported to have an impact on the level of ACE2 by several studies (14, 20). To further control for potential confounders, data on the use of statins, thiazolidinediones and other antihypertensive agents (α receptor blocking agents, β receptor blocking agents, calcium channel blockers and diuretics) prior to admission in each group were calculated within 90 days (6).

Two researchers also independently reviewed the data collection forms to double check the data collected. Any missing or uncertain records of the epidemiological, medication and symptom data were collected and clarified through direct communication with patients and their families.

We compared the two groups in terms of the above aspects to identify the differences between current users and non-users prior to admission. Then, among the current users of ACEIs/ARBs, an analysis was conducted by comparing the dynamic changes in indicators involved in immune status and inflammatory reactions, as well as the outcomes between patients who continued and terminated medication during hospitalization. As hypertension itself could activate the RAS, patients with hypertension were excluded to avoid potential confounders. A comparison of the immune status, inflammatory reactions and outcomes between the ACEI/ARB and control groups in patients without hypertension was conducted.

Cytokine and Chemokine Measurement

To evaluate the impact of coronavirus and additional ACE inhibitors or ARBs on the production of cytokines or chemokines in the acute phase of the illness, plasma cytokines and chemokines [interleukin 1β (IL-1β), IL-2R, IL-6, IL-8, IL-10, and tumor necrosis factor α (TNF-α)] were measured using chemiluminescent immunoassays (CLIAs) (CFDA approved) by Siemens IMMULITE 1000 for patients according to the manufacturer's instructions.

Definitions

Medications classified as ACE inhibitors were benazepril, perindopril and fosinopril, while the ARBs of the included patients were candesartan, irbesartan, valsartan, olmesartan, telmisartan, and losartan.

Patients were considered a current user of medication if they had a supply of medication to last until the date of hospitalization assuming an 80% compliance rate (6, 21). The patients who did not meet the definition were regarded as non-current users. ACE inhibitors or ARBs were considered to be continued if they were given more than 50% of the days during hospitalization (8); otherwise, they were considered to be terminated.

In-hospital progression was defined as a decline in PaO_2/FiO_2 of more than 100 mmHg or the need for invasive positive pressure ventilation (IPPV) and/or extracorporeal membrane oxygenation (ECMO) during hospitalization.

The duration of viral shedding was defined as the duration of the SARS-CoV-2 RNA test result becoming negative from positive. All patients were routinely reexamined for SARS-CoV-2 nucleic acid testing every 5 days to assess whether it had turned negative.

Shock was defined according to the interim guidance of the WHO for novel coronavirus (22). Acute kidney injury (AKI) was identified and classified on the basis of the highest serum creatinine level or urine output criteria according to the Kidney Disease Improving Global Outcomes Classification (KDIGO) (22, 23). Respiratory failure, coagulation and liver failure were

defined as a Sequential Organ Failure Assessment (SOFA) score greater than or equal to two points.

Statistical Analysis

Descriptive statistics included proportions for categorical variables and the mean (standard deviation) or median (interquartile range) for continuous variables. Data were unadjusted unless specifically stated otherwise.

Processing of Missing Data

When the missing rate of vital variables involved in our study was <15%, we used SAS predictive mean matching imputation to replace missing values within each variable, while the variables were abandoned when the missing rate reached 20%.

Processing of the Unbalanced Sample Size: Propensity Score Matching

The propensity score matching (PSM) method was applied at a ratio of 1:3 between the ACEI/ARB group and the control group. The Sequential Organ Failure Assessment (SOFA) score, Charlson's comorbidity index (CCI), and body mass index (BMI) were matched variables in PSM to derive the cohort. The overall balance test was conducted to confirm that the baseline data of the two groups matched successfully.

Proportions were compared using χ^2 or Fisher's exact tests, and continuous variables were compared using the t-test or Wilcoxon rank sum test, as appropriate. Statistical significance was defined as a two-tailed P-value of ≤ 0.05. SAS software, version 9.4 (SAS Institute Inc.) was used for all analyses.

RESULTS

From February 15, 2020 to March 25, 2020, a total of 229 patients with confirmed cases of COVID-19 were admitted; 51 patients were current users of ACEIs/ARBs, while the other 178 patients were non-current users of the medication. The PSM method was applied at a ratio of 1:3 between the ACEI/ARB group ($n = 38$) and the control group ($n = 114$). The SOFA score and CCI were matched variables in PSM to derive the cohort. Thirteen cases in the ACEI/ARB group and 64 cases in the control group were not matched successfully. The overall balance test was with no significant difference between the two groups ($P = 0.872$). Among the patients with ACEI/ARB medication, 18 continued medication during hospitalization, while the other 20 terminated medication (**Figure 1**). The mean age was 57 ± 12 years, male patients accounted for 52% ($n = 79$), the SOFA score was 1.5 (1–2.3) points, and the CCI was 1 (1–2) prior to admission.

Comparisons of Baseline Prior Hospitalization Between the ACEI/ARB and Control Groups

The ACEI/ARB group included more patients with hypertension (67 vs. 22%, $P < 0.01$) than the control group. The demographic characteristics, other comorbidities, severity of the condition and possible medication histories might have influenced the ACE2 level but did not differ significantly between the two groups. No significant difference was found between the two groups in

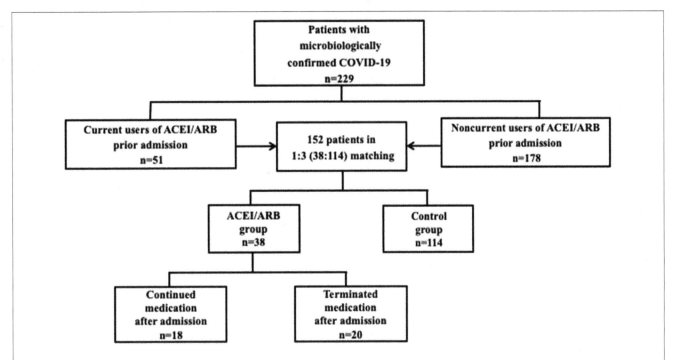

FIGURE 1 | Flowchart. A flowchart illustrated the enrollment of patients in our study. From February 15, 2020 to March 25, 2020, a total of 229 patients with confirmed cases of COVID-19 were admitted; 51 patients were current users of ACEIs/ARBs, while the other 178 patients were non-current users of the medication. The PSM method was applied at a ratio of 1:3 between the ACEI/ARB group (n = 38) and the control group (n = 114). The SOFA score and CCI were matched variables in PSM to derive the cohort. Among the patients with ACEI/ARB medication, 18 continued medication during hospitalization, while the other 20 terminated medication.

time from onset to hospitalization and to COVID-19 diagnosis (**Table 1**).

Comparisons of Clinical Symptoms, Laboratory Examinations, and Radiological Manifestations on Admission Between the ACEI/ARB and Control Groups

The symptoms, including fever, cough, hemoptysis, dyspnea, fatigue/myalgia and diarrhea, as well as vital signs, with the exception of systolic blood pressure, were not significantly different between the ACEI/ARB group and the control group. Although systolic blood pressure was lower in the study group (116 ± 14 vs. 124 ± 13 mmHg, $P = 0.031$), it was within the normal range. For laboratory examinations, patients with ACE inhibitor or ARB medication had lower lymphocyte counts [(0.76 ± 0.31) vs. (1.01 ± 0.45) $*10^9$/L, $P = 0.027$] than the control group (**Table 2**).

The first measurements of the inflammatory factors, including IL-1β, IL-2R, IL-6, IL-8, IL-10, and TNFα, were taken within 3 days of admission; while the most (97%, 147/152) were within 24 h. The time from COVID-19 diagnose to measurements was (3 ± 2) days. Besides, as the missing rate reached 12–15%, SAS predictive mean matching imputation was applied to replace missing values in each group. The missing rates of IL-2R, serum ferritin, erythrocyte sedimentation rate (ESR) and C-reactive protein (CRP) were as high as 25–35%; therefore, they were abandoned in the statistical analysis. Patients in the

ACEI/ARB group had slightly lower levels of proinflammatory cytokines, including IL-1β [(6.20 ± 0.38) vs. (9.30 ± 0.31) pg/ml, $P = 0.020$], IL-6 [(31.86 ± 4.07) vs. (48.47 ± 3.11) pg/ml, $P = 0.041$], IL-8 [(34.66 ± 1.90) vs. (47.93 ± 1.21) pg/ml, $P = 0.027$], and TNF-α [(6.11 ± 0.88) vs. (12.73 ± 0.26) pg/ml, $P < 0.01$], and higher levels of the anti-inflammatory cytokine IL-10 [(9.91 ± 0.42) vs. (5.26 ± 0.21) pg/ml, $P = 0.012$] than the control group (**Table 2**).

Comparison of Organ Function, Treatment and Outcomes During Hospitalization Between the ACEI/ARB and Control Groups

Current users of ACEIs/ARBs seemed to have a higher rate of vasoconstrictive agent application (18 vs. 7%, $P < 0.01$) than the control group; however, the percentages of respiratory failure, shock, AKI, coagulation failure, and liver failure were not different between the two groups. In addition, the necessities for invasive IPPV and ECMO were not decreased in the ACEI/ARB group (**Table 3**).

The duration of viral shedding [(24 ± 5) vs. (18 ± 5) days, $P = 0.034$], length of hospital stay [(24 ± 11) vs. (15 ± 7) days, $P < 0.01$], and time from onset to death or discharge [(32 ± 10) vs. (25 ± 7) days, $P < 0.01$] were longer in the ACEI/ARB group than in the control group, while no difference was found in the rate of in-hospital progression or death (**Table 3**).

TABLE 1 | Baseline variables in the two groups prior to admission.

	All (n = 152)	ACEI/ARB group (n = 38)	Control group (n = 114)	P
Age, years, mean ± SD	57 ± 12	57 ± 11	58 ± 18	0.671
Gender (men), number (%)	79 (52%)	19 (51%)	60 (53%)	0.533
Body mass index, kg/m², mean ± SD	21.0 ± 6.9	21.1 ± 6.4	21.0 ± 7.0	0.838
Comorbidities, number (%)				
Hypertension	55 (36%)	30 (67%)	25 (22%)	<0.001[b]
Diabetes	37 (24%)	10 (27%)	27 (24%)	0.217
Coronary heart disease	17 (11%)	6 (16%)	11 (10%)	0.071
Chronic heart failure	6 (4%)	2 (5%)	4 (4%)	0.622
Underlying lung disease	18 (12%)	7 (18%)	11 (10%)	0.094
Chronic kidney disease	2 (1%)	1 (3%)	1 (1%)	0.512
Chronic liver dysfunction	3 (2%)	0 (0%)	3 (3%)	0.425
Malignancy	3 (2%)	0 (0%)	3 (3%)	0.186
History of smoking, number (%)	23 (15%)	8 (21%)	15 (13%)	0.081
Other medication history within 90 days, number (%)				
Corticosteroids	0 (0%)	0 (0%)	0 (0%)	1
Immunosuppressants	0 (0%)	0 (0%)	0 (0%)	1
Statins	21 (14%)	6 (16%)	15 (13%)	0.214
Thiazolidinediones	1 (1%)	0 (0%)	1 (1%)	0.996
α receptor blocking agent	4 (3%)	1 (3%)	3 (3%)	0.820
β receptor blocking agent	19 (13%)	5 (13%)	14 (12%)	0.731
CCB	19 (13%)	5 (13%)	14 (12%)	0.731
Diuretics	16 (11%)	4 (11%)	12 (11%)	1
SOFA Score, points (IQR)	1.5 (1–2.3)	1.5 (1–2.5)	1.5 (1–2)	0.879
CCI, points (IQR)	1 (1–2)	1 (1–2)	1 (1–2)	1
Treatment before hospital, number (%)				
Methylprednisolone	10 (7%)	3 (8%)	7 (6%)	0.091
Antibiotic therapy	92 (61%)	22 (58%)	70 (61%)	0.429
Antiviral therapy	102 (67%)	22 (57%)	80 (70%)	0.239
Time from onset to hospital admission, days, mean ± SD	10 ± 6	11 ± 3	10 ± 6	0.296
Time from onset to diagnosis, days, mean ± SD	7 ± 5	7 ± 5	7 ± 2	0.8

[b]$P < 0.01$; CCB, calcium channel blocker; SOFA, Sequential Organ Failure Assessment; CCI, Charlson's Comorbidity Index (18).

Subgroup Analyses: Comparison Between Patients Who Continued and Terminated Medication During Hospitalization

Among the patients in the ACEI/ARB group, 18 continued medication during hospitalization, while the other 20 terminated medication for several reasons. The baseline variables were with no significant difference between the two groups (**Supplementary Table 1**). The dynamic changes in lymphocytes and inflammatory factors at the first, seventh, and fourteenth days after hospitalization as well as the outcomes were compared between the two groups. The missing rates of IL-2R and IL-8 at seven days and 14 days after admission were extremely high and were not included in the analysis. Patients with continued use of ACEIs/ARBs had consistently lower levels of lymphocytes, IL-1β, IL-6, and TNF-α but maintained higher levels of IL-10 on the seventh and fourteenth days than patients who terminated medication during hospitalization. However, the patients who terminated the medication had a trend of elevated lymphocyte counts [day 1, day 7, day 14: (0.82 ± 0.47) vs. (1.41 ± 0.74) vs. (1.69 ± 0.45)*10⁹/L, $P = 0.029$] and IL-1β [day 1, day 7, day 14: (6.03 ± 3.19) vs. (10.78 ± 6.88) vs. (13.75 ± 5.26) pg/ml,

$P < 0.01$] from the first day to the fourteenth day (**Figure 2, Supplementary Table 2**).

The duration of viral shedding [(27 ± 4) vs. (21 ± 5) days, $P = 0.032$], length of hospital stay [(26 ± 10) vs. (20 ± 3) days, $P = 0.044$], and time from onset to death or discharge [(34 ± 9) vs. (29 ± 10) days, $P = 0.019$] were longer in the continued medication group than in the terminated medication group. The rates of in-hospital progression and death were not significantly different between the two groups (**Table 4**).

Subgroup Analyses: A Comparison of the Immune Status, Inflammatory Reactions and Outcomes Between the ACEI/ARB and Control Groups in Patients With Hypertension

Among 55 patients with hypertension, 30 patients were divided into the study group (ACEI/ARB group), and the other 25 patients were in the control group.

Compared with the control group, the patients in the study group had lower levels of IL-1β [(6.33 ± 0.56) vs. (8.27 ± 0.14)

TABLE 2 | Clinical, laboratory findings, and radiological manifestations in the two groups on admission.

	All (n = 152)	ACEI/ARB group (n = 38)	Control group (n = 114)	P
Initial symptoms, number (%)				
Fever ($\geq$37.3°C)	140 (92%)	35 (92%)	105 (92%)	0.981
Cough	109 (72%)	27 (70%)	82 (72%)	0.866
Productive cough	60 (39%)	16 (42%)	44 (39%)	0.605
Hemoptysis	3 (2%)	1 (3%)	2 (2%)	0.263
Dyspnea	78 (51%)	20 (53%)	58 (51%)	0.432
Fatigue or myalgia	67 (44%)	16 (43%)	51 (45%)	0.619
Diarrhea	46 (30%)	12 (31%)	34 (30%)	0.764
Initial signs, mean $\pm$ SD				
Highest temperature, °C	38.4 $\pm$ 0.7	38.5 $\pm$ 1.1	38.3 $\pm$ 0.4	0.461
Respiratory rate, breaths/min	23 $\pm$ 3	22 $\pm$ 3	23 $\pm$ 3	0.709
Heart rate, beats/min	96 $\pm$ 11	97 $\pm$ 8	96 $\pm$ 14	0.338
Systolic blood pressure, mmHg	123 $\pm$ 10	116 $\pm$ 14	124 $\pm$ 13	0.031[a]
SpO_2, %	94 $\pm$ 4	93 $\pm$ 3	94 $\pm$ 4	0.741
FiO_2, %	40 $\pm$ 18	42 $\pm$ 15	40 $\pm$ 17	0.302
Laboratory examination, mean $\pm$ SD				
Blood routine				
WBC, *10^9/L	5.94 $\pm$ 3.00	6.27 $\pm$ 3.21	5.80 $\pm$ 2.97	0.085
Neutrophil count, *10^9/L	4.40 $\pm$ 2.99	5.21 $\pm$ 3.29	4.39 $\pm$ 3.01	0.097
Lymphocytes, *10^9/L	0.89 $\pm$ 0.40	0.76 $\pm$ 0.31	1.01 $\pm$ 0.45	0.027[a]
Biochemical examination				
ALT, U/L	43 $\pm$ 4	42 $\pm$ 4	43 $\pm$ 4	0.747
AST, U/L	40 $\pm$ 5	44 $\pm$ 4	40 $\pm$ 5	0.841
TBIL, mmol/L	11.3 $\pm$ 5.2	11.0 $\pm$ 5.9	11.4 $\pm$ 5.0	0.660
Scr, μmol/L	79.2 $\pm$ 2.7	77.5 $\pm$ 2.2	80.1 $\pm$ 3.6	0.915
LDH, U/L	295 $\pm$ 89	301 $\pm$ 77	294 $\pm$ 91	0.617
TnT, pg/ml	11 $\pm$ 1	12 $\pm$ 1	11 $\pm$ 1	0.770
NT-proBNP, pg/ml	401 $\pm$ 55	411 $\pm$ 55	397 $\pm$ 51	0.528
Inflammatory factors				
IL-1β, pg/ml	8.02 $\pm$ 0.33	6.20 $\pm$ 0.38	9.30 $\pm$ 0.31	0.020[a]
IL-2R, U/ml	796.02 $\pm$ 27.40	724.25 $\pm$ 52.30	807.23 $\pm$ 26.21	0.246
IL-6, pg/ml	47.11 $\pm$ 3.26	31.86 $\pm$ 4.07	48.47 $\pm$ 3.11	0.041[a]
IL-8, pg/ml	46.03 $\pm$ 1.85	34.66 $\pm$ 1.90	47.93 $\pm$ 1.21	0.027[a]
IL-10, pg/ml	6.37 $\pm$ 0.37	9.91 $\pm$ 0.42	5.26 $\pm$ 0.21	0.012[b]
TNF-α, pg/ml	11.21 $\pm$ 0.44	6.11 $\pm$ 0.88	12.73 $\pm$ 0.26	<0.001[b]
PCT, ng/ml	0.27 $\pm$ 0.07	0.26 $\pm$ 0.03	0.29 $\pm$ 0.08	0.619
Coagulation function				
PT, s	14 $\pm$ 3	14 $\pm$ 1	14 $\pm$ 1	0.995
APTT, s	42 $\pm$ 5	44 $\pm$ 3	42 $\pm$ 5	0.881
D-Dimer, μg/ml	2.19 $\pm$ 0.44	2.33 $\pm$ 0.47	2.12 $\pm$ 0.46	0.448
Chest CT manifestations, number (%)				
Bilateral lesion	82 (54%)	19 (49%)	63 (55%)	0.374
GGO	89 (59%)	19 (49%)	70 (61%)	0.310
Consolidation	36 (24%)	11 (29%)	25 (22%)	0.229

[a]P < 0.05; [b]P < 0.01; SpO2, saturation of peripheral oxygen; FiO2, fraction of inspiration; ALT, alanine aminotransferase; AST, aspartate aminotransferase; TBIL, total bilirubin; Scr, creatinine; LDH, lactate dehydrogenase; TnT, troponin T; NT-proBNP, N-terminal pro-brain natriuretic peptide; IL-1β, interleukin-1β; IL-2R, interleukin-2R; IL-6, interleukin-6; IL-8, interleukin-8; IL-10, interleukin-10; TNF-α, tumor necrosis factor-α; PCT, procalcitonin; PT, prothrombin time; APTT, activated partial thromboplastin time; GGO, ground-glass opacity.

pg/ml, $P = 0.026$], IL-6 [(40.16 $\pm$ 12.59) vs. (52.33 $\pm$ 14.09) pg/ml, $P = 0.030$], and IL-8 [(31.60 $\pm$ 2.97) vs. (42.83 $\pm$ 3.27) pg/ml, $P = 0.030$] on admission. Regarding clinical outcomes, the duration of viral shedding [(26 $\pm$ 6) vs. (19 $\pm$ 4) days, $P = 0.029$] and time from onset to death or discharge [(30 $\pm$ 10) vs. (24 $\pm$ 8) days, $P = 0.031$] were longer in the study group than in the

TABLE 3 | Organ function, treatments and outcomes in the two groups during hospitalization.

	All (n = 152)	ACEI/ARB group (n = 38)	Control group (n = 114)	P
Organ failure*, number (%)				
Respiratory failure	25 (16%)	8 (20%)	17 (15%)	0.092
Shock	13 (9%)	4 (11%)	8 (7%)	0.060
AKI	15 (10%)	4 (11%)	11 (10%)	0.829
Coagulation failure	3 (2%)	1 (3%)	2 (2%)	0.664
Liver failure	15 (10%)	4 (11%)	11 (10%)	0.796
Treatment, number (%)				
Antibiotics	105 (69%)	24 (64%)	81 (71%)	0.461
Antiviral treatment	145 (95%)	36 (92%)	109 (96%)	0.334
Glucocorticoids	49 (32%)	11 (30%)	38 (33%)	0.612
Intravenous immunoglobin	36 (24%)	9 (23%)	27 (24%)	0.552
Standard oxygen therapy	132 (87%)	35 (92%)	97 (85%)	0.080
HFNO	28 (18%)	7 (18%)	21 (18%)	0.927
NPPV	18 (12%)	5 (12%)	13 (11%)	0.327
IPPV	17 (11%)	4 (11%)	13 (11%)	0.629
ECMO	4 (3%)	1 (3%)	3 (3%)	0.994
Vasoconstrictive agents	15 (10%)	7 (18%)	8 (7%)	<0.01[b]
Outcome				
In-hospital progression[#], number (%)	28 (18%)	6 (16%)	22 (19%)	0.326
In-hospital death, number (%)	15 (10%)	4 (10%)	11 (10%)	0.983
Hospital length of stay, days, mean ± SD	17 ± 8	24 ± 11	15 ± 7	<0.01[b]
Duration of viral shedding, days, mean ± SD	19 ± 3	24 ± 5	18 ± 5	0.034[a]
Time from onset to death or discharge, days, mean ± SD	27 ± 9	32 ± 10	25 ± 7	<0.01[b]

[a]P < 0.05; [b]P < 0.01; *Shock was defined according to the interim guidance of the WHO for novel coronavirus (22, 23). AKI was identified and classified on the basis of the highest serum creatinine level or urine output criteria according to kidney disease, improving global outcome classification (23, 24). Respiratory failure, coagulation and liver failure were defined as a SOFA score greater than or equal to two points. [#]Defined as a decline in $PaO_2/FiO_2 > 100$ mmHg or the need for IPPV and/or ECMO during hospitalization. AKI, acute kidney injury; HFNO, high flow nasal oxygenation; NPPV, noninvasive positive pressure ventilation; IPPV, invasive positive pressure ventilation; ECMO, extracorporeal membrane oxygenation.

control group; however, no difference was detected in the rate of in-hospital progression and death between the two groups.

DISCUSSION

To our knowledge, this is the first study to thoroughly evaluate the inflammatory responses and viral clearance of COVID-19 patients treated with ACEIs/ARBs by a multicenter, retrospective cohort control study and to allow dynamic observation of inflammatory responses by continuous monitoring from the first to the fourteenth day after admission.

The major findings of our study were that ACEIs/ARBs inhibited the proinflammatory response but promoted the anti-inflammatory response and persistently decreased lymphocytes, thus extending the duration of viral shedding and the length of hospital stay. Antiviral treatments should be enforced in those patients. In addition, since current users of ACEIs/ARBs seem to have a higher necessity of vasoconstrictive agents, hemodynamics should be monitored closely during medication use. The message to the physician was that the influence on the ACEI/ARB treatment was limited, and they should not be withdrawn if there was no formal contraindication.

Inflammation is mediated by proinflammatory cytokines and anti-inflammatory cytokines. Inappropriate elevated

expression of proinflammatory cytokines can result in sepsis, tissue destruction, or death (21, 24). Our study revealed that the plasma levels of IL-1β, IL-6, IL-8, and TNF-α in patients taking ACEI/ARBs were lower than those in patients not without medication; in addition, persistently lower levels of proinflammatory factors were maintained in patients who continued medication during hospitalization, which was consistent with the previous experimental results by Gullestad et al. (25) with the conclusion that high-dose enalapril was associated with a significant decrease in IL-6 activity in patients with severe chronic heart failure. The specific organ and systemic inflammatory responses were postulated to attenuate through a reduction in the level of cytokines, which might be explained by the attenuating effects of ACE inhibitors through the deactivation of the ACE-AngII-AT1 axis but the stimulation of the ACE2-Ang-(1-7)-Mas axis in a feedback mechanism (9, 26, 27) as a negative regulator with attenuated cytokines and thus protecting the patients from organ injury. Consequently, some authors (28, 29) have speculated that the use of ACEIs/ARBs might actually be a potentially beneficial intervention in those with COVID-19.

Apart from organ protection by attenuating the inflammatory response, basic investigation has shown that bradykinin and substance P produced by ACE inhibitors sensitize the sensory

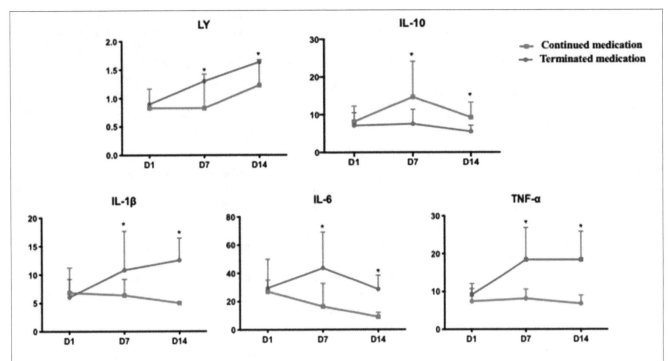

FIGURE 2 | The dynamic changes in the lymphocyte counts and inflammatory factors between patients who continued and those who terminated ACEIs/ARBs during hospitalization. Patients with continued use of ACEIs/ARBs had consistently lower levels of lymphocytes, IL-1β, IL-6, and TNF-α but maintained higher levels of IL-10 on the seventh and fourteenth days than patients who terminated medication during hospitalization. However, the patients who terminated the medication had a trend of elevated lymphocyte counts and IL-1β from the first day to the fourteenth day. *$p < 0.01$.

TABLE 4 | Outcomes in patients who continued and those who terminated ACEIs/ARBs during hospitalization.

Outcomes	Continued ACEIs/ARBs ($n = 18$)	Terminated ACEIs/ARBs ($n = 20$)	P
In-hospital progression[#]	3 (17%)	3 (15%)	0.611
In-hospital death	2 (11%)	2 (10%)	0.709
Duration of viral shedding, days	27 ± 4	20 ± 5	0.032[a]
Hospital length of stay, days	26 ± 10	20 ± 3	0.044[a]
Time from onset to death or discharge, days	34 ± 9	29 ± 10	0.019[a]

[a]$P < 0.05$; [#]Defined as a decline in $PaO_2/FiO_2 > 100$ mmHg or the need for IPPV and/or ECMO during hospitalization.

nerves of the airways and enhance the cough reflex (30, 31), which plays a protective role against pathogens. These two mechanics made it possible to improve the outcome in patients with pneumonia. Mortensen et al. (6) found a significant decrease in mortality, the length of hospital stay, and mechanical ventilation in patients taking ACE/ARBs who were hospitalized with pneumonia compared to a matched cohort. A meta-analysis (32) that included 19 studies noted that patients taking ACE inhibitors were associated with a significant approximately one-third reduction in the risk of pneumonia compared with controls. In addition, a recent study (8) by Christopher Henry also observed lower rates of death and intubation with continued use of ACE inhibitors than with terminated use (OR = 0.25; 95% CI, 0.09–0.64) throughout the hospital stay in cases of viral pneumonia not due to coronavirus. Unfortunately, our study did not find decreased mortality in patients with current use of ACEI/ARBs, even though we analyzed patients with

continued medication during hospitalization and combined with hypertension to avoid potential confounding factors. The most likely explanation was that our study included a small number of patients, while most of their patients had mild cases as determined by SOFA scores and without excessive inflammatory reactions, which was the target for ACE inhibitors or ARBs.

What noteworthy was that ACEI/ARBs increased the necessity of vasoconstrictive agents. It could be explained by the nature of the antihypertensive agents and came as a revelation to us that the hemodynamics should be monitored closely during medication.

Our research also revealed that ACE inhibitors or ARBs led to prolonged viral shedding and extended the length of hospitalization. SARS-CoV-2 appears to bind to its target cells through angiotensin-converting enzyme 2 (ACE2). ACE inhibitors or ARBs upregulate ACE2 receptor expression in humans (33) by blocking the classic ACE pathway; thus, it is theoretically possible that the pre-existing use of these drugs might predispose a person to infection with a greater viral load of SARS-CoV-2 (13). This hypothesis was supported by the evidence of Ferrario that there was a 4.7-fold increase in cardiac ACE2 mRNA by an ACE inhibitor (34). Decreased lymphocyte counts and elevated plasma levels of IL-10 were also important discoveries in patients with ACEI/ARBs. Moreover, the lymphocyte counts in patients with continued use of medication during hospitalization recovered slowly, as observed by successive monitoring on the first to fourteenth days. The immune status was weakened by lymphocytopenia and elevated anti-inflammatory cytokines in patients taking ACEI/ARBs, which might be another reason for the slow viral clearance. As the important criterion for discharge was the negative conversion of the SARS-CoV-2, prolonged viral shedding led to an extended length of hospitalization. This might be the defect of the ACEI/ARBs and might explain the mixed results and controversy about their prescription in COVID-19 patients. For this reason, antiviral therapy in patients taking ACEI/ARBs should be reinforced, and their viral load should be monitored closely.

An autopsy report revealed that mononuclear inflammatory infiltration dominated by lymphocytes was observed in the lungs, but no virus inclusion bodies were found (35). We could then propose a hypothesis that cytokines released by inflammatory storms secondary to viral infection might be more important in the death of critically ill patients with COVID-19 than the viral infection itself in a certain period. From this perspective, it is possible that ACEI/ARBs might improve the outcome in critically ill patients with excessive inflammatory responses or severe multiple organ failure; when the inflammatory storm gradually diminishes, the focus of therapy should be on clearance of the virus and the enhancement of the immune system. Prospective

cohort and randomized controlled trials are needed to confirm this hypothesis and examine potential mechanisms of action.

Our study was limited by the small number of patients included and by not strictly excluding confounding factors. We especially noticed that the number of patients with hypertension was much higher in the ACEI/ARB group, which might be an important confounding factor. However, by subgroup analyze in patients with hypertension, we found similar results. The prospective randomized controlled studies designed by increasing the sample size and strictly excluding potential confounders to explore the impact of ACE/ARBs on inflammatory responses, viral clearance and the mortality in COVID-19 patients should be encouraged in the future.

AUTHOR CONTRIBUTIONS

All authors made substantial contributions to the conception and design of the study or to the data acquisition, analysis, or interpretation, reviewed and approved the final manuscript, and significantly contributed to this study. QZ took full responsibility for the integrity of the submission and publication and was involved in the study design. LHuang and ZC involved in data collection, had full access to all of the data in the study, took responsibility for the integrity of the data and were responsible for data verification, as well as the drafting of the manuscript. LHua took the responsibility for statistical analysis and the accuracy of the data analysis. Others involved in data collection, had full access to all of the data in the study, and took responsibility for the integrity of the data.

REFERENCES

1. Yang X, Yu Y, Xu J, Shu H, Xia J, Liu H, et al. Clinical course and outcomes of critically ill patients with SARS-CoV-2 pneumonia in Wuhan, China: a single-centered, retrospective, observational study. *Lancet Respir Med.* (2020) 8:e26. doi: 10.1016/S2213-2600(20)30079-5
2. Guan WJ, Ni ZY, Hu Y, Liang WH, Ou CQ, He JX, et al. Clinical characteristics of Covid-19 in China. *N Engl J Med.* (2020) 382:1859–62. doi: 10.1056/NEJMc2005203
3. Zhang JJ, Dong X, Cao YY, Yuan YD, Yang YB, Yan YQ, et al. Clinical characteristics of 140 patients infected with SARS-CoV-2 in Wuhan, China. *Allergy.* (2020) 75:1730–41. doi: 10.1111/all.14238
4. Wu C, Chen X, Cai Y, Xia J, Zhou X, Xu S, et al. Risk factors associated with acute respiratory distress syndrome and death in patients with coronavirus disease 2019 pneumonia in Wuhan, China. *JAMA Intern Med.* (2020) 180:934–43. doi: 10.1001/jamainternmed.2020.0994
5. Zhou F, Yu T, Du R, Fan G, Liu Y, Liu Z, et al. Clinical course and risk factors for mortality of adult inpatients with COVID-19 in Wuhan, China: a retrospective cohort study. *Lancet.* (2020) 395:1054–62. doi: 10.1016/S0140-6736(20)30566-3
6. Mortensen EM, Pugh MJ, Copeland LA, Restrepo MI, Cornell JE, Anzueto A, et al. Impact of statins and angiotensin-converting enzyme inhibitors on mortality of subjects hospitalised with pneumonia. *The Eur Respir J.* (2008) 31:611–7. doi: 10.1183/09031936.00162006
7. Wu A, Good C, Downs JR, Fine MJ, Pugh MJ, Anzueto A, et al. The association

of cardioprotective medications with pneumonia-related outcomes. *PLoS ONE.* (2014) 9:e85797. doi: 10.1371/journal.pone.0085797
8. Henry C, Zaizafoun M, Stock E, Ghamande S, Arroliga AC, White HD. Impact of angiotensin-converting enzyme inhibitors and statins on viral pneumonia. *Proceedings.* (2018) 31:419–23. doi: 10.1080/08998280.2018.1499293
9. Tan WSD, Liao W, Zhou S, Mei D, Wong WF. Targeting the renin-angiotensin system as novel therapeutic strategy for pulmonary diseases. *Curr Opin Pharmacol.* (2018) 40:9–17. doi: 10.1016/j.coph.2017.12.002
10. Walls AC, Park YJ, Tortorici MA, Wall A, McGuire AT, Veesler D. Structure, function, and antigenicity of the SARS-CoV-2 spike glycoprotein. *Cell.* (2020) 181:281–92.e6. doi: 10.1016/j.cell.2020.02.058
11. Hoffmann M, Kleine-Weber H, Schroeder S, Kruger N, Herrler T, Erichsen S, et al. SARS-CoV-2 cell entry depends on ACE2 and TMPRSS2 and is blocked by a clinically proven protease inhibitor. *Cell.* (2020) 181:271–80.e8. doi: 10.1016/j.cell.2020.02.052
12. Li XC, Zhang J, Zhuo JL. The vasoprotective axes of the renin-angiotensin system: physiological relevance and therapeutic implications in cardiovascular, hypertensive and kidney diseases. *Pharmacological Res.* (2017) 125(Pt A):21–38. doi: 10.1016/j.phrs.2017.06.005
13. Thomson G. COVID-19: social distancing, ACE2 receptors, protease inhibitors and beyond? *Int J Clin Pract.* (2020) 74:e13503. doi: 10.1111/ijcp.13503
14. Fang L, Karakiulakis G, Roth M. Are patients with hypertension and diabetes mellitus at increased risk for COVID-19 infection? *Lancet Respir Med.* (2020) 8:e21. doi: 10.1016/S2213-2600(20)30116-8

15. Okaishi K, Morimoto S, Fukuo K, Niinobu T, Hata S, Onishi T, et al. Reduction of risk of pneumonia associated with use of angiotensin I converting enzyme inhibitors in elderly inpatients. *Am J Hypertens.* (1999) 12(8 Pt 1):778–83. doi: 10.1016/S0895-7061(99)00035-7

16. Van de Garde EM, Souverein PC, van den Bosch JM, Deneer VH, Leufkens HG. Angiotensin-converting enzyme inhibitor use and pneumonia risk in a general population. *Eur Respir J.* (2006) 27:1217–22. doi: 10.1183/09031936.06.00110005

17. World Health Organization. *Clinical Management of Severe Acute Respiratory Infection When Novel Coronavirus (nCoV) Infection is Suspected: Interim Guidance.* (2020). Available online at: https://www.who.int/publications-detail/clinical-management-of-severe-acute-respiratory-infection-when-novel-coronavirus-(ncov)-infection-is-suspected

18. National Health Commission of the People's Republic of China. *Chinese Management Guideline for COVID-19 (Version 7.0).* (2020). Available online at: http://211.136.65.146/cache/www.nhc.gov.cn/yzygj/s7653p/202003/46c9294a7dfe4cef80dc7f5912eb1989/files/ce3e6945832a438eaae415350a8ce964.pdf?ich_args2=65-11155015043898_f32a0b9f969d8670abb9ee3d42d8e898_10001002_9c896c2ad2caf0d59239518939a83798_0ad7c3e0d3161a7f69a04f61b3ce861b.

19. Chopra V, Rogers MA, Buist M, Govindan S, Lindenauer PK, Saint S, et al. Is statin use associated with reduced mortality after pneumonia? A systematic review and meta-analysis. *Am J Med.* (2012) 125:1111–23. doi: 10.1016/j.amjmed.2012.04.011

20. Wan Y, Shang J, Graham R, Baric RS, Li F. Receptor recognition by the novel coronavirus from Wuhan: an analysis based on decade-long structural studies of SARS coronavirus. *J Virol.* (2020) 94:e00127-20. doi: 10.1128/JVI.00127-20

21. Mortensen EM, Nakashima B, Cornell J, Copeland LA, Pugh MJ, Anzueto A, et al. Population-based study of statins, angiotensin II receptor blockers, and angiotensin-converting enzyme inhibitors on pneumonia-related outcomes. *Clin Infect Dis.* (2012) 55:1466–73. doi: 10.1093/cid/cis733

22. Huang C, Wang Y, Li X, Ren L, Zhao J, Hu Y, et al. Clinical features of patients infected with 2019 novel coronavirus in Wuhan, China. *Lancet.* (2020) 395:497–506. doi: 10.1016/S0140-6736(20)30183-5

23. Kidney Disease: Improving Global Outcomes (KDIGO) Acute Kidney Injury Work Group. *KDIGO Clinical Practice Guideline for Acute Kidney Injury.* (2012). Available online at: https://kdigo.org/wp-content/uploads/2016/10/KDIGO-2012-AKI-Guideline-English.pdf (accessed January 23, 2020).

24. Nathan C. Points of control in inflammation. *Nature.* (2002) 420:846–52. doi: 10.1038/nature01320

25. Gullestad L, Aukrust P, Ueland T, Espevik T, Yee G, Vagelos R, et al. Effect of high- versus low-dose angiotensin converting enzyme inhibition on cytokine levels in chronic heart failure. *J Am Coll Cardiol.* (1999) 34:2061–7. doi: 10.1016/S0735-1097(99)00495-7

26. Duprez DA. Role of the renin-angiotensin-aldosterone system in vascular remodeling and inflammation: a clinical review. *J Hypertension.* (2006) 24:983–91. doi: 10.1097/01.hjh.0000226182.60321.69

27. Marchesi C, Paradis P, Schiffrin EL. Role of the renin-angiotensin system in vascular inflammation. *Trends Pharmacol Sci.* (2008) 29:367–74. doi: 10.1016/j.tips.2008.05.003

28. Liu Y, Yang Y, Zhang C, Huang F, Wang F, Yuan J, et al. Clinical and biochemical indexes from 2019-nCoV infected patients linked to viral loads and lung injury. *Sci China Life Sci.* (2020) 63:364–74. doi: 10.1007/s11427-020-1643-8

29. Sun M, Yang JM, Sun YP, Su GH. Inhibitors of RAS might be a good choice for the therapy of COVID-19 pneumonia. *Zhonghua Jie He He Hu Xi Za Zhi.* (2020) 43:219–22. doi: 10.3760/cma.j.issn.1001-0939.2020.03.016

30. Fox AJ, Lalloo UG, Belvisi MG, Bernareggi M, Chung KF, Barnes PJ. Bradykinin-evoked sensitization of airway sensory nerves: a mechanism for ACE-inhibitor cough. *Nat Med.* (1996) 2:814–7. doi: 10.1038/nm0796-814

31. Tomaki M, Ichinose M, Miura M, Hirayama Y, Kageyama N, Yamauchi H, et al. Angiotensin converting enzyme (ACE) inhibitor-induced cough and substance P. *Thorax.* (1996) 51:199–201. doi: 10.1136/thx.51.2.199

32. Caldeira D, Alarcao J, Vaz-Carneiro A, Costa J. Risk of pneumonia associated with use of angiotensin converting enzyme inhibitors and angiotensin receptor blockers: systematic review and meta-analysis. *BMJ.* (2012) 345:e4260. doi: 10.1136/bmj.e4260

33. Vuille-dit-Bille RN, Camargo SM, Emmenegger L, Sasse T, Kummer E, Jando J, et al. Human intestine luminal ACE2 and amino acid transporter expression increased by ACE-inhibitors. *Amino Acids.* (2015) 47:693–705. doi: 10.1007/s00726-014-1889-6

34. Turgeon RD, Kolber MR, Loewen P, Ellis U, McCormack JP. Higher versus lower doses of ACE inhibitors, angiotensin-2 receptor blockers and beta-blockers in heart failure with reduced ejection fraction: systematic review and meta-analysis. *PLoS ONE.* (2019) 14:e0212907. doi: 10.1371/journal.pone.0212907

35. Wang H-j, Du S-h, Yue X, Chen C-x. Review and prospect of pathological features of corona virus disease. *Fa Yi Xue Za Zhi.* (2020) 36:16–20. doi: 10.12116/j.issn.1004-5619.2020.01.004

Permissions

All chapters in this book were first published by Frontiers; hereby published with permission under the Creative Commons Attribution License or equivalent. Every chapter published in this book has been scrutinized by our experts. Their significance has been extensively debated. The topics covered herein carry significant findings which will fuel the growth of the discipline. They may even be implemented as practical applications or may be referred to as a beginning point for another development.

The contributors of this book come from diverse backgrounds, making this book a truly international effort. This book will bring forth new frontiers with its revolutionizing research information and detailed analysis of the nascent developments around the world.

We would like to thank all the contributing authors for lending their expertise to make the book truly unique. They have played a crucial role in the development of this book. Without their invaluable contributions this book wouldn't have been possible. They have made vital efforts to compile up to date information on the varied aspects of this subject to make this book a valuable addition to the collection of many professionals and students.

This book was conceptualized with the vision of imparting up-to-date information and advanced data in this field. To ensure the same, a matchless editorial board was set up. Every individual on the board went through rigorous rounds of assessment to prove their worth. After which they invested a large part of their time researching and compiling the most relevant data for our readers.

The editorial board has been involved in producing this book since its inception. They have spent rigorous hours researching and exploring the diverse topics which have resulted in the successful publishing of this book. They have passed on their knowledge of decades through this book. To expedite this challenging task, the publisher supported the team at every step. A small team of assistant editors was also appointed to further simplify the editing procedure and attain best results for the readers.

Apart from the editorial board, the designing team has also invested a significant amount of their time in understanding the subject and creating the most relevant covers. They scrutinized every image to scout for the most suitable representation of the subject and create an appropriate cover for the book.

The publishing team has been an ardent support to the editorial, designing and production team. Their endless efforts to recruit the best for this project, has resulted in the accomplishment of this book. They are a veteran in the field of academics and their pool of knowledge is as vast as their experience in printing. Their expertise and guidance has proved useful at every step. Their uncompromising quality standards have made this book an exceptional effort. Their encouragement from time to time has been an inspiration for everyone.

The publisher and the editorial board hope that this book will prove to be a valuable piece of knowledge for researchers, students, practitioners and scholars across the globe.

List of Contributors

Carlotta Sciaccaluga, Flavio D'Ascenzi, Matteo Cameli, Maddalena Gallotta, Daniele Menci, Giovanni Antonelli, Veronica Mochi, Serafina Valente and Marta Focardi
Division of Cardiology, Department of Medical Biotechnologies, University of Siena, Siena, Italy

Benedetta Banchi
Unit of Diagnostic Imaging, University Hospital Santa Maria alle Scotte, Siena, Italy

Chia-Tung Wu and Pao-Hsien Chu
Department of Cardiology, Linkou Medical Center, Chang Gung Memorial Hospital, Taoyuan City, Taiwan

Shy-Chyi Chin
Department of Medical Imaging and Intervention, Chang Gung Memorial Hospital, Linkou Medical Center and Chang Gung University College of Medicine, Taoyuan City, Taiwan

Claudia Meier, Dennis Korthals, Michael Bietenbeck, Bishwas Chamling, Stefanos Drakos, Volker Vehof, Philipp Stalling and Ali Yilmaz
Division of Cardiovascular Imaging, Department of Cardiology I, University Hospital Münster, Münster, Germany

Jef Van den Eynde and Wouter Oosterlinck
Department of Cardiovascular Diseases, University Hospitals Leuven, Leuven, Belgium

Karen De Vos
Faculty of Law, KU Leuven, Leuven, Belgium

Kim R. Van Daalen
Cardiovascular Epidemiology Unit, Department of Public Health and Primary Care, University of Cambridge, Cambridge, United Kingdom

Runyu Liu and Junbing Pan
Department of General Surgery (Vascular Surgery), The Affiliated Hospital of Southwest Medical University, Luzhou, China

Chunxiang Zhang
Key Laboratory of Medical Electrophysiology, Ministry of Education and Medical Electrophysiological Key Laboratory of Sichuan Province, Collaborative Innovation Center for Prevention and Treatment of Cardiovascular Disease of Sichuan Province, Institute of Cardiovascular Research, Southwest Medical University, Luzhou, China
Cardiovascular and Metabolic Diseases Key Laboratory of Luzhou, Luzhou, China
Nucleic Acid Medicine of Luzhou Key Laboratory, Southwest Medical University, Luzhou, China

Xiaolei Sun
Department of General Surgery (Vascular Surgery), The Affiliated Hospital of Southwest Medical University, Luzhou, China
Key Laboratory of Medical Electrophysiology, Ministry of Education and Medical Electrophysiological Key Laboratory of Sichuan Province, Collaborative Innovation Center for Prevention and Treatment of Cardiovascular Disease of Sichuan Province, Institute of Cardiovascular Research, Southwest Medical University, Luzhou, China
Cardiovascular and Metabolic Diseases Key Laboratory of Luzhou, Luzhou, China
Nucleic Acid Medicine of Luzhou Key Laboratory, Southwest Medical University, Luzhou, China
Department of Interventional Medicine, The Affiliated Hospital of Southwest Medical University, Luzhou, China
King's College London British Heart Foundation Centre of Research Excellence, School of Cardiovascular Medicine and Sciences, Faculty of Life Science and Medicine, King's College London, London, United Kingdom

Yi-Ping Gao, Wei Zhou, Pei-Na Huang, Hong-Yun Liu, Xiao-Jun Bi, Ying Zhu, Jie Sun, Qiao-Ying Tang, Li Li, Jun Zhang, Rui-Ying Sun, Xue-Qing Cheng, Ya-Ni Liu and You-Bin Deng
Department of Medical Ultrasound, Tongji Hospital, Tongji Medical College, Huazhong University of Science and Technology, Wuhan, China

Cheng Li, Mu Chen, Mohan Li, Haicheng Wang, Xiaoliang Hu, Qunshan Wang, Jian Sun and Mei Yang
Department of Cardiology, Xinhua Hospital, School of Medicine, Shanghai Jiao Tong University, Shanghai, China

Xiangjun Qiu, Baohong Zhou and Min Chen
Shanghai Siwei Medical Co. Ltd., Shanghai, China

Yuling Zhu, Xia Liu, Yuelin Zhao, Mingzhen Shen and Jinkang Huang
Medical Information Telemonitoring Center, School of Medicine, Shanghai Jiao Tong University, Shanghai, China

Peng Liao and Li Luo
School of Public Health, Fudan University, Shanghai,
China

Hong Wu
Shanghai Health Commission, Shanghai, China

Yi-Gang Li
Department of Cardiology, Xinhua Hospital, School of
Medicine, Shanghai Jiao Tong University, Shanghai,
China
Medical Information Telemonitoring Center, School of
Medicine, Shanghai Jiao Tong University, Shanghai,
China

Hayder M. Al-kuraishy and Ali I. Al-Gareeb
Department of Clinical Pharmacology and Medicine,
College of Medicine, Al-Mustansiriya University,
Baghdad, Iraq

Saleh M. Abdullah
Department of Medical Laboratory Technology,
Faculty of Applied Medical Sciences, Jazan University,
Jazan, Saudi Arabia

Natália Cruz-Martins
Faculty of Medicine, University of Porto, Porto, Portugal
Department of Metabolism, Nutrition and
Endocrinology, Institute for Research and Innovation
in Health (i3S), University of Porto, Porto, Portugal
Laboratory of Neuropsychophysiology, Faculty of
Psychology and Education Sciences, University of
Porto, Porto, Portugal

Gaber El-Saber Batiha
Department of Pharmacology and Therapeutics,
Faculty of Veterinary Medicine, Damanhour University,
Damanhour, Egypt

**Karina Carvalho Marques, Camilla Costa Silva, Pedro
Fernando da Costa Vasconcelos, Juarez Antônio
Simões Quaresma and Luiz Fábio Magno Falcão**
Postgraduate Program in Parasitic Biology
in the Amazon, Laboratory of Infectious and
Cardiopulmonary Diseases, Long COVID Program,
Centre for Biological and Health Sciences, Pará State
University, Belém, Brazil

Steffany da Silva Trindade
Laboratory of Infectious and Cardiopulmonary Diseases,
Long COVID Program, Centre for Biological and Health
Sciences, Pará State University, Belém, Brazil

Márcio Clementino de Souza Santos
Department of Human Movement Sciences, Centre for
Biological and Health Sciences, Pará State University,
Belém, Brazil

Rodrigo Santiago Barbosa Rocha
Centre for Biological and Health Sciences, Pará State
University, Belém, Brazil

Marco Ferlini and Luigi Oltrona Visconti
Division of Cardiology, Fondazione IRCCS Policlinico
San Matteo, Pavia, Italy

Diego Castini
Cardiology Department, ASST Santi Paolo e Carlo,
Milan, Italy

Giulia Ferrante and Stefano Carugo
Department of Clinical Sciences and Community
Health, Division of Cardiology, University of Milan,
Fondazione IRCCS Cà Granda Ospedale Maggiore
Policlinico, Milan, Italy

Giancarlo Marenzi
IRCCS Centro Cardiologico Monzino, University of
Milan, Milan, Italy

Matteo Montorfano
Interventional Cardiology Unit, IRCCS San Raffaele,
Milan, Italy

Stefano Savonitto
Cardiology Department, Manzoni Hospital, Lecco, Italy

Maurizio D'Urbano
Cardiology Department, Legnano Hospital, ASST
Ovest Milanese, Legnano, Italy

Corrado Lettieri
Cardiology Department, Carlo Poma Hospital, ASST
Mantova, Mantua, Italy

Claudio Cuccia
Cardiology Department, Poliambulanza Hospital,
Brescia, Italy

Marcello Marino
Cardiology Department, Ospedale Maggiore di Crema,
ASST Crema, Crema, Italy

Philipp Jud and Marianne Brodmann
Division of Angiology, Department of Internal
Medicine, Medical University of Graz, Graz, Austria

Harald H. Kessler
Diagnostic and Research Institute of Hygiene,
Microbiology, and Environmental Medicine, Medical
University of Graz, Graz, Austria

**Chaoqun Ma, Dingyuan Tu, Qiang Xu, Pan Hou, Hong
Wu, Zhifu Guo, Yuan Bai, Xianxian Zhao and Pan Li**
Department of Cardiology, Changhai Hospital, Naval
Medical University, Shanghai, China

Jiawei Gu
Department of General Surgery, The Fifth People's Hospital of Shanghai, Fudan University, Shanghai, China

Ching Chee Law, Brett D. Hambly and Shisan Bao
School of Biomedical Engineering, The University of Sydney, Sydney, NSW, Australia

Rajesh Puranik
Department of Cardiology, Royal Prince Alfred Hospital, Sydney, NSW, Australia

Jingchun Fan
School of Public Health, Gansu University of Chinese Medicine, Lanzhou, China

Jian Fei
Shanghai Engineering Research Centre for Model Organisms, SMOC, Shanghai, China

Thorsten Kessler, Jens Wiebe, Heribert Schunkert, Adnan Kastrati and Hendrik B. Sager
Deutsches Herzzentrum München, Klinik für Herz- und Kreislauferkrankungen, Technische Universität München, Deutsches Zentrum für Herz-Kreislauf-Forschung (DZHK) e.V., Partner Site Munich Heart Alliance, Munich, Germany

Tobias Graf
Universitätsklinikum Schleswig-Holstein, Medizinische Klinik II, Deutsches Zentrum für Herz-Kreislauf-Forschung (DZHK) e.V, Partner Site Hamburg/Kiel/Lübeck, Lübeck, Germany

Liang Tang, Zhao-jun Wang, Xin-qun Hu, Zhen-fei Fang and Sheng-hua Zhou
Department of Cardiology, The Second Xiangya Hospital of Central South University, Changsha, China

Zhao-fen Zheng
Hunan Provincial People's Hospital, The First Affiliated Hospital of Hunan Normal University, Changsha, China

Jian-ping Zeng
Xiangtan Central Hospital, Xiangtan, China

Lu-ping Jiang
Changsha Central Hospital, Changsha, China

Fan Ouyang
Zhuzhou Central Hospital, Zhuzhou, China

Chang-hui Liu
The First Affiliated Hospital of University of South China, Hengyang, China

Gao-feng Zeng
The Second Affiliated Hospital of University of South China, Hengyang, China

Yong-hong Guo
Department of Geriatric, The Second Xiangya Hospital of Central South University, Changsha, China

Helena Angelica Pereira Batatinha and José Cesar Rosa Neto
Immunometabolism Research Group, Biomedical Science Institute, University of São Paulo, São Paulo, Brazil

Karsten Krüger
Department of Exercise Physiology and Sports Therapy, University of Giessen, Giessen, Germany

Sher May Ng
St. Bartholomew's Hospital, London, United Kingdom

Jiliu Pan
Royal Brompton and Harefield Hospitals, London, United Kingdom

Kyriacos Mouyis
Royal Free London NHS Foundation Trust, London, United Kingdom

Sreenivasa Rao Kondapally Seshasai
Cardiovascular Clinical Academic Group, Molecular and Clinical Sciences Research Institute, St. George's University of London, St. George's University Hospitals NHS Foundation Trust, London, United Kingdom

Vikas Kapil and Ajay K. Gupta
William Harvey Research Institute, Queen Mary University London, London, United Kingdom

Kenneth M. Rice
Department of Biostatistics, University of Washington, Seattle, WA, United States

Sizhong Xing
Shenzhen Bao'an District Traditional Chinese Medicine Hospital, Shenzhen, China

Yanjiao Wang and Linlin Kang
Shenzhen Bao'an District Traditional Chinese Medicine Hospital, Shenzhen, China
Institute for Hospital Management, Tsing Hua University, Shenzhen, China

Ching-Wen Chien, Jiawen Xu and Peng You
Institute for Hospital Management, Tsing Hua University, Shenzhen, China

Tao-Hsin Tung
Evidence-Based Medicine Center, Taizhou Hospital of Zhejiang Province Affiliated to Wenzhou Medical University, Linhai, China

Dongqiong Xiao, Fajuan Tang, Lin Chen, Hu Gao and Xihong Li
Department of Emergency, West China Second University Hospital, Sichuan University, Chengdu, China
Key Laboratory of Birth Defects and Related Diseases of Women and Children (Sichuan University), Ministry of Education, Chengdu, China

Yaliu Yang and Mengwen Yan
Department of Cardiology, China-Japan Friendship Hospital, Beijing, China

Thomas Menter and Alexandar Tzankov
Department of Pathology, Institute of Medical Genetics and Pathology, University Hospital Basel, University of Basel, Basel, Switzerland

Nadine Cueni and Eva Caroline Gebhard
Intensive Care Unit, University Hospital Basel, Basel, Switzerland

Justin Y. Lu, Alexandra Buczek, Roman Fleysher, Wouter S. Hoogenboom and Tim Q. Duong
Department of Radiology, Montefiore Medical Center, Albert Einstein College of Medicine, Bronx, NY, United States

Wei Hou
Department of Family, Population and Preventive Medicine, Stony Brook Medicine, New York, NY, United States

Carlos J. Rodriguez
Cardiology Division, Department of Medicine, Montefiore Medical Center, Albert Einstein College of Medicine, Bronx, NY, United States

Molly C. Fisher
Nephrology Division, Department of Medicine, Montefiore Medical Center, Albert Einstein College of Medicine, Bronx, NY, United States

Alpo Vuorio
Mehiläinen Airport Health Centre, Vantaa, Finland
Department of Forensic Medicine, University of Helsinki, Helsinki, Finland

Frederick Raal
Faculty of Health Sciences, University of Witwatersrand, Johannesburg, South Africa

Petri T. Kovanen
Atherosclerosis Laboratory, Wihuri Research Institute, Helsinki, Finland

Ralph Ryback
Mindful Health Foundation, Naples, FL, United States

Alfonso Eirin
Department of Internal Medicine, Division of Nephrology and Hypertension, Mayo Clinic, Rochester, MN, United States

Arthur Shiyovich, Guy Witberg, Yaron Aviv, Ran Kornowski and Ashraf Hamdan
Department of Cardiology, Rabin Medical Center, Tel Aviv University, Tel Aviv, Israel

Guanglin Cui, Rui Li, Chunxia Zhao and Dao Wen Wang
Division of Cardiology, Department of Internal Medicine, Tongji Hospital, Tongji Medical College, Huazhong University of Science and Technology, Wuhan, China
Hubei Province Key Laboratory of Genetics and Molecular Mechanisms of Cardiological Disorders, Wuhan, China

Audrey A. Y. Zhang, Nicholas W. S. Chew, Yin Nwe Aye and Kalyar Saw
Department of Cardiology, National University Heart Centre, National University Health System, Singapore, Singapore

Cheng Han Ng, Aaron Mai and Gwyneth Kong
Yong Loo Lin School of Medicine, National University of Singapore, Singapore, Singapore

Kailun Phua
Department of Medicine, National University Hospital, Singapore

Raymond C. C. Wong, William K. F. Kong, Kian-Keong Poh, Koo-Hui Chan, Adrian Fatt-Hoe Low, Chi-Hang Lee, Mark Yan-Yee Chan, Ping Chai, James Yip, Tiong-Cheng Yeo, Huay-Cheem Tan and Poay-Huan Loh
Department of Cardiology, National University Heart Centre, National University Health System, Singapore, Singapore
Yong Loo Lin School of Medicine, National University of Singapore, Singapore, Singapore

Linna Huang, Xiaojing Wu, Xu Huang, Xiaoyang Cui, Ye Tian, Zeyu Zhang and Qingyuan Zhan
Center for Respiratory Diseases, China-Japan Friendship Hospital, Beijing, China
Department of Pulmonary and Critical Care Medicine, China-Japan Friendship Hospital, Beijing, China
National Clinical Research Center for Respiratory Diseases, Beijing, China

Ziying Chen
Center for Respiratory Diseases, China-Japan Friendship Hospital, Beijing, China
Department of Pulmonary and Critical Care Medicine, China-Japan Friendship Hospital, Beijing, China
National Clinical Research Center for Respiratory Diseases, Beijing, China
Peking University Health Science Center, Beijing, China

Lan Ni
Department of Pulmonary and Critical Care Medicine, Zhongnan Hospital of Wuhan University, Wuhan, China

Lei Chen
Department of Pulmonary and Critical Care Medicine, Tongji Hospital, Tongji Medical College, Huazhong University of Science and Technology, Wuhan, China

Changzhi Zhou
Department of Pulmonary and Critical Care Medicine, The Central Hospital of Wuhan, Wuhan, China

Chang Gao
Department of Critical Care Medicine, The First Affiliated Hospital of Soochow University, Suzhou, China

Lin Hua
School of Biomedical Engineering, Capital Medical University, Beijing, China

Index

Printed in the USA
CPSIA information can be obtained
at www.ICGtesting.com
JSHW051403091023
49903JS00006B/249